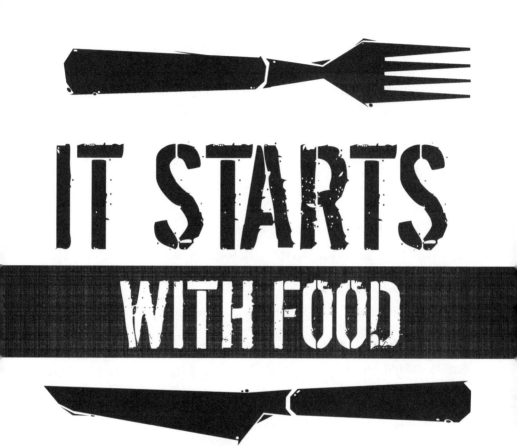

IT STARTS

WITH FOOD

DALLAS & MELISSA HARTWIG

VICTORY BELT PUBLISHING INC
LAS VEGAS

This book is dedicated to the memory of Wayne Hartwig.

First Published in 2012 by Victory Belt Publishing Inc.

ISBN 13: 978-1-936608-89-8

The information included in this book is for educational purposes only. It is not intended nor implied to be a substitute for professional medical advice. The reader should always consult his or her healthcare provider to determine the appropriateness of the information for their own situation or if they have any questions regarding a medical condition or treatment plan. Reading the information in this book does not create a physician-patient relationship.

Victory Belt ® is a registered trademark of Victory Belt Publishing Inc.

Whole30 ® is a registered trademark of Whole9 Life LLC.

Printed in the USA

Cover and interior design by Kathleen Shannon

Illustrations by Greg White

Author photo by R. Sean Galloway

Meal Map created by Melissa Joulwan

Food photography by Dave Humphreys

RRD 05-13

TABLE OF CONTENTS

PART 5: LET'S EAT!

PART 6: THE WHOLE30

PART 7: WHOLE30, WHOLE LIFE

APPENDIX A: THE MEAL MAP

APPENDIX B: RESOURCES

ENDORSEMENTS

"The Whole30 program is completely safe, healthy, and effective. The changes I have experienced have led me to promote these dietary changes to many of my patients as the first step in medical treatment, and the results they have seen have been equally amazing. What I have learned from the Whole30 is that diet can make some drastic improvements to people's health—I look at food as medicine now."

—Matthew Mechtenberg, DO

"I have done the Whole30 and prescribe it to my patients. The Whole30 dietary program is safe and healthy for the following reasons: First, it is based on whole, unprocessed foods, thus making it very nutrient-dense. Second, it is anti-inflammatory. Third, it helps to regulate insulin metabolism. And fourth, the Whole30 eliminates most of the foods known to cause allergies and intolerances."

—Luc Readinger, MD

"I have personally experienced the benefits of the Whole30 program, and I wholeheartedly recommend the Whole30 plan to optimize a woman's health during pregnancy and lactation. The nutrient-dense foods recommended provide ample vitamins and minerals without the need for the standard prenatal supplement. This healthy eating program will also help regulate blood sugars, alleviating hypoglycemic spells common in pregnancy. In addition, the Whole30 will reduce the likelihood of gestational diabetes and excess pregnancy weight gain."

—Michele Blackwell, MD, OB-GYN

"As a doctor who started with a love for 'food as medicine,' I counsel every patient I see on nutrition due to its powerful ability to heal and restore. I can attest to the safety and efficacy of the Whole30 program, particularly in the area of food sensitivities, autoimmune diseases and digestive disorders like IBS and IBD. The plan is organized, doable and easy to follow. Every patient with these disorders should show this program to their doctor and give it a try."

—*Lauren Noel, ND*

"The Whole30 program is a great tool to get people motivated and on track. Its focus is real, whole, high-quality foods. This is not some fad diet that cuts calories to a ridiculous level and prescribes pills and powders—there is nothing for sale but health. If done correctly it is safe, effective, sustainable, and includes nothing outlandish, expensive or hazardous—just the basic tenets of good nutrition and health."

—*Amy Kubal, RD, LN*

"I have done the Whole30 myself, have been using the Whole30 with my patients, and have seen some amazing and exciting results. One patient lost twenty pounds in three months, and her most recent labs show a normal A1c, increased HDL cholesterol, and lower overall cholesterol and LDL-C. She also was able to completely resolve her non-ulcer dyspepsia without the need for medications. I have seen similar results in those patients compliant with the recommended program."

—*Chad Potteiger, DO*

"The Whole30 is by far one of the best programs available to help individuals learn how and why to make the best food choices. While Dallas and Melissa's information is based on credible scientific references, the information is presented in an easy-to-understand and captivating manner. There are thousands of testimonials available that give credit to this program's success, and I highly recommend it."

—*Stephanie Greunke, RD*

FOREWORD

Luc Readinger, MD

I first heard of Dallas and Melissa Hartwig (and the Whole9 community) while listening to their interview on Robb Wolf's *Paleo Solution* podcast. After the interview, I visited the Whole9 Web site and found a gem called the Whole30, Dallas and Melissa's original thirty-day nutrition program. It is part diet guide, part tough-love behavioral coaching, and I have witnessed the way it has transformed the lives and health of many.

I was working at an integrative family medical practice in a rural town. From day one, I realized my patients could benefit from dietary changes. Often a complete overhaul was in order. On both a personal and professional level, I knew many of these people would benefit from Dallas and Melissa's healthy eating plan.

There are several good books on the subject, many of which I recommended. But it really came down to making it as easy as possible for people. I knew the diet I was recommending probably sounded unappealing, intimidating, or downright challenging and that only the super-motivated would follow through with purchasing a book. So to facilitate compliance with this lifestyle change, I printed copies of the Whole30 program from the Web site and began handing it out to those patients needing an intervention. They left my office with four pages in hand that contained everything they needed, freshly motivated by the program's admonition to *start right now*.

I did not have a lot of hope at first. The changes I was asking people to make could be perceived as radical and even, in some cases, near impossible. To my surprise, people started returning to my office feeling better—

often amazingly so. They had followed through! They had made drastic changes in how they ate and were reaping the results.

Almost all had lost weight and reported improved energy and mood. Patients were able to stop their blood-pressure medications after just thirty days on this plan. One diabetic's hemoglobin A1c (a marker for average blood sugars over a four-month period) dropped by three points in three months, an unheard of improvement using oral medications alone. Another diabetic's insulin requirements decreased by 80 percent. Asthma improved, rashes went away, chronic infectious diseases abated, chronic pain diminished, and health and well-being increased.

One day, my secretary told me that Melissa Hartwig had called. "Uh-oh," I thought, "she's found out that I've been printing the Whole30 off their Web site and handing it out to patients. A cease-and-desist order must be close at hand." A patient who had experienced the tremendous benefits of the program had reached out to her and given her my contact information. To my relief, the Hartwigs were thrilled that I had been able to apply their material in my clinical practice and told me of other health-care providers who have had similar experiences with their patients as a result of the program.

Not only does the food we eat have a substantial impact on our health—a fact vastly underrated in today's conventional medical community—it is the very *cornerstone* of good health. Out of all of the tools in my medical arsenal, the Whole30 is by far the most powerful and the most applicable across a wide range of ills. It is a potent antidote to the chronic diseases of modern society and can be used both as prevention and as treatment.

This book will take you through the Whole30 and beyond, going further into the practical application of the Hartwigs' healthy eating plan. It elucidates a sustainable way to eat to maintain lifelong health, wellness, and physical performance. I hope the work you now hold in your hands leads you to a life of optimal health and vitality, as it has for my patients.

Luc Readinger, MD | January 2012

PREFACE

"We eat real food—fresh, natural food, like meat, vegetables, and fruit. We choose foods that are nutrient-dense, with lots of naturally occurring vitamins and minerals, over foods that have more calories but less nutrition. And food quality is important—we are careful about where our meat, seafood, and eggs come from, and we buy organic, local produce as often as possible.

"This is not a 'diet'—we eat as much as we need to maintain strength, energy and a healthy body weight. We aim for well-balanced nutrition, so we eat both plants and animals. We get all the carbohydrates we need from vegetables and fruits, while healthy fats like avocado, coconut, and olive oil provide us with another excellent source of energy.

"Eating like this allows us to maintain a healthy metabolism and keeps our immune system in balance. It's good for body composition, energy levels, sleep quality, mood, attention span, and quality of life. It helps eliminate sugar cravings and reestablishes a healthy relationship with food. It also works to minimize our risk for most lifestyle-related diseases and conditions, like diabetes, cardiovascular disease, stroke, and autoimmune conditions."

—Dallas and Melissa Hartwig, "Nutrition in 60 Seconds"

If you've purchased this book for yourself, congratulations! You clearly care about your health and would like to take the necessary steps to becoming the healthiest version of you. Making changes is never easy, but what we've laid out for you here is an approachable path to a new, healthy relationship with food and sustainable, satisfying nutritional habits. Keep an open mind and be proud of yourself for taking the first—and most important—step toward changing your life.

If you've received this book as a gift, it means you are loved. Someone cares about you and your health so much that they are willing to facilitate your transformation and support you along the way. We think you'll find our approach sensible, manageable, and, most important, immediately applicable to your situation, regardless of your age, health status, or habits. Use this book as a means to make permanent changes to your diet and lifestyle and jump-start your journey to optimal health. It is possible. The person who gave you this book believes in our methods—but more important, he or she believes in *you*.

And if at any point you begin to doubt your ability to make these changes in your own life, we want you to remember one very important thing:

You've already begun.

Because whatever you are seeking—improvement in energy, mood, focus, sleep, athletic performance, symptoms, medical conditions, body composition, or quality of life …

It starts with food.

Your partners in health,
Dallas and Melissa Hartwig

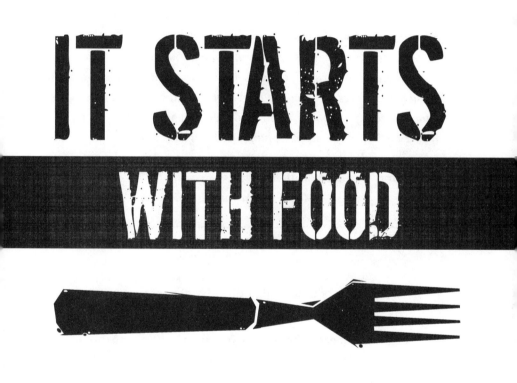

CHAPTER 1:

FOOD SHOULD MAKE YOU HEALTHY

"I read up on the Whole30 and decided to participate. I have type 2 diabetes and, after hearing about the side effects of the medicine I was taking, decided that I wanted to stop my meds. By the fifth day of my program, my blood sugar was in the normal range! I can't believe how fast it's gone down with just the dietary changes. I completed my Whole30 and lost about six pounds … but the best part for me was feeling healthier, dropping a pant size, reducing my A1c levels by a point and a half, and being able to control my blood sugar! I've been off my diabetes medication since completing the program, and my doctor is very happy with the results."
—*Maricel B., Sugar Land, Texas*

We have a theory about food that directly influences the rest of this book.

The food you eat either makes you *more* healthy or *less* healthy. Those are your options.

There is no food neutral; there is no food Switzerland—every single thing you put in your mouth is either making you *more* healthy or *less* healthy.

It should be simple then, right? Just eat the foods that make you more healthy.

Well, it is and it isn't.

See, making good food choices isn't just about knowing what's healthy. If that was the case, we'd just give you a copy of our shopping list and send you on your merry way (shortest book ever!). No, the way we choose the foods we eat is much more complicated and nuanced than that.

Food is highly emotional, in ways that go far beyond your conscious awareness.

Food is sneaky, affecting you in subtle ways you would never connect to your diet.

And by any definition, today's modern food landscape is enormously confusing.

So, it's actually not that easy.

We are going to make it easy.

We're going to share our views on food. We'll share our personal experiences. We'll give you testimonials from others who have changed their lives just by changing the food on their plate. And we'll give you the science—the studies, experiments, and conclusions that form the basis for all of our recommendations.

And then we'll say, "Don't just take our word for it."

We are going to teach you how to turn yourself into a scientific experiment of one, so you can figure out for yourself, once and for all, whether the foods you are eating are making you more healthy or less healthy. And that's worth more than *any* scientific findings you read about—because there hasn't been a single scientific experiment that includes *you* as a subject.

Until now.

When you complete our Whole30 program, you'll see for *yourself* the effects of more healthy and less healthy foods. By the time the program is over, you'll know in no uncertain terms which foods are improving the quality of your life and which are detracting from your health. In just thirty days, you will have gained that incredibly powerful knowledge. Why is this knowledge so valuable?

Because it will change your life.

After implementing our program, you won't have to wonder whether the foods you are eating are healthy for *you*. You'll be able to make educated, informed food choices for the rest of your life. And you'll know how to enjoy treats, sweets, and other "less healthy" foods in a way that is always moving you toward better health, fitness, and quality of life.

Sounds pretty amazing, doesn't it? We don't take the promise to change your life lightly.

Finally, by the time you turn the last page, you'll know more than just why you should eat this way—you will know *how* to eat this way for the rest of your life. We'll show you how to break free of unhealthy cravings, restore your body's natural hunger mechanism, eat to satiety while still losing weight, and eliminate the symptoms of any number of lifestyle-related diseases and conditions—forever.

It starts with food.

OUR STORIES

Our story starts in 2006, when Dallas (a licensed physical therapist) was reading research relevant to his sister Amber's rheumatoid arthritis. In Dallas' own words:

I've always enjoyed life sciences, and as strange as it may sound, I actually think of scientific studies as "pleasure reading." So it was not unusual for me to read an article in the British Journal of Nutrition *about dietary factors that were of special relevance for individuals with rheumatoid arthritis (RA). I tried to keep up with current research about RA for my sister, but during that same period of time, I had been struggling with a stubborn case of tendonitis. My shoulder had been bothering me for almost eighteen months, partly because I played competitive volleyball and hadn't let it rest long enough to fully heal after a minor injury. After I played at USAV Nationals, I swore that I would let my shoulder heal. And I did rest it, but it didn't get better.*

Being a physical therapist with a special interest in athletics, I knew a thing or two about facilitating the healing of connective tissue. I consulted with other therapists and two orthopedists and ended up getting a series of MRIs that revealed no structural damage to my shoulder. Something was promoting ongoing inflammation in my shoulder's connective tissues, but I didn't know what.

The research paper I was reading outlined a theory about how certain dietary proteins (in this case, those from legumes) may exacerbate rheumatoid arthritis by stimulating the immune system into overactivity. I knew from my physiology training that abnormal immune activity was the root cause of chronic inflammation, so the idea that something I was eating might be contributing to the inflammation in my shoulder caught my attention. I decided to read more research from that paper's lead author, Dr. Loren Cordain.

At this time in my life, I was eating a plant-based omnivorous diet—small amounts of meat and eggs and lots of grains, legumes, vegetables, fruit, and nuts. I thought, "If something I'm eating might be causing inflammation in my shoulder, why don't I just avoid that food for a while and see what happens?" So I did. I cut out all legumes and grains, and six weeks later my shoulder pain was gone—eighteen months of pain and limited functionality gone in six weeks. That got my attention! (Six years later, I haven't had a single twinge in my shoulder.)

I was eager to learn more about how diet affected inflammatory conditions like RA and tendonitis. I read Dr. Cordain's book The Paleo Diet *and everything else I could find on the topic of food-induced chronic inflammation. I was able to share what I'd learned with patients, friends, family, and Melissa. My sister eventually adopted our dietary guidelines, and almost all of her rheumatoid arthritis symptoms have disappeared.*

So how did this experience lead us to create our Whole30 program? Fast-forward to April 2009 when, in Melissa's own words:

Dallas' shoulder was still pain-free, and we were both eating pretty well, but an aggressive training schedule, lack of sleep, and some serious stress (working full-time jobs while managing a fast-growing strength and conditioning facility) had both of us feeling kind of run-down. While eating lunch after a particularly grueling Olympic lifting session, I wondered aloud whether cleaning up our diets even more would make a difference in how we felt.

Remembering something we'd heard at a Robb Wolf seminar—you need at least thirty days of dedication to make a real difference—Dallas proposed that we adopt a 100 percent clean, no cheats, no slips Paleo diet for the next thirty days. We started hashing out our "rules," and when we had a plan outlined, I asked when we should start. Dallas (with a devilish look in his eye) proposed that we start immediately. Now. Like, RIGHT now.

I looked longingly at my Thin Mints, sighed, and accepted his challenge.

During those thirty days, I went through a lot of ups and downs. It was easy. It was impossible. I was tired. I had boundless energy. I tossed and turned. I slept like a baby. But by the third week, something shifted. It was as dramatic as flipping a switch—and my life would never be the same.

My energy levels skyrocketed—and stabilized. I felt just as peppy at 6 a.m. as I did at noon as I did at 6 p.m. I started losing body fat without even trying. My performance in the gym, which had plateaued, suddenly started improving again. I was falling asleep easier, staying asleep longer, and waking up without an alarm clock. As the days went on, I realized just how not-great I'd been feeling, compared to how clean and fresh and amazing I was feeling now.

But the most remarkable thing was how this thirty-day adventure completely changed my relationship with food and eating.

I'd always had an unhealthy relationship with food. Food was my best friend and my worst enemy. It was punishment or reward, control or powerlessness. I went through stages of extreme dieting and extreme exercise. But after just thirty days on this new plan, my relationship with food was different. For the first time in my life, food made me feel good. (And not just the quick-and-dirty "good" that comes with the first few bites of ice cream, followed by a full day's worth of guilt, shame, and anxiety. Wholesome good. Lasting good. Good good.)

My sugar cravings disappeared. The urge to eat junk food when I was upset, bored, angry, or frustrated just … vanished. My skin was clear, my hair was shiny, my stomach was flatter, and people said I was "glowing." I had more energy, smiled more, was friendlier to co-workers. All of a sudden, I was indescribably happy.

The remarkable realization I had was that, after all of my complicated multi-step self-improvement initiatives, all I had to do was change the food I put on my plate. For thirty days, I ate nothing but food that made me healthier, as much as I wanted, no counting calories or measuring portions. And those thirty days changed my life in a very real, very positive way.

To this day, I have been able to maintain a healthy and satisfying relationship with food, eating, and my body… all because, for those thirty days, I changed what I put on my plate.

From these revelations, the Whole30 was born.

Dallas' experience with his thirty days was no less eye-opening, and although he didn't have the same emotional issues with food, this experiment brought to light the impact of removing *all* of the potentially harmful foods and beverages in his diet for an extended period of time.

We decided to share our experience with our blog readers in July 2009. We called the post "Change Your Life in 30 Days" and outlined the full rules of the program we had followed in April. We invited our readers to participate and asked them to let us know if they were on board.

We had no idea how many people would take us up on this challenge.

During that first iteration, several hundred people worked through our program and reported their results. We were thrilled to hear that most experienced the same kind of "miracles" we had—effortless weight loss, better sleep, consistent energy, improved mood, and increased athletic performance. Many reported the elimination of sugar cravings and a healthier relationship with food, allowing them to pass up desserts and sweets they used to find irresistible. But what impressed us the most were the number of people who told us the program had improved or completely eliminated their physical ailments. Seasonal allergies—gone. Asthma—not a single attack. Blood pressure—back to normal. Cholesterol—improved by an astonishing degree. Heartburn—vanquished. Stubborn tendonitis—healed. (OK, that one didn't surprise us!)

Since that inception in July 2009, we've freely offered our Whole30 program on our Web site. The program has spread virally through word-of-mouth, and over the past three years, tens of thousands of people all around the world have completed the program and have reported that the Whole30 did, in fact, change their life.

CHANGE YOUR LIFE? It's funny how many of our testimonials start with, "When you told me the Whole30 was going to change my life, I thought, 'Yeah right. Whatever.' But it totally did!" Our own stories were pretty dramatic, and we have hundreds of readers' stories and testimonials on our Web site (http://whole9life.com), but if you're still skeptical about the whole "life changing" thing, that's OK. Just keep reading.

CHAPTER 2:
OUR NUTRITIONAL FRAMEWORK

"I'm 46 years old and have lost the same fifty pounds over and over again, only to gain it back—and more. At the beginning of the year, my cholesterol was so high I was sure I'd need to go on medication. But by the end of my Whole30, my overall cholesterol level dropped 83 points, triglycerides dropped 82 points, LDL dropped 63 points, and HDL rose 3 points. Plus I lost ten pounds and over seven inches. Thank you!"
—Patty M., Boise, Idaho

The framework for our Whole30 program and general recommendations are built on what we've learned from some very smart people—one in particular. Robb Wolf, the *New York Times* bestselling author of *The Paleo Solution* and one of the world's leading experts on the Paleo lifestyle, has been a friend and mentor for several years now. Robb has influenced our program and the way we work with our clients tremendously. In fact, his "thirty-day elimination" approach formed the foundation of our Whole30 program.

As a result, the basics of our food recommendations look a lot like the fundamental tenets of the Paleo diet. You've probably heard of it by now—you know, that "caveman diet" the media has been talking about? Its recommendations are based on the diet consumed by man during the Paleolithic era—a 2.6-million-year period of time that ended about 10,000 years ago with the advent of agriculture. The theory is that we are genetically adapted to the diet of our Paleolithic ancestors, and that genetic disposition hasn't changed much in the last 10,000 years—which means we are not genetically suited to our modern, industrially-produced, agriculture-based diet. Paleo diet advocates believe that the healthiest diet for people today should resemble the diets of our hunter-gatherer ancestors.

PALEO, DEMYSTIFIED Before we go any further, let's debunk some myths about the Paleo diet. First, it's not about recreating the existence of cavemen. No one wants you to go without electricity, hot showers, or your beloved iPhone. And yes, cavemen didn't always have a long life span, but that's not because of their food choices—it was more likely the lack of antibiotics, the abundance of predators, and harsh living conditions. Second, it's not a carnivorous diet—the moderate amount of high-quality meat is balanced with *tons* of plant matter (vegetables and fruit). Third, the fat you eat as part of a Paleo diet will *not* clog your arteries because fat all by itself is not the culprit in that scenario. (Really. More on that later.) Finally, the diet is not carb-phobic; it's *100 percent sustainable* from day one, and it's really not that radical—unless you consider eating nutrient-dense, unprocessed food radical. Which, in today's microwave-dinner-fast-food-low-fat era, might very well be the case.

Now, we agree that foods advocated by the Paleo diet are the healthiest choices in today's modern age. The research and experience of folks like Dr. Loren Cordain and Robb Wolf heavily influenced our own experimentation, and the results we achieved after eating this way were hard to ignore. But please, hear us clearly on this one subject:

We are far more concerned with *health* than we are with *history*.

We aren't recommending meat and vegetables because we think that's what our ancestors ate; we don't say cheesecake is a poor choice because cavemen didn't eat cheesecake; and we're *certainly* not about to debate whether any one food is "technically Paleo." While the Paleo diet is backed by solid scientific research (refer to our references), we generally don't get all hung up on what Paleolithic man may or may not have eaten.

We care about what is making us, here and now, more or less healthy.

And we suspect that's what you care about too.

CREATIONISTS WELCOME If our program's evolutionary perspective resonates with you, fabulous. But if you're not interested in the history or you don't believe in evolution at all, that's OK too. You don't have to buy into Darwinian evolutionary theory to participate because we'll just be concentrating on biology and natural patterns of behavior. There are some things for which we are simply hardwired, like being active during the day and sleeping at night, liking sweet tastes, and experiencing thirst when we are dehydrated. In the natural world, these primal urges are designed to keep us safe, fed, hydrated, and healthy. But in today's modern world, these biological signals don't always work the same way—and our ability to override them often gets us into trouble. Understanding the biological purpose of these signals and how to hear them over all the noise in today's busy world is one of the keys to optimal health.

Now is a good time to address one of our most commonly heard questions: Do you have the science to back this stuff up? The answer, of course, is yes. We will reference a ton of technical information—what we call "science-y stuff"—and we promise to translate any complicated material into easy-to-understand concepts. We have references galore in our appendix: peer-reviewed, credible research that we've used to back up the program we present here. We don't recommend anything that we don't believe is true, based on the findings of the scientific research community.

But relying on science *alone* is tricky.

Many of these nutritional theories aren't as rock-solid as, say, the theory of gravity. There is still a lot the scientific community doesn't know about food, nutrition, and health. Which means that for every finding we present, you can consult the Source of All Knowledge (the Internet) and find studies that suggest the opposite.

Coffee is good for everyone!

Coffee may increase your risk of cancer!

Which one is right? Maybe neither, maybe both—it's hard to know. But one thing is certain—in the case of nutrition and health, the science can be confusing, and can lead to "paralysis by analysis" (a state in which you take *no* action because you're not sure *what* to do).

In the absence of enough conclusive science, what else can we rely on? Observation, experience, and clinically-based evidence. Our recommendations are based on the protocols that have been effective for our clients. Getting positive results from one client is good, but getting similar positive results from a thousand clients truly confirms the efficacy of the protocols and suggests that they will produce reliable results for other people with similar health conditions.

The trouble is, we can't rely exclusively on observation, experience, or clinically-based evidence. Despite loads of experience and careful observation, it can be difficult to pinpoint the exact cause and effect of any one behavior on a population. For example, consider the following statement:

When ice cream sales are high, the frequency of shark attacks increases. Therefore, sharks attack in response to rising ice cream sales.

Obviously, those two things are merely *correlated* and not cause and effect. (The two variables exhibit a common trait—the warm season—when people are more likely to both eat ice cream and swim in the ocean.) Yet it's easy to confuse *correlation* with *causation* when you are relying solely on observational data.

So, how did we come up with our dietary recommendations?

We combined scientific research with clinical experience.

We have scientific studies to back up our recommendations. We have years of experience and documented Whole30 results to confirm that we're on the right track. It's the best of both worlds—the academic evidence and the boots-on-the-ground experience that comes from working with thousands of people and getting amazing results. Win-win.

But none of those published studies take into account *your* life, *your* history, *your* context. The most relevant form of experimentation for you is *self-experimentation,* so you can figure out for yourself, once and for all, how certain factors affect *you.*

And that is exactly what we are proposing here, with our Whole30 program.

Grounded in science, based on thousands of observations and proven results, and anchored with a thirty-day structured self-experiment.

Win-win-win.

SCIENTIFIC RESEARCH + CLINICAL EXPERIENCE + SELF-EXPERIMENTATION

CHOOSE YOUR OWN ADVENTURE We're about to dive into some of the most technical information in the book—the "science-y stuff." In Chapters 3 through 7, we'll outline our four Good Food standards and talk about the ways that less-healthy foods mess with your brain, hormones, gut, and immune system. We'll do our best to keep the science accessible and use lots of analogies to help you understand the way things work in the body.

If you're the kind of person who needs to know not just the *how*, but also the *why*, these chapters are a must-read. If you don't care about the science and just want to know what to eat, how much to eat, and how to create lifelong healthy eating habits, feel free to skip straight to the food in Chapter 8.

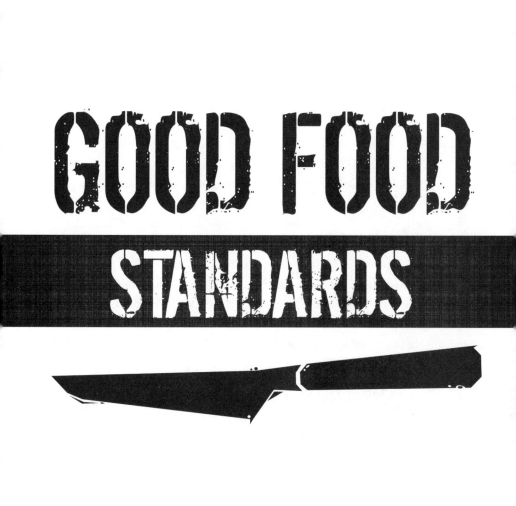

GOOD FOOD

STANDARDS

CHAPTER 3:
WHAT IS FOOD?

"My wife and I have had terrible seasonal allergies for several years. Now our allergies have all disappeared. We are off all allergy meds, which we used to take like candy. As for our four-year-old daughter, we are two weeks into her Whole30, and I am amazed to report that her allergy symptoms are virtually gone. No sneezing. No runny nose. After taking both pills and nose spray for much of her life, her allergy symptoms are better now than they have ever been."

—Brian C., Burnsville, Minnesota

We choose our foods by following four Good Food standards. We're pretty picky about this: all the foods we recommend have to satisfy all four criteria. Not three, not most … all. We'll explain them in more detail in the coming chapters, but here are the basics.

OUR GOOD FOOD STANDARDS

The food that we eat should:

1. Promote a healthy psychological response.
2. Promote a healthy hormonal response.
3. Support a healthy gut.
4. Support immune function and minimize inflammation.

Before we get into each of the Good Food standards, however, we need some general background on food.

WHAT IS FOOD?

Food is composed of a multitude of complex molecules. Some provide energy, some provide structural components, some interact with various receptors and transmit signals to our bodies, and some are relatively inert. People sometimes oversimplify food, and say things like, "I eat whole grains for *fiber*" or "I drink milk for *calcium*," but the reality is that all whole, unprocessed food is a rich, complex blend of nutrients. We broadly organize these components into two major classifications: micronutrients and macronutrients.

A *micronutrient* is defined as an essential compound needed only in relatively small amounts. A micronutrient's purpose is not to generate energy but to serve a wide variety of important biological functions, including: protection against free radicals, enhancing immune response, and repairing DNA. There are hundreds of different micronutrients, but some you've probably heard of include vitamins (like vitamin C), minerals (like calcium), and phytonutrients (like beta-carotene). Selecting foods with the right amounts and a wide variety of micronutrients is critical for our long-term health.

A *macronutrient* is defined as a group of chemical compounds consumed in large amounts and necessary for normal growth, metabolism, and other bodily functions. Macronutrients are used to supply energy and, in some cases, are used as structural components. In humans, the three macronutrients are carbohydrate, protein, and fat.

THE MACRO VIEW

Carbohydrates include several types of sugars, multiple types of starches, and dietary fiber. All carbohydrates, whether they come from a carrot, brown rice, or a Pop-Tart, break down into simple sugars in the body. Complex carbohydrates are simply a bunch of sugars linked together, and those chains of sugars are broken into their individual "links" upon digestion. Simple carbohydrates, specifically glucose, are a universal energy source that is easily used by most cells in the body. Glucose is fuel for intense activity and fuel for your brain cells.

CARB CONVERSION Even if you don't eat any carbohydrates, your body can manufacture them from certain amino acids (and to a small extent, from fat) in order to supply an adequate amount to your brain. This is why some people say that there is no dietary requirement for carbohydrate.

Proteins are made up of long chains of amino acids, which are the building blocks for all sorts of biological structures. The amino acids in proteins are necessary for building, maintaining, and repairing muscles, connective tissue like tendons and ligaments, skin, hair, and even your bones and teeth. In addition, most enzymes and many hormones in the body are actually proteins.

Fats are either in free form (free fatty acids) or built into complexes. Fatty acids belong to one of three types or families: saturated, monounsaturated, or polyunsaturated. Fats allow you to absorb fat-soluble vitamins and essential nutrients from food, help to transport nutrients across cell membranes, and are critical to maintaining proper immune function. Dietary fats are also the building blocks for brain tissue, nerve fibers, reproductive and stress hormones, immune messengers, and cellular membranes. Finally, fat is also an excellent slow-burning energy source, perfect for supporting lower intensity activity.

The energy contained within each type of macronutrient is measured in calories. Carbohydrates and protein each contain four calories per gram; fat contains nine calories per gram. Diet books and experts have long attributed weight problems to simply eating too many calories, and specifically, too much fat. After all, fat is more than *twice* as calorie-dense as either protein or carbs!

If only it were that easy.

While calories do count for something, good health depends on far more complex factors—and simply reducing calories (or fat) isn't the answer. The foods you eat exert a powerful psychological influence, stronger than any act of willpower. They influence your hormones, silently directing your metabolism. They affect your digestive tract, your body's first line of defense. And they impact your immune system and your risk for any number of diseases and conditions.

Your good health starts with the foods you eat. And determining which foods make you more healthy starts with our four Good Food standards.

SNEAK PEEK

Chapter 4: Your Brain on Food
Chapter 5: Healthy Hormones, Healthy You
Chapter 6: The Guts of the Matter
Chapter 7: Inflammation: No One is Immune

We're about to introduce our four Good Food standards. They're in this order for a reason—because we think this is generally how things start going wrong. First, you overconsume nutrient-poor foods, because of their psychological effect on you. Overconsumption (and the kinds of foods you tend to overconsume) then leads to hormonal, gut, and immune-system disruption—and all of the symptoms, conditions and diseases that may follow. These chapters will lay the groundwork for the discussion on food, and make it that much easier for you to understand *why* we'll be asking you to remove certain foods from your plate. We'll also wrap up each of these four chapters with a summary to make it easier for you to refresh your memory when we do start talking about food.

CHAPTER 4:
YOUR BRAIN ON FOOD

"This program has shown results that I didn't think were possible. Prior to the Whole30, I recognized that I had severe difficulties dealing with food cravings and knowing when to stop eating. Cheat meals turned into cheat feasts and cheat weekends. My frustration with controlling my cravings and urges skyrocketed. Daily I asked myself, 'How can I get these urges under control? Why do I feel like I need these bad foods? Where should I go for help?' Whole30 is the answer. I haven't felt the deep desire to binge since I've submerged myself into this program. I don't feel like I have to struggle to make decisions when trying to decide what to eat. The way I eat now is how I honestly desire to feed myself."

—Aubrey H., Manassas, Virginia

Surprised that we're leading off with psychology and not calories, energy, or metabolism? Stay with us, because we suspect this section is going to resonate with you. As a rule, we think the foods that are good for your body should also not mess with your mind. And we think the *psychological* effects of your food choices are perhaps the most important factors to consider during your healthy-eating transformation.

How many times have you tried a new plan, bought new foods, and stuck to the new menu for a few weeks, only to fall right back into your old habits—and old waistline? (Every time you've tried to "diet," we suspect.) Want to know why your previous efforts have failed?

Dieting doesn't work.

But you knew that already, didn't you?

Calorie-restrictive plans have been found to help folks lose weight, but only in the short term. Most folks can't sustain their new dietary habits, and after a year or two, the vast majority end up gaining back even more weight than they lost. (Kind of a bummer, right?) The truth is, simply reducing your calories isn't likely to change or alleviate your food cravings, even if you do lose weight. And we'll show how your cravings, habits, and patterns are critical to your long-term success.

In addition, creating healthy dietary habits isn't just about restricting or eliminating certain foods. You already *know* that fast food, junk food, and sweets aren't good for you. You *know* you shouldn't eat them if you want to lose weight, get off your medication, or be healthier.

Yet you continue to eat them.

You struggle with food cravings, bad habits, compulsions, and addictions. You know you shouldn't, but you feel compelled to eat these foods. Sometimes, you don't even *want* them, but you eat them anyway. And you have a hard time stopping.

All of which makes you feel guilty and stressed—and more likely to comfort yourself with even more unhealthy food.

We're here to tell you:

It's not your fault.

You are not lacking willpower. You are not lazy. And *it's not your fault* that you can't stop eating these foods.

Now we're not trying to say that the choices you make aren't your own or that you don't have any responsibility for your current health status (or waistline). But what you have to understand is that these unhealthy foods have an unfair advantage. They are *designed* to mess with your brain. They are *built* to make you crave them. They *make* it hard for you to give them up.

And until you know their dirty little secrets, you will never be able to leave these foods, and your cravings, habits, and patterns, behind.

We are going to spill their secrets.

We are going to help you understand *why* you crave the foods you do and explain how these unhealthy foods trick you into eating them. Then we'll show you how to outsmart your cravings once and for all.

HARD TO RESIST

Food craving can be defined as "an intense desire to consume a particular food (or type of food) that is difficult to resist." Cravings aren't merely about your *behavior* related to the food in question—they're about your emotional motivation and the conditioning (habit) that is created with repeated satisfaction. You don't even have to be hungry to experience cravings—in fact, they're more closely related to moods like anger, sadness, or frustration than to hunger. In addition, your capacity to visualize the food and imagine its taste are strongly correlated with craving strength—so the more you fantasize about indulging, the less likely you are to resist.

Specific food *cravings* can turn into poor eating *habits* in just a few days, leaving us stuck in a cycle of relentless urges, short-term satisfaction, and long-term guilt, shame, anxiety, and weight gain. To effectively change our relationship with food (and maintain new, healthy habits forever), we need to understand what is behind our cravings, habits, and patterns.

It all starts with biology and nature.

ANCIENT SIGNALS IN A MODERN WORLD

If we were hunting and foraging our food in nature, our bodies would need some way to signal to us that we'd found something useful. For example, bitter tastes signify toxic foods while sweet tastes signify a safer choice. Thanks to nature and our biology, our brains have been hardwired to appreciate three basic tastes: sweet (a safe source of energy), fatty (a dense source of calories), and salty (a means of conserving fluid). When we came across these flavors, neurotransmitters in our brain would help us remember that these foods were good choices by sending us signals of pleasure and reward, reinforcing the experience in our memories. These important signals from nature helped us select the foods best suited to our health.

But there is one very important point to keep in mind with respect to these signals from nature. They weren't designed to tell us which foods were *delicious*—they were designed to tell us which foods were *nutritious*.

In nature, pleasure and reward signals led us to vital nutrition.

The trouble is that in today's world, the ancient signals persist —but the foods that relay them are anything but good sources of nutrition. And that creates a major disruption in our bodies and in our brains.

Over the last fifty years, the makeup of our foods has dramatically changed. Our grocery stores and health food markets are packed with shelves of processed, refined *food-like* products—which no longer look anything like the plant or animal from which they were derived.

Food scientists caught on to the fact that our brains respond strongly to specific flavors (such as the aforementioned sweet, fatty, and salty), and armed with this knowledge, they began to modify our whole foods. They sucked out the water, the fiber, and the nutrients, and replaced them with ingredients like corn syrup, MSG, seed oils, and artificial sweeteners, colors, and flavors. All of this with the specific intention of inducing cravings, overconsumption and bigger profits for food manufacturers.

They've turned real food into *Franken*-food.

These foods light up pleasure and reward centers in the brain for a different reason than nature intended—not because they provide vital nutrition, but because they are *scientifically designed* to stimulate our taste buds. The effect is a total disconnection between pleasurable, rewarding tastes (sweet, fatty, and salty) and the nutrition that *always* accompanies them in nature.

In nature, sweet tastes usually came from seasonal raw fruit, rich in vitamins, minerals, and phytonutrients. Today, sweet flavors come from artificial sweeteners, refined sugars, and high fructose corn syrup. In nature, fatty tastes usually came from meats, especially nutrient-packed organ meats. In modern times, fats come from a deep-fryer or a tub of "spread." In nature, precious electrolytes like sodium came from sea life, or from the animals we ate. In modern times, salt comes from a shaker.

Do you see the problem with this?

Modern technology has stripped the nutrition from these foods, replacing it with empty calories and synthetic chemicals *that fool our bodies into giving us the same powerful biological signals to keep eating.*

This means we are eating more calories with less nutrition.

Persistent biological signals lead us to overeat sweet, fatty, salty foods while keeping us malnourished.

These Franken-foods are ridiculously cheap to produce.

They unnaturally electrify our taste buds.

They contain little, if any, nutrition.

And they mess with our brains in a major way.

VIVA LAS VEGAS "Supernormal stimulus" is the science-y term for something so exaggerated that we prefer it to reality—even when we know it's fake. A supernormal food stimulus arouses our taste receptors more intensely than anything found in nature. Candy is far sweeter than fruit. Onion rings are fattier and saltier than onions. Sweet-and-sour pork is sweeter, fattier, and saltier than actual pork. And Franken-foods like Twinkies and Oreos outcompete any taste found in nature, which is, of course, *exactly* why we prefer them. These supernormal stimuli are like the Las Vegas Strip of foods. Dazzling! Exotic! Extreme! But entirely contrived. Not at all realistic. Totally overwhelming. (And if you take a good, hard look in the light of day—i.e., read your ingredients—you'll see that they're actually cheap, dirty, and kind of gross.) But the over-the-top flavors found in these foods (and the extra-strong connections they forge in your brain) make it hard to stop eating them—and make natural, whole foods look bland and boring by comparison.

You may be thinking, "If these foods taste so good that I can't stop eating them, maybe I should just stop eating foods that taste good." But that just sounds miserable to us—and flavor restriction would probably be just as unsuccessful long-term as caloric restriction! Thankfully, this strategy is wholly unnecessary. The problem isn't that these foods are *delicious*.

The problem is that these foods are supernormally stimulating *in the absence of nutrition and satiety*.

They are the essence of empty calories—foods with *no brakes*.

PRIME RIB AND OREOS

The idea of food brakes can be explained by *satiety* and *satiation*. They sound the same, but biologically speaking they are two separate and distinct concepts.

Satiety occurs in your digestive tract—specifically, in your intestines. When you've digested and absorbed enough calories and nutrients to satisfy your body's needs, hormones signal to your brain that "I am well nourished now," which decreases your desire for more food. Satiety can't be fooled or faked, as it is dependent on the *actual nutrition* in your food. But since digestion is slow, these signals may take several hours to be transmitted, which means they can't do a very good job all by themselves to keep you from overeating.

That's where satiation comes in.

Satiation is regulated in the brain and provides more timely motivation to stop eating. It's based on the taste, smell, and texture of food, the perception of "fullness," even your knowledge of how many calories are in a meal. As you eat, you perceive various sensations ("This is delicious," "I shouldn't eat the whole bag" or "I'm getting pretty full"), all of which send your brain status updates to help you determine whether you still want more. But unlike satiety, satiation is an *estimate* dependent on your perceptions, not an absolute measurement.

Ideally, the brain would signal us to stop eating when our bodies have sensed that we've digested and absorbed enough nutrition to support our health. In this case, satiation and satiety would be one and the same. Let's use the example of a prime rib dinner.

Prime rib contains complete protein, the most satiating of all the macronutrients, and naturally occurring fat, which makes protein even more satiating. As you eat your prime rib, you'll find yourself wanting prime rib less and less with every bite. The first bite was amazing, the second fantastic, but by your tenth bite, the texture, smell, and flavor are less appealing. And by the twentieth bite, you've had enough, and you no longer desire the flavor or texture of the meat—so down goes your fork.

This is satiation.

Prime rib also takes longer to eat than processed food (as you actually have to chew and swallow), which gives your brain a chance to catch up with your stomach. As you eat and start to digest the meat, your body recognizes that the dense nutrition in that prime rib is adequate for your energy and caloric needs. This sends a "we're getting nourishment" signal to your brain while you're still working on your plate, which also reduces your "want" for more food.

This is satiety.

This scenario plays out differently for foods lacking the satiation factors of adequate nutrition—complete protein, natural fats and essential nutrients. Let's compare prime rib to a tray of Oreos.

Oreos are a highly processed food containing almost no protein, saturated with sugar and flavor-enhancing chemicals, and filled with added fats. As we eat the Oreos (generally at a much faster rate than prime rib), they move through us quickly and don't provide enough nutrition to induce satiation *or* satiety. So unlike the prime rib, there are no "brakes" to decrease our want. We *want* the tenth Oreo just as much as the first. And we never *stop* wanting more because even though we've eaten plenty of calories, our bodies know that we are still seriously lacking in nutrition. So we eat the whole darn package because *satiety can't be fooled.*

In the case of Oreos, the only reason to stop eating is when our bellies are physically full, and we realize we're about to make ourselves sick from overconsumption.

Those aren't brakes at all—that's just an emergency ejection seat.

LET US SUMMARIZE These scientifically designed foods artificially concentrate highly palatable flavors (sweet, fatty, and salty) that stimulate our pleasure centers with a far bigger "hit" than we could ever get from nature. This processing removes any nutrition once found in the food but still leaves all the calories. The final concoction (we can't really call it "food" at this point) offers a staggering variety of over-the-top flavor sensations in every single bite—but your body knows there is no nutrition there, so you continue to *want* more food, even past the point of fullness.

If we stopped right here, we'd have made our point. Clearly, these foods violate our first Good Food standard by provoking an unhealthy psychological response—heck, they were designed to do just that!

Unfortunately, there's more.

Chronic consumption of these foods doesn't just affect our taste buds, our perceptions, and our waistlines.

Over time, they literally rewire our brains.

PLEASURE, REWARD, EMOTION, AND HABIT

Pleasure, reward, and emotion are all interconnected in our brains. Reward circuitry is integrated with parts of the brain that enrich a pleasurable experience with emotion, making it more powerful, and easier to remember. The combination of pleasure, reward, and emotion pushes you *toward* rewarding stimuli—including food.

The foods in question—supernormally stimulating without adequate nutrition to invoke satiation or satiety—tell the brain to release dopamine, the neurotransmitter associated with the pleasure center. Dopamine motivates your behavior, reinforces food-seeking ("wanting") and energizes your feeding. It gives you that rush of anticipation before you've even taken your first bite. (You're daydreaming at work and start thinking about your favorite cookie from the downtown bakery. You're visualizing the taste, the smell, the texture. You start to get excited and happy at the thought of picking up cookies on the way home. You *want* those cookies. That's dopamine talking.)

On the way home, you stop at the bakery, pick up a dozen cookies, and take your first bite before you've even pulled out of the parking lot. (Of course, because that cookie is supernormally stimulating, but lacking in nutrients that satiate, you don't stop at just one.) Immediately, the brain releases opioids (endorphins—the body's own "feel good" compounds), which also have a rewarding effect. The release of opioids brings pleasure and emotional relief, releases stress, and generally makes you feel good.

Over time and with continued reinforcement, those dopamine pathways begin to light up at the mere suggestion of the food, like when you're driving past that bakery, see someone else eating a similar-looking cookie, or watch a commercial for cookies on television. This preemptive dopamine response (and the memory of the reward you'll experience when you indulge) makes it all but impossible to resist the urge to satisfy that craving. Your *want* has turned into a *need*.

The kicker?

You don't even have to be hungry—because it's not about satisfying your *hunger*. It's about satisfying the *craving*.

After just a few trips to the bakery, your memory circuits tell your reward circuits that the cookie will bring you joy. Dopamine promises satisfaction, if you only give in to your urge. You can't resist, so you eat the cookie(s) and your endorphins help you feel good (for a while). And so the vicious cycle serves only to reinforce itself until you have developed a *habitual* response—the automatic craving for a specific food in response to certain triggers.

Automatic cravings do not sound psychologically healthy to us.

THE STRESS EFFECT

Stress is another factor that promotes the reinforcement of these unhealthy patterns. We don't need a scientific study to tell us that many people eat when they're stressed to distract themselves from the situation and help themselves relax. The trouble is, chronic stress (whether it stems from anxiety or worry, lack of sleep, over-exercise, or poor nutritional habits) is driving us—via our biology—to overeat.

Stress affects the activation of reward pathways and impairs your attempts to control your eating habits. Did you catch that?

Stress makes it even harder for us to resist our cravings.

When you are under stress, the urge to "pleasure eat" (eating for reward) is strong—and you are far more likely to overeat. Stress also causes you to change the *type* of foods you eat, moving away from healthier choices toward—you guessed it—highly palatable foods that are sweet, salty, and high in fat. (Who craves grilled chicken and steamed broccoli when they're stressed?) And when you finally, inevitably, indulge, one thing is true:

Eating sugary, salty, fatty foods makes you feel less stressed.

This works via the same old mechanism we've been talking about—dopamine and opioid pathways in the brain. We experience stress, we eat the cookies, and we really *do* feel better.

This creates two problems, however. The first is that, during stress, these strong opioid and dopamine responses in the reward center of your brain promote the encoding of habits. Future stress triggers you to remember the relief you experienced the last time you ate those cookies. Memories of these responses are stored in your brain and you quickly establish a learned behavior—a "want" for more cookies. Which means that the next time you're stressed, you'll find yourself *automatically* reaching for the cookies.

CRANKY COOKIE Stress eating can promote habit-driven overeating *even in the absence of active stress.* So as a result of the stress-related habits you've created, you may find yourself reaching for the cookies when you're feeling tired, cranky, or just kind of down. (Remember, cravings are strongly tied to emotion.) Over time, as your brain continues to create new links between "cookie" and "feeling better," the association—and your wanting for more—only continues to grow stronger.

The last nail in your stress-cookie coffin: The stressed brain expresses both a strong drive to eat and *an impaired capacity to inhibit eating.* You may not even want to eat the cookie, but because your ability to not eat it is impaired, you sort of *have* to. You tell yourself you'll have only one, but under stress, you'll probably end up eating the whole bag—which, in turn, makes you pretty stressed-out.

It's a vicious cycle—and you probably didn't even realize you were stuck in it.

Until now.

Of course, we can't always eliminate stress in our lives—that half of the equation may, unfortunately, be here to stay. Our only recourse is to concentrate on the other half by eliminating the foods that *play into* this unhealthy stress response.

Not coincidentally, they're the same highly processed, supernormally stimulating, non-nutritive foods that have been causing us trouble all along.

It's all the same story.

GET ME OUT OF HERE

By now you probably agree that the food you eat shouldn't mess with your head. You may even be a little bit mad at the way some of the things you've been eating have manipulated you into cravings and overconsumption. And we bet if we said, "Let's kick all of these sneaky, tricky foods off our plates forever and eat only *naturally* delicious, nutritious, satiety-inducing foods," you'd probably throw up your hands and say, "Hurrah!" Theoretically, that is. There's just one small problem with this plan.

These unhealthy foods are really hard to give up.

First, it's difficult to radically change your diet when you have so many powerful emotional associations with the foods you're eating—especially if you're eating as a coping mechanism, instead of from hunger.

Second, these foods are designed to be hard to give up. Through the misuse of biological and natural cues, our modern technology has made these foods supernormally stimulating, rewiring the reward, emotion, and pleasure pathways in our brains to create an artificial demand for more. And when we tell you which foods are the worst offenders, which ones you'll be kicking to the curb, that's when the real trouble will start.

You may panic.

You may think, "No way can I do this."

You may say to yourself, "I cannot live without [fill in food]."

We assure you, you can. And you will. We'll walk you through it. And when you're done, three things will happen.

First, you will once again be able to appreciate the natural, delicious flavors (including sweet, fatty, and salty) found in whole foods.

Second, the pleasure and reward you experience when eating that delicious food will once again be closely tied with good nutrition, satiation, and satiety—you'll be able to stop eating because you're satisfied, not just because you're "full."

Third, *you will never again be controlled by your food.*

Freedom.

THE SCIENCE-Y SUMMARY

- The food choices you make should promote a healthy psychological response.
- Sweet, fatty, and salty tastes send pleasure and reward signals to the brain. In nature, these signals were designed to lead us to valuable nutrition and survival.
- Today, these flavor sensations are unnaturally concentrated in food, which is simultaneously stripped of valuable nutrition.
- This creates food-with-no-brakes—supernormally stimulating, carbohydrate-dense, nutrient-poor foods with all the pleasure and reward signals to keep us overeating, but none of the satiety signals to tell us to stop.
- These foods rewire pleasure, reward, and emotion pathways in the brain, promoting hard-to-resist cravings and automatic consumption. Stress and inadequate sleep only reinforce these patterns.
- Reconnecting delicious, rewarding food with the nutrition and satiety that nature intended is the key to changing these habits.

CHAPTER 5:
HEALTHY HORMONES, HEALTHY YOU

"Just finished my Whole30, and my (diagnosed type 2 diabetic) blood sugar levels are now normal—completely normal. I have cut my diabetes medications in half, and my blood pressure is in the normal range too. All of my pain, stiffness, soreness, and puffiness is gone... and I lost twenty-five pounds. The Whole30 has changed my life."
—*Alan H., East Bremerton, Washington*

Our second Good Food standard states that the food you eat should produce a healthy hormonal response in the body. This is probably the most science-y section of the whole book, but as promised, we'll use a lot of analogies and examples to make the science easy to understand. We're also going to simplify things quite a bit, because you don't need to understand how *everything* works to know how to apply it.

Let's start with some basics.

HORMONES

Hormones are chemical messengers that are usually transported in your bloodstream. They are secreted by cells in one part of the body and bind to receptors in another part of the body. (Think of a courier carrying a message from one person to another.) Hormones have many roles, but one essential function is to keep things in balance.

Essentially all biological processes have regulatory mechanisms designed to keep systems operating within safe, healthy parameters and maintain homeostasis (equilibrium) in the body. Think of the thermostat in your house. The furnace kicks on to keep the temperature above the lowest point set, but as the temperature rises to the top end of the range, the thermostat turns on your fan or air conditioner. Much as your thermostat keeps your house within a "healthy" temperature range, hormones work in delicate, intertwined ways to maintain homeostasis in your body.

Hormones also respond to any external factor that tips the scales out of balance. To go back to our thermostat analogy, opening a window in wintertime will push the temperature in your home off balance. The act of opening a window sends a message ("It's getting cold in here!") to your thermostat, which reacts to that stimulus with an internal correction (firing up your furnace). When the temperature reaches the normal range again, your furnace then turns off.

When you eat and digest food, various biochemical components of the food trigger multiple hormonal responses in the body. These hormonal responses control the use, storage, and availability of nutrients—where they go and what happens when they get there. Different nutrients cause different hormonal responses, but *all* of those responses are intended to correct the shift in balance caused by the influx of digested food particles.

ONE BIG TEAM

While there are a lot of hormonal players, for the sake of simplicity, we're going to talk about only four in detail:

Insulin, leptin, glucagon, and cortisol.

These four hormones (along with many others) form a complex, elegant—but not indestructible—web of feedback loops that influence all body systems. They all interact with one another's functions, behaving like a team in the body. These hormones are neither "bad" nor "good" in the right amounts. Things get ugly, however, when you've got too much or not enough of any given hormone.

Let's start with both insulin and leptin, as it's hard to separate these two.

INSULIN

Summary: An anabolic ("building, storing") hormone secreted by the beta cells of the pancreas in response to ingestion of energy, most notably from carbohydrate. Insulin facilitates the moving of macronutrients (protein, fat, and carbohydrate) from the bloodstream into cells for immediate or future use, and coordinates the metabolic shift from predominantly burning one fuel source (carbohydrate) to the other (fat). Chronically elevated insulin levels are correlated with leptin resistance and indirectly related to elevated cortisol levels.

Insulin is about as close to a "master hormone" as you can get. It acts on virtually all cells in the body and directly controls or influences energy storage, cell growth and repair, reproductive function, and, most important, blood sugar levels.

Insulin "unlocks" a one-way door into cells so they can store or use nutrients. Insulin effectively stores all macronutrients—protein, fat and carbohydrates—but its secretion is most closely tied with carbohydrate ingestion.*

When we eat carbohydrate, it is broken down in our bodies into simple sugars and then absorbed into the bloodstream. This leads to a rise in the amount of circulating blood sugar (glucose).

To be optimally healthy, our blood glucose levels *must* be kept within a normal range—not too low, not too high. Remember, just as in the thermostat analogy, "normal" is pretty much synonymous with "healthy." In the case of regulating blood sugar, your pancreas is the primary thermostat, and insulin is like your air conditioner, keeping blood sugar levels from remaining too high.

A rise in blood sugar is sensed by beta cells in the pancreas, which then secrete insulin into the bloodstream. Insulin signals cells in the body to pull glucose out of the bloodstream and move it into storage, bringing blood sugar levels back to a normal, healthy range. Elevated insulin levels also have a satiety function, reducing hunger.

INSULIN SENSITIVITY

The scenario we just described is called *insulin sensitivity*. If you have a healthy metabolism, when you eat a healthy meal, your blood sugar levels rise moderately—not too much, and not too fast. When blood sugar increases, the pancreas dispatches just enough insulin to communicate to the cells exactly how much blood sugar needs to be stored. Insulin's message is,

---

Protein sources (like beef, fish, eggs and milk) also trigger insulin secretion to varying degrees. We'll discuss this in more detail when we talk about dairy.

"Store these nutrients." The cells, which are *sensitive* to the insulin message, hear the request and respond appropriately by pulling blood sugar out of the bloodstream and storing it, thereby returning blood glucose levels to normal.* Insulin sensitivity is indicative of a nice, normal, healthy relationship between the pancreas and most tissues in the body.

Insulin's management of blood sugar serves a very important function, as chronically elevated blood glucose levels are highly damaging to many body systems, including the liver, pancreas, kidneys, blood vessels, brain and peripheral nerves. Got that?

Chronically high levels of blood sugar (hyperglycemia) are harmful, so managing blood sugar is critical for long-term health.

Once cells have taken glucose out of the bloodstream, that glucose can either be used for energy or stored for future use. The primary place to store glucose is in the liver and muscles, as a complex carbohydrate called *glycogen*. If stored in the liver, glycogen can easily be converted back into glucose and released back into the bloodstream when energy is needed. However, glycogen stored in muscle cells can't be emptied back into the bloodstream—it stays there, to provide fuel for your muscles. (Which is good, because your muscles can do a lot of hard work!)

GLYCOGEN STORES Your body's storage tanks for carbohydrates (the liver and muscles) are kind of like the gas tank in your car. When your gas tank is full, it's full. It can't get any bigger, and you can't make it any fuller. Your body's carbohydrate fuel tank, however, isn't very big—you can store only enough glycogen to maintain hard, continuous activity for about 90 minutes. And because carbohydrate is fuel for *intense* activity, you don't tap into your glycogen stores in any meaningful way while you're sitting at your desk at work, watching television, or puttering around the house. In other words, it's really easy to

---

There is always a small amount of insulin circulating in the blood, directing small amounts of sugar into vital tissues like your brain. Insulin secretion is not a black-or-white, on-or-off proposition: it's a trickle, a flow, or a flood. In a healthy metabolism, how much insulin is secreted is proportionate to the quantity of glucose and the rate at which it has entered your bloodstream.

fill your tank up with carbohydrates—but if you're not doing lots of high-intensity activity, you're not really using much fuel!

Your hormonal troubles start with "overcarbsumption": the chronic overconsumption of supernormally stimulating, nutrient-poor, carbohydrate-rich foods.

To begin with, a constant excess supply of carbohydrates will tilt your metabolic "preference" toward burning what's most plentiful—sugar—when fuel is needed. If there is an overabundance of sugar, the sugar takes precedence over fat as a source of energy in many metabolic processes, and stored fat doesn't get burned for energy.

If less fat is being burned for fuel, then it accumulates, and body fat levels tend to increase.

In addition, all that excess glucose poses a storage problem in the body. If there's space available in the liver and muscle cells, they'll happily uptake glucose. However, if those cells are already full of glycogen, they will politely decline any additional nutrition (essentially putting up a No Vacancy sign). When there is no room in the liver and muscle cells, the body shifts fuel storage to Plan B.

You will not like Plan B.

When the liver and muscle glycogen stores are full, the liver (and your fat cells) converts the extra glucose into a type of saturated fat called palmitic acid, which can then bind together in groups of three (with glycerol) to form *triglycerides*.

These two processes combined—the preferential burning of carbohydrate over fat for fuel and the creation of triglycerides—lead to increased body fat and increased triglycerides and free fatty acids in the blood, neither of which is desirable or healthy. And this pileup of sugar and triglycerides in the blood pushes another hormone, leptin, out of balance.

LEPTIN

Summary: An "energy balance" hormone that is secreted primarily by fat cells and is released in proportion to the amount of fat stored. Leptin tells the brain how much body fat is stored and regulates both energy intake and energy expenditure to keep body fat levels in balance. Overconsumption of nutrient-poor, supernormally stimulating carbohydrates leads to chronically elevated triglycerides and blood sugar levels, which promotes leptin resistance and an increase in fat storage, accompanied by greater insulin resistance.

Leptin is sometimes referred to as a "satiety hormone," because higher leptin levels help to keep us full and satisfied. Leptin levels follow a normal daily cycle tied primarily to your eating schedule. Since you don't eat while you're asleep, leptin is pretty low first thing in the morning. This triggers the secretion of appetite-stimulating hormones and is one of the reasons we wake up hungry. When you're done eating for the day (typically after dinner), leptin levels are higher, helping you stay full and satisfied until bedtime.

However, leptin's primary job is to regulate your big-picture hunger and activity levels to help keep your body in "energy balance"—not too fat, not too lean. Body fat is not a bad thing—it's what allows us to survive long periods of food shortage (or to not eat for a few days when we have the flu). But our bodies are pessimists. Our DNA always expects, despite the surplus of readily available energy *right now*, that food will run out soon, and so the only way to survive this coming famine is to store some energy as fat. It's as natural as breathing.

24-7-365   For those of us in the developed world, the idea of a "food shortage" sounds silly. Maybe you're thinking, "Why hasn't my brain caught on to the fact that food is *everywhere* these days?" The fact is, for thousands of years, we worked hard for the food we ate—and there were no guarantees that our food supply could be taken for granted. We're back to ancient signals in a modern world, where the brain continues to send biologically appropriate messages to ensure your survival, despite the fact that you are now living in a wholly *unnatural* food landscape.

As fat is a storage depot for energy, it is important for your body to have a way to measure how much energy (fat) is available at any given moment. Fat cells do this by secreting leptin, as a way to communicate to your brain whether you are too fat, too lean, or just right. Based on leptin's critically important message, your brain constantly gives you subconscious directions, which drive your food-seeking behavior and physical activity levels.

If you have very little body fat—perhaps too little to survive a potential food shortage—leptin levels are low. The relative absence of leptin's message tells the brain, "I don't have enough body fat!" Your brain then tells you to eat more and move less, which serves to change your behavior until your body fat is within a safer range. You become hungrier (and probably eat more), your metabolism slows down (thanks in part to changes in your thyroid hormone levels) and you start to gain body fat.

As body fat continues to accumulate, leptin levels rise, and your fat cells start to send more messages to your brain—"OK, we've got enough energy stored now!" If that message is properly received (i.e., you are *sensitive* to the leptin message), your brain then tells you to increase your activity and makes you less hungry, so you move a little more and eat a little less, and don't gain too much weight.

Although it's much more complicated than this simple summary, this energy-balance system is naturally designed to keep your body fat levels "just right." The trouble starts, though, when the foods you're eating promote an unhealthy psychological response, leading to chronic overcarbsumption.

Shall we recap?

When you chronically overconsume food-with-no-brakes, it floods your system with glucose. With sugar in such large supply, it is burned first for energy—which means fat takes a metabolic back seat and accumulates. This leads to a buildup of triglycerides in the liver, and increased glucose and triglyceride levels in the bloodstream. But how does this lead to problems with leptin?

The excess glucose and triglycerides in the bloodstream make their way to parts of your brain and start impairing your brain's ability to "hear" the leptin message. This leads to a condition called *leptin resistance*.

THE SKINNY-FAT

If you're overweight, it's very likely that you're leptin resistant—but you don't have to appear overweight to fall into this camp. Accumulation of visceral fat (fat stored in and around your organs) is enough to promote hormonal dysfunction, including leptin resistance. We call these folks "skinny fat": not visibly overweight, they still have an unhealthy amount of body fat, comparatively little muscle mass, and a serious degree of hormonal dysfunction, including out-of-whack thyroid and reproductive hormones.

Leptin resistance is like a hormonal conversation gone haywire. Normally, when you've accumulated adequate body fat, your fat cells send a message (via leptin) to your brain that says, "Hey, we've got enough energy stored, so you should eat less and move more." But when receptors in the brain and other tissues become less sensitive to leptin, those messages don't get through. Your brain doesn't hear leptin say that you've got enough body fat stored.

Which means your brain thinks you're *too skinny*.

Imagine that your brain is blind, unable to see your chubby reflection in the mirror or the creeping number on the scale. It *needs* leptin to give it the facts it can't see. So until the brain hears leptin say, "OK, we're fat enough," the brain is going to keep telling you to eat more and move less, to ensure your survival.

Remember, it's pessimistic. And without that leptin message, your subconscious brain will continue to direct your behaviors as if you were too lean—despite the fact that you *know* you're gaining too much weight.

NIGHT MUNCHIES Leptin's message (or lack thereof) is stronger than your willpower. You may see that you've gained some weight, and try to eat less … but the brain's directives are far more powerful. In fact, a hallmark of leptin resistance is uncontrollable cravings after dinner—you try to eat healthy all day, but come 8 p.m., your pantry or freezer is impossible to resist. This isn't a lack of willpower on your part—it's your brain responding to leptin's primal signals, and constantly undermining your conscious decisions.

Leptin resistance means that you are gaining fat and swimming in leptin—but your brain is clueless, so it turns your metabolism down to conserve fuel, and tells you to eat more. And isn't this all too easy to do when supernormally stimulating, nutrient-poor, carbohydrate-rich foods are whispering in your ear? Of course, overcarbsumption only promotes more sugar-burning for fuel, additional accumulation of body fat (and the conversion of excess carbohydrates to fat), and even-higher triglyceride levels in the blood.

Which makes your leptin resistance worse.

And … takes us back to insulin.

BACK TO THE START

Remember insulin sensitivity? This is when insulin's message to "store nutrients" is heard clearly by the cells, which remove glucose from the bloodstream and store it, keeping blood glucose levels from getting (or staying) high.

In contrast to insulin sensitivity, there is also a condition called *insulin resistance*. And …

Leptin resistance leads to insulin resistance.

Let's recap: You chronically overconsume, because supernormally stimulating, nutrient-poor food has no brakes. This makes you leptin resistant, which means your brain thinks you are too lean (even if the mirror tells you otherwise). This leads your brain to tell you to eat more and move less, which promotes further overconsumption. You are now metabolically reliant on sugar for energy, you continue to accumulate fat in the body and the liver, and have excess glucose and triglycerides in your bloodstream.

All of that excess glucose needs to be stored. The trouble is, jamming lots of energy into a cell causes damage. So to protect themselves from being "overfilled," the cells become insulin *resistant.* Once this occurs, the cells lose their sensitivity to insulin's message to store nutrients: the pancreas sends a message (via insulin) to "store," but the cells don't listen, and blood sugar levels remain high.

Since high levels of blood sugar are *very* unhealthy, the body really needs the cells to store that energy—so it responds with an even stronger message. Insulin resistance requires that the pancreas produce even *more* insulin, until the message is strong enough to *force* nutrients into the already-full cells. However, this "force-feeding" creates oxidative stress and elevated fat levels in the blood, which further damages the cells. The damaged cells continue to try to protect themselves, further increasing insulin resistance … and the cycle continues.

SYSTEMIC INFLAMMATION

These cells, overfilled and running mostly on sugar, produce "reactive oxygen species" (which you probably know as "free radicals"), which cause cellular damage. The response to this damage is a cascade of immune responses, including the release of inflammatory chemicals, as well as immune cells that show up as "first responders" to help repair the damaged tissue. This immune response is termed *systemic inflammation* (we'll get to this soon), and further increases insulin resistance.

At this point, you have excess glucose in a system that is insulin resistant. Blood sugar *remains* high because the cells are stuffed and resisting insulin's message to store. This creates ongoing hyperglycemia—chronically elevated levels of blood sugar. Which, as you recall, is very damaging—specifically to pancreatic beta cells, where insulin is produced.

Chronic hyperglycemia first causes beta cell adaptation, to allow the pancreas to produce progressively more insulin to manage the excess blood sugar. The pancreas can't adapt forever, however. Eventually, damaged by ongoing hyperglycemia, pancreatic beta cells start to disintegrate. Yes, they actually *die* from toxic levels of blood sugar and the resulting oxidative stress.

At this point, you lose the ability to produce enough insulin to manage blood sugar—which is how toxic levels of blood sugar and insulin resistance can lead to type 2 diabetes.

However, there are consequences to your health *long* before you get to diabetes. Hyperglycemia (chronically high levels of blood sugar) is damaging, but hyperinsulinemia (chronically high levels of insulin) is *profoundly* damaging, and a clear risk factor for major lifestyle-related diseases and conditions, like diabetes, obesity, heart attack, stroke, and Alzheimer's disease.

Chronically high levels of insulin are harmful, so
managing insulin levels is critical for long-term health.

MUST. EAT. SUGAR. When you are insulin resistant (and, thanks to leptin resistance, you continue to overcarbsume), the pancreas needs to secrete ever-increasing amounts of insulin to pull glucose out of the bloodstream. Since your blood sugar regulation mechanism no longer works properly, all that insulin can pull blood sugar levels too far in the *other* direction—what was *too high* is now *too low* (a condition often referred to as "reactive hypoglycemia"). Too low comes with its own set of side effects—cranky, tired, foggy, and, thanks to constant appetite dysregulation, *hungry*. To you, this translates as, "Must.

Eat. Sugar." Your body doesn't actually need calories, but thanks to the messed-up messages your body is sending—you're too lean, your blood sugar is too low—you give in to the same foods (supernormally stimulating and nutrient-poor) that got you into trouble in the first place. It's a vicious cycle—and it could be worse. If you don't change your eating habits pronto, insulin resistance very well could progress to type 2 diabetes.

Type 2 diabetes occurs when (because of the severity of insulin resistance and beta cell death) your body can no longer produce enough insulin to keep your blood sugar within healthy parameters.

This is very, *very* bad—especially if your diet still doesn't change.

Diabetes comes with its own list of side effects and related conditions: obesity, glaucoma and cataracts, hearing loss, impaired peripheral circulation, nerve damage, skin infections, high blood pressure, heart disease, and depression. Tens of thousands of people die of complications from diabetes every year.

Nobody wants diabetes. In fact, nobody wants *any* of this—the primary reliance on sugar for energy, the ongoing accumulation of body fat, ineffective hormonal messages, energy peaks and crashes, relentless hunger, long-term health consequences. ... *This* is why a healthy hormonal response is one of our four Good Food standards, and why we advocate for eliminating foods that promote an unhealthy metabolism.

But there's more to the story.

And we assure you, there is good news.

First, let's discuss glucagon.

GLUCAGON

Summary: A catabolic ("energy access") hormone secreted from the alpha cells of the pancreas in response to the demand for energy, either as a result of activity or after several hours without eating ("fasting"). Glucagon unlocks the one-way door out of storage cells (like liver and fat cells), and allows you to access the energy you've previously stored. Chronic stress, protein intake and low blood sugar levels stimulate glucagon release. Glucagon's function is inhibited by elevated insulin and free fatty acids in the blood.

THE THREE G'S Were the scientists who named this stuff *trying to confuse us?* Let's recap our three G's before we move on. *Glucose* is one form of sugar found in food and is also the type of sugar circulating in the bloodstream. *Glycogen* is the stored form of glucose, found in the liver and muscles. *Glucagon* is the energy access hormone, which triggers the conversion of glycogen in the liver back into glucose and releases it into the bloodstream for use as energy elsewhere in the body. Got it? Good.

There is normally about five grams (a teaspoon) of blood sugar circulating in your bloodstream at any given time. However, for various reasons—when we're under stress, when we haven't eaten in a long time, or when we've had the low blood sugar rebound previously described—our blood sugar "temperature" can get too low. (The science-y term for this is "hypoglycemia.") Since glucose supply to the brain is literally a matter of life or death—you'll go into a coma if blood glucose levels dip extremely low—your body has multiple fail-safe mechanisms to ensure that doesn't happen. One of these mechanisms works via a hormone called *glucagon.*

Just as insulin is the "air conditioner" for safe blood glucose levels, glucagon functions as the "heater," preventing blood sugar levels from falling too low and giving us access to energy we've previously stored. When the body senses a dip in normal blood sugar levels, alpha cells in the pancreas release glucagon. Glucagon then tells the body to break down stored fat and convert stored liver glycogen (and, if necessary, protein from your muscles) into glucose, trickling it into the bloodstream to provide you with energy and keep blood sugar levels normal.

There is a caveat.

Glucagon can tell the cells to release stored energy—and use body fat—*only* when there's not a lot of circulating insulin. After all, if insulin is elevated, nutrients are being stored as fast as they're being mobilized—or faster. Which means that when insulin levels are elevated (even moderately), the net effect is more energy storage than energy access.

When you are insulin resistant and eat a high-carb meal, insulin levels stay high and "echo" throughout the body for a few hours. Between meals, when you should be tapping into your fat stores for fuel, you can't—because insulin is *still* talking, and glucagon can't get a word in edgewise.

Strike seventeen against dietary habits that chronically elevate blood sugar and, in turn, promote leptin and insulin resistance. The takeaway:

Glucagon can't help us stabilize blood sugar and access fat for energy if insulin levels are chronically elevated.

We're almost done, so hang in there. We just need to introduce yet another hormone related to overcarbsumption, insulin resistance, and … stress. Say hello to cortisol.

CORTISOL

Summary: The "stress hormone" secreted from the adrenal glands to help the body recover from an acute fight-or-flight stress response. It is secreted in response to low blood sugar, physical or psychosocial stress, intense and prolonged exercise, and sleep deprivation. Cortisol plays a key role in salt metabolism, blood pressure, immune function (having immunosuppressive and anti-inflammatory effects), and energy regulation. It raises blood sugar by stimulating glycogen breakdown. Chronically elevated cortisol promotes insulin resistance and tends to elevate leptin levels.

Cortisol has a circadian rhythm that coincides with the light-dark cycle. Cortisol is highest just before waking, functioning as a "get up and go" hormone during the early morning hours. It mobilizes energy for activity and helps to fire up your nervous system so that you (mentally) feel more like Einstein than like Homer Simpson. Cortisol levels then decline rapidly as the day progresses, remaining low in the late evening and overnight, helping you to relax before bed and sleep well until morning.

LIGHTS OUT It's normal to have higher cortisol levels first thing in the morning, but artificial light (including the light from your TV, computer, and mobile phone) after dark tells your body it's still daytime. This does not allow you to hormonally "wind down" in the evening, which promotes that "tired but wired" effect. Sending your brain daytime messages right before bed also upsets normal hormonal responses (like melatonin secretion) when you're sleeping, so you don't get adequate deep, restorative sleep. That sleep, and normal cortisol rhythms, are important for memory formation and future access. Now, where did you put your highlighter?

Cortisol secretion is tied to many factors (like sleep, exercise, and psychological stress) but is also influenced by your eating habits. One of cortisol's jobs is to help glucagon keep blood sugar within a healthy range. When your body senses that blood sugar is too low (like when you haven't eaten for a very long time) or if it crashes too fast (as they tend to do following a blood sugar spike when you're insulin resistant), it reacts to that stressful situation by releasing cortisol. Cortisol then prompts glucagon to get to work, breaking down energy stored as liver glycogen (or muscle tissue) and flooding it into the bloodstream as a response to your volatile blood sugar levels.

The trouble comes when your actions (dietary or otherwise) tell your body that you're very stressed *all the time*. This causes your adrenals to release cortisol *all the time*. And when cortisol gets rowdy, it creates all sorts of trouble—some of which is going to sound awfully familiar.

Being chronically underslept, constantly over-exercising, or experiencing chronic psychological stress—a hallmark of modern life—can all trigger unhealthy levels of cortisol in the body. But so can prolonged periods of not eating (extended fasting), or eating too little (excessive calorie restriction).

Fasting—when you don't eat for eight, twelve, sixteen hours—is somewhat stressful to the body and may elevate cortisol levels, which only adds more stress to your already overstressed system. Cutting too many calories (which we're pretty sure you've done before) is also profoundly stressful and also elevates cortisol levels.

Want to know another reason that skipping meals and restricting your calories doesn't work for long-term weight loss? Because chronically elevated cortisol sends a variety of messages via different hormonal pathways, all designed to do one thing—*preserve body fat*. In fact, chronically elevated cortisol levels actually erode your muscle mass, leaving you with more fat and less muscle.

Now we have your attention.

Chronically elevated cortisol impairs glucose uptake from the bloodstream *and* enhances the breakdown of glycogen in the liver—both leading to more glucose in the blood. To make matters worse, cortisol also inhibits insulin secretion from the pancreas.

Translation?

**Chronically elevated cortisol levels increase blood
sugar levels, which may contribute to insulin resistance.**

Elevated cortisol also contributes to weight gain by inducing stress-related overeating. (Remember this from the last chapter?) Cortisol stimulates the drive to eat supernormally stimulating, nutrient-poor, carbohydrate-dense foods, which may reduce your stress … but increases your girth.

Elevated cortisol levels preferentially direct body fat to the abdominal region (instead of, say, the buttocks or thighs). Excessive abdominal fat (also called *central obesity*) is part of *metabolic syndrome*, a collection of highly correlated symptoms: obesity, high blood pressure, insulin resistance/hyperinsulinemia, hyperglycemia, elevated triglycerides, and low HDL ("good") cholesterol. Increased central obesity is also a direct risk factor for conditions like heart disease, stroke, atherosclerosis, and kidney disease.

Finally, as a weight-gain triple-whammy, elevated cortisol messes with normal thyroid function, leading to a metabolic slowdown that makes it that much easier for you to pack on the pounds.

So if you have an intimate relationship with food-with-no-brakes, *and* you're leptin resistant, *and* you're insulin resistant, *and* you're chronically stressed …

Is it any wonder you can't lose weight, even on your low-fat, calorie-restricted diet?

We think we can summarize our case right here:

It's all about hormones.

In real life, these hormones ebb and flow in reaction to various external stimuli: eating, physical activity, sleeping, reacting to stressful situations, and other more subtle influences. There are not enough pages in this book to examine all those influences in detail, but since our book is called *It Starts With Food*, we are going to explore the effects of *eating*—the right stuff, the wrong stuff, not enough, and too much—by outlining a few real-life scenarios. These examples will show you why it's vitally important that the foods you eat provoke a healthy hormonal response—and what can happen when they don't.

Ready?

First, let's talk about a prototypical good day.

HEALTHY HORMONES: A GOOD DAY

You are relatively lean and have a healthy diet and lifestyle, and good sleep habits. You don't overconsume highly rewarding, nutrient-poor foods and your hormones are all in a good, healthy balance. For you, nearly every day is a good day.

Around 6 a.m., cortisol levels (which were very low throughout the night) rise dramatically, helping you wake up a half-hour later feeling like one of those "morning people."

Thanks in part to appropriately low leptin levels, you also wake up hungry. By 7, you're sitting down to a simple meal—three eggs scrambled with onion, peppers, and spinach, half an avocado, some fresh blueberries, and a cup of coffee.

There's not a lot of carbohydrate in this meal, so your blood sugar rises modestly. Your pancreas secretes a proportional amount of insulin in response to the rise in blood sugar, which sends a gentle message to your liver and muscles to take up the circulating blood glucose and store it as glycogen. Because you exercise regularly, there's some room in your glycogen "tanks," and because you're insulin sensitive, the glucose, amino acids, and fats are efficiently transported into cells to start doing their respective jobs.

Over the next few hours, your blood glucose gradually declines, which triggers your pancreas to secrete some glucagon. Glucagon tells your liver to release some glucose back into the blood, keeping your blood sugar in a normal, healthy range. This give-and-take balance is constantly monitored and adjusted, helping to keep your energy levels and mental focus consistent throughout the day.

Around noon, your declining blood sugar and rising "hunger hormones" remind you it's time for lunch. You enjoy a hearty salad (mixed greens, roasted beets, sliced apples, grilled chicken breast, and walnuts) with an olive oil and balsamic dressing. Though you have only 30 minutes for lunch, you relax and enjoy your meal. The digestive and hormonal response to lunch is similar to that of breakfast—a modest, gradual rise in blood sugar, modest insulin response, and a gradual decline in blood sugar over the next few hours. Glucagon continues to allow you to tap into your glycogen and fat stores to keep you on an even keel.

As your afternoon progresses, things start to get crazy at work, and it suddenly looks like this is going to be a long day.

By 5 p.m., your blood sugar has dipped a little *too* low, which signals cortisol to use glucagon to release some stored energy, keeping blood sugar and energy levels pretty constant. Because you can use dietary fats (and body fat) as primary fuel and your insulin levels aren't elevated, you are able to access your fat stores to keep your energy up.

You finally arrive home at 6:30. You're hungry, but not cranky, light-headed, or lethargic. You dig into the stew (grass-fed beef with chunks of carrot, onion, and tomato) that's been in your slow cooker all day. This nutritious meal triggers the secretion of satiety hormones like leptin and insulin, leaving you full and satisfied after dinner. The moderate insulin response, as well as a glucagon response stimulated by the protein from the beef, ensure stable energy levels over the coming hours.

By 7:30, your cortisol levels are quite low (even though they were temporarily elevated earlier because of your stressful afternoon). Multiple satiety hormones (including leptin) are elevated, which help you remain satisfied after dinner.

At 8, you prepare your lunch for the next day, grab a good book and a cup of herbal tea and start to wind down before you head to bed around 9:30. You fall asleep quickly and sleep well through the night, facilitated by appropriately low cortisol and stable blood sugar levels.

Does this experience sound like *your* typical day?

Most likely not, we suspect.

Let's examine a more common scenario. It starts with the same early morning, but that morning is very different from the one we just described.

NOT SO HEALTHY HORMONES: A BAD DAY

At this point, thanks largely to your eating habits, you're a few pounds overweight, leptin resistant and somewhat insulin resistant, and your lifestyle and eating habits have disrupted your normal cortisol levels and daily rhythm.

Your alarm goes off at 7 a.m., and again at 7:09, and 7:18, at which point you head straight to the kitchen, ready for that first cup of coffee. Your cortisol levels are abnormally low in the morning (a dysfunctional situation created by an overly stressful life and worsened by unhealthy eating habits), which means you're not feeling very bright or perky. You grab a low-fat blueberry muffin, a banana, and some orange juice on your way out the door, and stop at your favorite coffee shop for a large soy latte.

Since your breakfast is almost exclusively fast-digesting carbohydrate (and sugar!), it quickly raises your blood sugar and insulin, aggressively driving energy into your liver and muscles. The high levels of blood sugar give you a kick-start, but by 10 a.m. lots of insulin has pulled too much sugar out of your bloodstream—which means you're now experiencing the crash that often follows a sugar spike when you're insulin resistant. This stressful blood sugar crash prompts a cortisol response, which uses glucagon to get your blood sugar back to normal. Glucagon breaks down liver glycogen and increases blood sugar, but since you're metabolically over-reliant on glucose for energy, you can't use fat efficiently for fuel.

Your brain translates these events as, "Need energy now!"—so you have another cup of coffee, plus half a bagel with peanut butter. Since you're generally sedentary, your liver and muscles are still full. Some of the carbohydrate from the bagel is used for fuel, but the excess fuel is stored (or remains circulating in the bloodstream).

At noon, you grab a small turkey sub (whole-wheat bread, turkey, low-fat cheese, and mustard), a small bag of baked potato chips, and a diet soda from the deli next door. Again, your carb-dense meal drives blood sugar and insulin levels up, and the caffeine in your soda also prompts a cortisol (stress) response, both of which serve to give you a short burst of energy. Even though there is some protein in the turkey, glucagon's attempt to releasing stored energy is overshadowed by elevated insulin levels, so once again the sugar is used as fuel, while fat is stored and blood (and liver) triglycerides accumulate.

A few hours later, all of that insulin has driven blood sugar levels too low—again—which means that by 3 p.m. you've hit the midafternoon trifecta: you're tired, hungry, and mentally foggy. Luckily, you've stashed some healthy snacks for just such occasions and come up with a granola bar and a low-fat strawberry yogurt. Once again, your carbohydrate-rich snack serves to temporarily prop up your energy levels and mostly stave off your hunger.

Work is busy, and you're totally brain-dead by 4, so you grab a small iced coffee (with skim milk and a teaspoon of sugar) to get you through the rest of the day. The caffeine in the coffee provokes another cortisol response, which increases blood sugar to give you some energy. That works for a while, but by the time you head home at 5:30, you're stressed, exhausted, and cranky.

You resist the urge to call for pizza delivery and make chicken parmigiana, with low-fat cheese and whole-wheat pasta, and a side salad. To help you deal with the stress of your day, you also have a glass of red wine. Thanks to leptin resistance, you eat more than you really need, feeling stuffed when you finally put down your fork.

Just two hours later, however, you find yourself craving something sweet. You forage for a pint of frozen yogurt in the freezer and settle in front of the television. By 9, half the pint is gone.

You're exhausted from your day, but because of your blood sugar volatility and caffeine intake (all provoking a stress response), as well as your poor sleep habits, your cortisol is higher than it should be. You can't seem to wind down, so you stay up until 11:30, watching the news and sending a few emails. You don't sleep well, tossing and turning for hours, until your alarm blasts you awake again the next morning.

Thanks to overconsumption, leptin resistance, insulin resistance, weight gain, hunger dysregulation, and energy spikes and slumps, your day wasn't quite so pleasant.

What happens in the evening is highly indicative of aspects of your hormonal dysfunction. At the end of your day, leptin resistance and elevated cortisol (thanks to your volatile blood sugar levels and regular caffeine "bumps") promote hunger and sugar cravings even after you've eaten a filling dinner, and make it hard for you to go to sleep (and stay asleep). But even though the day we just described wasn't so great, it wasn't *that* bad, right? You still ate pretty "healthy" food, you still feel pretty good overall, and maybe you're just a few pounds overweight, so things must be OK.

Or maybe not—because the hormonal disruptions are *invisible*. Due in large part to your diet, they are occurring beneath your radar. You aren't necessarily aware of their effects today, but that won't be the case forever. Let's see how this eating scenario plays out over months or even years.

After all, this is a "typical day" for most of us.

NOT SO HEALTHY HORMONES: THREE YEARS LATER

You've gained fifteen (OK, twenty) pounds in the last three years. Your doctor says that your blood pressure is high, and that you also have pre-diabetes. You're not sure how all of this has happened, because you're still avoiding junk food and eating low-fat meals and snacks. But you've been stuck in the cycle of overconsumption, worsening leptin resistance, worsening insulin resistance, and an even more disrupted cortisol rhythm. Things are Not Good.

After another rotten night's sleep, the alarm goes off. Thanks in part to your chronic poor-eating habits, cortisol levels are still abnormally low in the morning, making it even harder to drag yourself out of bed. A cup of coffee gets you motivated enough to shower.

Your out-of-whack cortisol keeps you from being hungry for breakfast, but you force yourself to eat a bowl of shredded wheat with skim milk, a piece of whole-wheat toast with margarine, and more artificially-sweetened coffee. You head to work, stopping on the way for a "skinny" caramel macchiato, your treat for the day.

Your high-carb, low-fat, protein-sparse breakfast yields rapid and prolonged elevated blood sugar levels and a disproportionately high insulin response (because you're still insulin resistant). These high levels of blood sugar and insulin create "silent" damage in the body and increase your risk for a number of lifestyle-related diseases and conditions.

And that's just breakfast.

By midmorning, your blood sugar has crashed (cue cortisol to tell glucagon you need blood sugar stat!) and you're raging hungry, so you grab a low-fat blueberry muffin and a juice drink. Once again, large amounts of sugar begets large(r) amounts of insulin, and you jump on the energy-focus-mood-hunger roller coaster and take another ride. Since you're eating high-carb foods every few hours, your insulin levels stay elevated, so glucagon rarely has the need to ask cells to tap into fat stores for energy—not that you could, since you are so heavily reliant on sugar.

Your lunch (leftover spaghetti-and-meatballs and a glass of skim milk) recreates the same pattern for the third time today—blood sugar spikes and crashes, provoking a cortisol response. By 3 p.m., you're hungry again. A fig bar and a small iced coffee stave off hunger until you head home.

When you get home, you're cranky, lethargic, and totally beat, but you still take the time to prepare a healthy dinner (brown rice, a lean steak, some honey-glazed carrots, and a whole-wheat dinner roll). Since your brain is leptin-resistant (and can't tell that you're already overweight), you still have room for a fruit salad with yogurt and granola for dessert.

Later in the evening, the serious cravings start. You prowl through the pantry and freezer on autopilot, looking for more fat, salt, and *especially* sugar. You settle on a pint of specialty ice cream and the rest of a bag of pretzels—both highly processed, supernormally stimulating and nutrient-poor (all of which, as we've been trying to tell you, promote overconsumption and worsening leptin resistance and insulin resistance over the long term).

You're exhausted, but your cortisol levels are abnormally high, so you can't wind down until after the last late-night talk show—and you're in for another fitful night of sleep.

The worst part?

It starts all over again tomorrow.

In this scenario, those "invisible" hormonal disruptions are finally up close and center. Those additional twenty pounds of body fat are immunologically active—and secreting a lot of leptin. Since leptin's satiety signal isn't registering in your brain, you chronically overeat—especially food-with-no-brakes, because it *tastes so good.*

Your less-than-active lifestyle and continuous overreliance on sugar and carb-dense processed foods has kept your blood sugar and insulin levels chronically elevated for *years*: you've progressed well into insulin resistance—diabetes could be right around the corner. You continue to gradually accumulate body fat, glucagon has no opportunity to tell the cells to use fat as fuel, and you're desperately reliant on sugar for energy.

Thanks in part to cortisol dysregulation, your body stubbornly holds on to your belly fat even when you try to cut calories—making weight loss *even harder.*

BUT I EAT SO HEALTHY!

This hormonal dysregulation is really powerful, making it very difficult to overcome your addiction to supernormally stimulating foods and *not* to gain fat, and virtually impossible to be healthy in the long-term.

So you're probably thinking, "I must need to exercise more."

But you'd be wrong.

And you've probably tried that already, haven't you?

You cannot "out-exercise" poor food choices and the resulting hormonal disruption.

Remember that *hormones* create and perpetuate these dysfunctions. And the single largest factor in the balance and function of these hormones is food.

So maybe now you're thinking, "Then I must need to eat less."

Wrong again.

You've already tried that, too, with all of the low-fat, low-calorie "health foods" you've been eating. But consider the food choices you've made in these last two symbolic days. We didn't have the hypothetical you binging on pizza, cheeseburgers, or Cool Ranch Doritos. Why? Because we can easily make our point with granola bars, bagels, and low-fat yogurt. Surprised that candy, cakes, and cookies aren't the only foods-with-no-brakes? Processed foods that add or concentrate carbohydrates, sugar, salt, and/or fat—even the "healthy" ones—more than meet the criteria.

Which leads to overconsumption. Which leads to leptin resistance, insulin resistance, and a disrupted cortisol cycle. All of which further promote overconsumption.

Given all this, I wonder if you're thinking what we're thinking?

The "healthy" diet you've been eating isn't really all that healthy after all.

And simply eating less of the same foods isn't going to improve your hormonal responses. (In fact, cut calories too much and you'll make your cortisol situation even *worse.*)

If you need to take a breather right now, go right ahead. This is new information for a lot of people, but we hope it switches on some light bulbs.

Why do I crave sweets late at night?

Why can't I lose weight, even when I eat less?

Why do I get that 3 o'clock slump every afternoon?

Why do I wake up at 2 or 3 a.m. every single night?

Why do I get so cranky if I don't eat every two hours?

Where did this spare tire come from—I eat so healthy!

If this sounds like you, take comfort in two simple facts.

Now you know why.

And we will help you fix it.

THE GOOD NEWS

There is some good news. (About time, right?)

The good news is that even after decades of poor eating habits and hormonal dysfunction, all the way through leptin resistance, insulin resistance and, in many cases, a diagnosis of type 2 diabetes, your health condition is *highly reversible.*

You can stop overconsuming, dial all the way back to insulin and leptin sensitivity, retrain your body to burn fat and, to a significant degree, restore normal cortisol levels, by doing one simple thing:

Changing the food you put on your plate.

Read on, please.

THE SCIENCE-Y SUMMARY

- The food choices you make should promote a healthy hormonal response in the body.
- Chronic "overcarbsumption" of food-with-no-brakes leads to reliance on sugar for fuel, an accumulation of body fat, triglyceride buildup in the liver, and an excess of glucose and triglycerides in the bloodstream.
- Excess glucose and triglycerides in the bloodstream promote leptin resistance in the brain.

- Leptin resistance means your brain doesn't hear the leptin message and thinks you're still too lean. This promotes further overconsumption, and the down-regulation of your metabolism (in part, via your thyroid).
- Leptin resistance promotes insulin resistance, in which cells are no longer sensitive to insulin's message to store. Forcing nutrients into cells creates damage and inflammation and leads to chronically elevated blood sugar and insulin levels.
- Chronically elevated blood sugar and insulin levels are contributing factors to type 2 diabetes and a number of other lifestyle-related diseases and conditions.
- Glucagon can help you stabilize blood sugar and use fat for fuel, but only when insulin levels aren't elevated.
- Cortisol is a stress hormone. Periods of fasting or excessive caloric restriction, along with lack of adequate sleep or too much stress, may contribute to chronically elevated cortisol levels.
- Chronically elevated cortisol levels increase blood sugar, which may contribute to insulin resistance and promotes weight gain in the abdominal region, a component of metabolic syndrome.

CHAPTER 6:
THE GUTS OF THE MATTER

"Because of my Crohn's disease, I was in so much pain that I couldn't stand up straight. Every time I ate something, it hurt. In 1999, I had surgery to remove two and a half feet of intestine, including part of my colon. The surgery relieved the severe pain, but I still dealt with intestinal spasms and gut pain after eating. I completed my first Whole30 in March 2010. Through the process, the intestinal pain, gas, and bloating completely went away—and did not return. The constant underlying fear of Crohn's returning is gone because now I understand its root cause."
—Sarah G., Fort Collins, Colorado

Our third Good Food standard evaluates the effect of certain foods on the digestive tract. We believe you should consume only foods (and drinks) that support normal, healthy digestive function; eating anything that impairs the integrity of your gut impairs the integrity of your health.

Let's discuss normal gut function first, and then talk about how your food choices can disrupt it.

THE GUT

The purpose of your digestive tract (or gut) is to absorb nutrients from food, but it is also a prominent part of the immune system. (Didn't know that, did you?) These two functions—digestive and immune—are inextricably intertwined, though the gut's critical role in regulating immune response often goes underappreciated. We'll talk more about that in the next chapter.

You're probably already familiar with the major components of the digestive system: the stomach, small intestine, and large intestine. Let's take a digestion road trip, shall we?

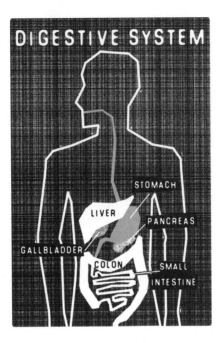

You take a bite of food and start chewing. Chewing breaks your food (i.e., the mishmash of macronutrients, water, fiber, and micronutrients) into smaller pieces, and an enzyme in your saliva starts to break the carbohydrates down into simple sugars.

When you swallow that food, it moves into your stomach. Essentially nothing happens to carbohydrate and fat in the stomach, but protein gets some attention—the acidic environment of the stomach, plus some digestive enzymes, start to break the protein down into smaller pieces.

Your stomach also acts as a sensor for satiety, talking to your brain through both the nervous system and hormones. The stomach's message that you've eaten also tells your brain to allow more energy to be used.

Your stomach then releases a controlled flow of this mixture of food and digestive enzymes into your small intestine, where bile salts and pancreatic enzymes help break food down even further. The carbohydrates are completely broken down into individual sugars; smaller protein molecules are broken down into peptides or individual amino acids; fats are broken down into glycerol and fatty acids.

When everything is properly broken down, most of the useful parts are absorbed through the lining of the small intestine and eventually end up in the bloodstream, which is the primary means of transporting nutrients from place to place.

The remainder of your meal then passes into the large intestine, which reabsorbs water and some minerals. The rest of the solid waste is excreted via, well … you know.

THE LIVER AND GALLBLADDER

Almost everything that goes from your gut into your bloodstream then goes directly to your liver, a critical metabolic regulator and filtration system. One of your liver's many jobs is to detoxify compounds in your blood that managed to improperly pass through your gut barrier into your bloodstream *before* that blood goes to the rest of your body. For example, bacteria that manage to barge their way through your intestinal lining are mostly destroyed by your immune system, but some leftover (toxic) components of those cells can still make their way into your bloodstream. Your liver filters them out before they get into the rest of the body. Your liver is also responsible for producing bile (which is stored in the gallbladder and helps to digest fats) and cholesterol (which is critical for normal cellular and hormonal function). It also forms fats (triglycerides) out of excess dietary carbohydrate and stores important substances like vitamins A, D, and B_{12} and copper and iron.

INSIDE OUTSIDE

Your small intestine is the key to a healthy digestive tract. It is long and convoluted, with an enormous surface area. (In fact, if you stretched it all out, it would be the size of a tennis court!) The small intestine functions as a "holding tank," keeping your food in place until it's fully digested, but its most important job is to help you effectively absorb nutrients.

Think of the intestinal lining as similar to the skin on your body—a highly flexible, resilient, semi-permeable membrane that acts as a barrier between your insides and the outside world. Skin is designed to keep good stuff (fluids, tissues, etc.) *inside* your body and bad stuff (bacteria, viruses, etc.) *out.*

Your small intestine does pretty much the same thing—except on a much larger scale. Yep, your gut is your largest interface with the outside world, more so than your skin or respiratory tract. This is why your gut is so critical to your immune system.

IT STARTS IN YOUR GUT

About 70 percent to 80 percent of your entire immune system is stationed in your gut. That's because there are all kinds of nasty beasties that would love to use your body as base camp, and most of them come in with your food and drink. So your immune system fortifies your intestinal wall with immune cells, which seek out and destroy pathogens trying to get through the intestinal lining. Any bad guys who make it past these immune cells into the bloodstream then have to travel through the liver, where even more immune cells are on hand to protect you. If they get past *all* of those defenses and manage to infect other tissues, a full-body immune response is triggered.

Think of food that is still *inside* your small intestine (in the lumen) as technically still *outside* your body. That's right, until your food passes through the lining of your intestine and into your bloodstream, it is technically not yet *in* your body.

Here is another critical point: The entire process of digestion takes place while your food is still inside the long tube that passes from the one end of your digestive tract to the other. If undigested food somehow finds its way *into* the body, well, it's as good as wasted.

Useless.

And probably harmful.

Keeping the right stuff in and the wrong stuff out is critical to a healthy gut.

Let's go back to talking about skin. Think about what would happen if your skin was "leaky," for example, if you crashed your bike and had major road rash. That road rash would expose your unprotected insides to the outside world. If some bacteria found their way inside, they could cause a pretty ugly infection, which your immune system would then have to work hard to fight off.

Well, a similar thing could happen if your gut was damaged and "leaky," to the extent that it was no longer able to keep the bad stuff out. If that were the case, your immune system would (again) have to deal with the foreign invaders that got "inside," where they didn't belong.

LEAKY GUT SYNDROME Leaky gut syndrome is not generally recognized by mainstream medical practitioners, which is probably frustrating for those of you who experience the consequences on a daily basis. Leaky gut (a simple way of saying "ongoing increased intestinal permeability") occurs when the intestinal lining is abnormally permeable or structurally damaged, leaving the small intestine unable to do its job of nutrient absorption while maintaining inside-outside order. As a result, some bacteria and their toxins, undigested food, and waste may "leak" out of the intestines into the bloodstream, triggering an immune reaction. This is how leaky gut syndrome is related to immune-mediated problems in the body.

So if the lining of your gut is *the* physical barrier between your insides and the outside world, it should be clear why the integrity of this barrier is pretty darn important. You must be able to maintain control over what is allowed inside your body.

Without that control, there is chaos, which starts in your digestive tract and spreads throughout the body.

The good news is that a healthy gut is very well adapted to filtering out the bad guys while still absorbing the stuff from your food that you need. Let's use another analogy to show how a healthy intestinal lining manages the process of selective absorption.

THE PARTY IS ROCKIN' (SECURITY ON THE INSIDE)

Think of your body as an exclusive members-only nightclub in the rough part of town. At Club Body, there is a security force on patrol inside the club at all times (immune cells circulating throughout the body) that watches over the members and deals with any riffraff that happens to sneak in. But the big, muscular bouncers at the doors (a collection of immune cells that form a part of your intestinal barrier) are your first line of defense: they decide who can enter Club Body (members) and who can't (anyone else).

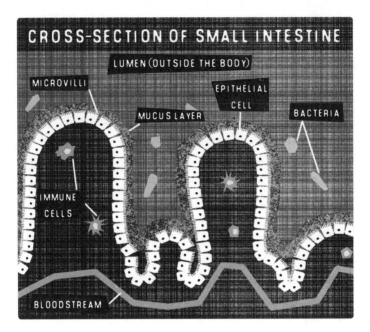

Some substances—properly digested food, for example—are recognized as members and allowed to come inside, while strangers and troublemakers (like bacteria and viruses) are denied entry. Other things we can't make use of inside, like undigested food and fiber, are also turned away.

The bouncers take their jobs very seriously, as experience has taught them that *all* outsiders have the potential to cause a lot of trouble if they get inside. There are only so many ways into the club, however, so as long as the bouncers guard all the doors and screen out any unsavory characters, things inside should (theoretically) stay healthy and safe.

BACTERIAL FRIENDS AND FOES

Since keeping your inside healthy and secure is so important, your body has assigned your security force some additional agents—a group of unlikely allies on the outside. Your body is home to trillions (yes, *trillions*) of bacteria, and most of them are in your gut. Over the course of a very long time, our immune system has developed a working relationship, an alliance of sorts, with some of these bacteria. Their presence does not trigger an immune response—they're considered trusted friends, and are a vital component of a healthy human body. We consider them our BBFs (Best Bacterial Friends), and we'd rather go without our big toes than give up these "friendlies"—they are *that* important.

Our alliance with these friendly bacteria is largely what helps regulate our delicately balanced immune activity. These bacterial undercover agents hang out in the intestine just outside the door to Club Body, helping your security staff by discouraging the bad guys from loitering and starting trouble. Friendly gut bacteria help us digest our food, absorb micronutrients, manufacture vitamins, stabilize immune function, and generally take up space that would otherwise be snapped up by pathogenic bacteria.

GOOD GUYS, BAD GUYS Researchers are rapidly growing to appreciate the centrality of the gut's bacterial population (microbiota) in determining many aspects of health, including metabolism, psychological well-being, and … immunity. Balanced gut bacteria (the right kinds, in the right amounts) help to promote balanced immune function, which leads to a more relaxed, finely-tuned immune system. If we compromise our population of good bacteria on the outside, the bad guys would have the opportunity to multiply. As the bad guys pile up just outside the doors, they put a lot of stress on our security team. Balance is key. It's a Goldilocks kind of situation: not too much, not too little … we need just the right amount.

HOW THINGS GO WRONG

So it seems as if your body (and your club) has a pretty good system for keeping itself healthy and safe. You've got the secure structure of the club itself (your intestinal lining), bouncers at the doors (immune cells in the lining), and a security force on the inside (circulating immune cells). Plus, you've got your friendly bacterial allies (BBFs) on the outside, helping to maintain law and order.

Your body's gut defense system generally works very well.

Until it doesn't.

There are a few ways bad guys can get into this exclusive nightclub. They might assault a bouncer, or wear a mask pretending to be a member, or pry open a locked (unused) door that was left unguarded. Or, if your

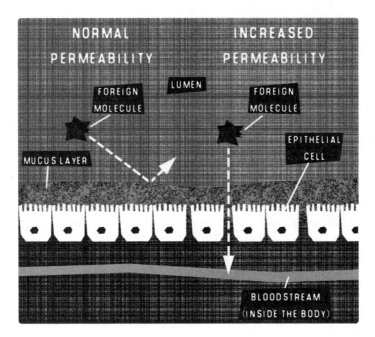

gut is leaky (picture a sieve), all the doors and windows are wide open, and there's no way to control who comes in. This spells big-time trouble for the in-house security force.

In this situation, your club is no longer healthy and safe. Letting bad guys in (through what should be tightly controlled entry points) leads to fights and destruction of property and could eventually overwhelm the rest of the security staff inside.

**The same thing happens inside your body if your
intestinal lining is compromised.**

Once they're in, the bad guys run rampant through the *whole body*.

And that is a very bad situation—but do you want to know the worst part?

Poor food choices are to blame.

Poor food choices flood your gut with bad guys, overwhelming your immune system. Bad food is what brings in the hoodlums, impersonators, and lock pickers, all of whom do what they are biologically designed to do—get in and wreak havoc. You create this condition of increased gut permeability, digestive distress, and systemic inflammation just by choosing the wrong foods. And it's not your fault, because you didn't even know you were doing it. (Not to worry—we'll explain which foods disrupt your gut in Part 3.)

WHY IT MATTERS

Some overly optimistic folks may wonder at this point if there could be an *advantage* to increased intestinal permeability. We get where they're coming from—like maybe if that barrier were a little more lenient, you could potentially absorb more nutrients, or digest your food a little bit faster. But that's not how the body is meant to work. Again, let's talk about skin. Is there *ever* a biological advantage to having an open wound? The answer is, of course, no.

Increased gut permeability is *always* a problem because it means your body no longer has control over what comes in and what stays out. Increased gut permeability (and the ensuing inflammatory chaos) is linked not only to intestinal inflammatory conditions like Crohn's disease, ulcerative colitis, and irritable bowel syndrome (IBS), but also chronic diseases like cardiovascular disease and diabetes, hypersensitivities like asthma and allergies, and autoimmune conditions like Hashimoto's thyroiditis, rheumatoid arthritis, and type 1 diabetes.

In fact, this third Good Food standard is directly linked to the fourth, because increased intestinal permeability provokes systemic inflammation. (You'll learn why that's bad soon enough.)

The importance of your gut as a healthy, intact barrier cannot be overstated.

One last thing—and the final nail in your leaky gut coffin. Remember how excessive abdominal fat (central obesity, or what the media calls being "apple shaped") is a clear risk factor for heart disease, high blood pressure, stroke, and diabetes?

Deposition of visceral fat (which contributes to that sexy apple shape) is one of the *direct* effects of increased gut permeability.

Over time, with ongoing gut leakage, your liver and surrounding fat deposits act like a spongy trap for some of the bad guys that get in. This leads to significant inflammation in those tissues, as well as excessive deposits of fat in both the liver and surrounding adipose tissue.

That means your leaky gut also plays a major role (along with cortisol) in your stubborn belly fat and directly contributes to your risk of conditions like heart disease, high blood pressure, stroke, and diabetes.

We should have your attention by now—but once again, there is good news. Much like with your hormones, even after decades of poor diet and in the face of a gut leaking like a sieve, in most cases, the situation is all *highly reversible*. You can heal your intestinal lining, reinstate a high-functioning security system, and restore a thriving population of healthy bacteria if you do the same simple thing:

Change the food you put on your plate.

THE SCIENCE-Y SUMMARY

- The food you eat should foster a healthy gut and digestive system.
- Maintaining a healthy gut barrier is critically important to your health.
- Certain foods can unbalance your healthy gut bacteria and/or promote intestinal permeability, compromising gut integrity.
- Compromised gut integrity and bacterial imbalance lead to digestive distress and can promote chronic disease, hypersensitivities, and autoimmune conditions in the body.
- Most of your immune system is located in your gut, which means our third and fourth Good Food standards are very closely linked.

CHAPTER 7:
INFLAMMATION: NO ONE IS IMMUNE

"The thought of resetting my system so it didn't crave sugar or carbs was my original Whole30 motivation. I had no clue that God would use the Whole30 to bring total alleviation of my pain! I've been diagnosed with fibromyalgia, osteoarthritis, IBS, and other issues. At one point, I was on four or five different medications! But by my third week of the Whole30, all of my joint pain, bone pain, and muscle pain was gone. My mind was clear. I was focused. I also happened to lose fourteen pounds and kicked my cravings, but those were minor compared to having complete relief from all of the other issues."
—*Bethann M., Pleasant Lake, Indiana*

Our final Good Food standard, clearly linked to the third standard, states that your food choices should support immune function and minimize inflammation.

When we say "support immune function," we mean that your food choices should result in a well-rested, highly-effective defense system. In other words, food should not cause excessive ongoing immune activity, also known as *systemic inflammation*. (More specifically, we're concerned with *chronic* systemic inflammation—the stuff that goes on for weeks, months, or even years.)

You might have heard of systemic inflammation before, in a headline or a media sound bite, but you probably don't have a very clear picture of what it actually is, or why it matters.

Let's tackle the first part.

INFLAMMATION—HERE, THERE, EVERYWHERE?

Inflammation, put simply, is the immune system doing its job—it is your body's protective attempt to stop injury in its tracks and initiate recovery. Inflammation indicates a mobilization of your immune system; it's a call to arms. Whether the damaged tissue is a result of infection from bacterial invaders, overuse, or physical trauma, the purpose of the inflammation that ensues is to prevent additional damage and repair the damage already done.

But what starts out as a healthy response can have adverse effects if it persists for too long or spreads too far. Since there are a few different subsets of inflammation (some healthy, some not so healthy), we'll give you the rundown here:

Related to *duration*

Acute	Chronic
Your body's initial, short-term response to damage. Think of acute inflammation as the cleanup before the rebuilding. It decreases quickly as your body begins the healing process. Acute inflammation is a good thing, and you wouldn't want to lose that function.	Chronic inflammation stretches the inflammatory response out over months or even years, which impairs the rebuilding of normal tissues and creates all sorts of health problems.

Related to *location*

Localized	Systemic
Mostly confined to a specific area of the body.	"Full body," characterized by a highly activated immune system circulating in your bloodstream and going *everywhere.*

So from here on out, when we say "inflammation," we're not talking about the kind of inflammation you get when you sprain your ankle (acute localized inflammation) or the kind you get when you have the flu (acute systemic inflammation). We're talking about the most damaging kind of inflammation—the unhealthy kind—*chronic* (long-term) *systemic* (full-body) inflammation.

GOT IMMUNITY?

Before we discuss how chronic systemic inflammation can be devastating to your health, let's go back to how the immune system controls inflammation, both good and bad. Your immune system is actually a highly interconnected complex of tissues and circulating cells that protect you from all the mean, ugly stuff out in the big, bad world: bacteria, parasites, fungi, viruses, and more. The world is chock-full of nasty little buggers that would love to use your insides as home sweet home, and your fork is the easiest vehicle for them to hitch a ride on.

In order for your immune system to properly protect you, it must be able to accurately differentiate between "you" and "not you." (Immunologists call it "self" and "non-self.") When your body senses something that is "non-self" where it doesn't belong, it will perform an immediate evaluation, which may then trigger one of two immune responses: a nonspecific suspicion of something unfamiliar or a specific, aggressive response to a known troublemaker.

Let's use another analogy.

If you woke up and found a strange man hanging out in your kitchen, you'd feel threatened and anxious. You'd be suspicious of his motives and would probably react in an anxious, defensive manner, asking him what the heck he's doing in your home, and then taking appropriate action—inviting him to stay if you discovered he was a family friend, or asking him to leave if he didn't belong there.

But if this man was in the process of vandalizing your kitchen, you'd immediately know he wasn't a good guy, and would respond strongly to his presence by calling the police or chasing him out with a golf club. And if you happened to see him in your kitchen again the next day (persistent, isn't he?), you'd immediately remember that he was a bad guy, and would launch an even more aggressive response to get him out of your house.

Your immune system operates in a similar fashion. Anything that doesn't belong in your body is assumed to be a threat, so it's trapped and assessed—questioned, if you will. If it's determined that the substance may cause you harm, it's immediately dealt with and "logged" as a troublemaker. Your immune system will then respond to future encounters with this same substance in a more specific, targeted fashion—with antibodies and a SWAT-team level of aggression.

So, identity matters. Being able to tell "you" from "not you" matters. Keeping things in their rightful places matters. This is where the third and fourth Good Food standards come back together.

Certain foods beat up, fool, or sneak past the "bouncers," finding a way out of your digestive tract and into your body. They create immune chaos, forcing your system to protect you from the downstream effects of what *should* be a normal bodily function—digesting food. They confuse your immune cells, causing them to create antibodies to fight what would normally be perfectly healthy and good. As a result of the immune system dysfunction that ensues, you can develop food sensitivities or allergies, systemic inflammation, and possibly an autoimmune condition.

Bad things happen when you confuse or overwork your immune system.

And to drive the point home, we'll show you exactly what that looks like.

FIGHT FIRES AND FIX FLAWS

Your immune system defends you against external invaders, but it also plays a critical role in recovery from injury and the repair and maintenance of various body structures. Your immune system has its priorities and tends to rank fighting off invaders above general repair and maintenance. (Getting the guy out of your kitchen is more important than doing the dishes.) But all of these jobs are important in the body—and if something doesn't get done, there will eventually be consequences.

Let's use another analogy.

Think of your immune system as a team of firefighters. Their top priority is to defend against potentially damaging threats—fires. But they also have to do routine maintenance and repair jobs, like fixing damaged tools, washing fire trucks, sleeping, and eating. Your firefighters work very hard when they're fighting a fire, but they also have periods of time when they

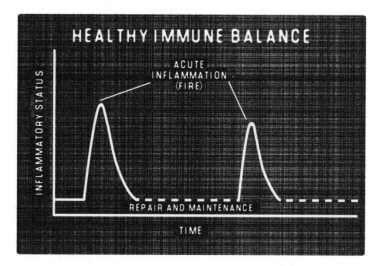

are relatively relaxed. There is a distinct difference between infrequent responses to fires (acute conditions, like a traumatic injury or short-term infection) and having to battle them 24-7 (chronic activation of your immune system, or systemic inflammation).

In the "healthy immune balance" example, your firefighters respond to a four-alarm fire. They fight the blaze, head back to the station, and have time to clean up and do some low-level repair and maintenance before they're expected to go all out again. In this situation, your firefighters (immune system) ramp *way* up for the fire (acute inflammation from traumatic injury, infection, etc.), but once the fire is out, immune activity decreases, allowing for repair, recovery and maintenance tasks to be performed.

This is normal, and represents a healthy, balanced response. Your immune system needs an "on" switch to be able to ramp up to a threat, but it also needs an "off" switch in order to allow for recovery and have the time and resources to complete important repair and maintenance chores.

In the "chronic systemic inflammation" example, however, as the firefighters are winding down from the acutely stressful and demanding fire, they're told that while they're still expected to fulfill their normal firehouse repair and maintenance obligations, their job parameters have expanded to include sweeping the city streets, collecting the garbage, teaching the school kids, and filling in potholes.

Whew.

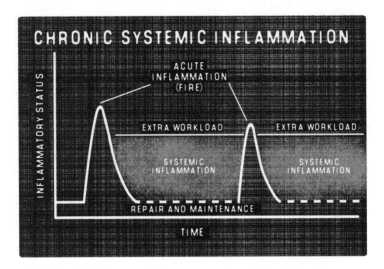

As if their original job description didn't entail enough responsibility, now they've got a lot more work to do. If this were a one-time event, they could manage—they'd do the extra work and eventually catch up on their repair and maintenance functions. But if this situation continues for any length of time, it causes serious trouble long-term.

An overworked, out-of-balance immune system is very unhealthy.

If certain factors (like your food choices) are overloading your immune system with too many tasks, it's going to be less effective at doing its *main* jobs, and something is going to be left undone, or done ineffectively.

Like fighting off that bug that's going around.

Or healing that stubborn tendonitis.

Or keeping your arteries clear of plaque.

All very important jobs, we think you'd agree.

WHY IT MATTERS

The reason we are so adamant about reducing chronic systemic inflammation is that it has been clearly implicated as a causative factor for most lifestyle-related diseases.

Medical researchers have long known that a cluster of symptoms (labeled "metabolic syndrome") were highly statistically correlated, often occurring together and increasing your risk of heart disease, stroke and diabetes. What they didn't know for a long time, however, was exactly how they were related. They used to think that obesity caused diabetes, that high cholesterol caused heart attack, that high blood pressure caused stroke, and that maybe diabetes caused obesity too, but there was no unified theory to put all of these pieces together.

Today, while there are still multiple theories about how to explain these associations, some significant relationships have been established. More specifically, we've learned that systemic inflammation contributes directly to insulin resistance and diabetes, cardiovascular disease, stroke, high blood pressure, high cholesterol, high triglycerides, chronic inflammatory diseases (like IBS and asthma), bone and joint disease (like osteoporosis and arthritis), neurological conditions (like Alzheimer's and Parkinson's), and most certainly weight gain.

This makes chronic systemic inflammation a *very* big deal.

Managing your inflammatory status profoundly impacts your quality of life.

Having any one of these symptoms or conditions—or more than one, which is all too common when it comes to metabolic syndrome—will seriously affect your quality of life today, tomorrow, and for years to come ... even if you exercise regularly, eat "pretty healthy" and aren't overweight. Remember, it's called *silent* inflammation. And it's why 40-year-old men drop dead of a heart attack while running marathons.

But what if you're young, healthy, active, and lean? Surely this stuff doesn't apply to you!

Of course it does, but you're probably too young to realize it. It's OK—when you're 20, conditions like heart disease and stroke don't even *register*—they're diseases "old people" get.

We were 20 once. We understand.

So let's bring this one home for you younger folks.

Chronic systemic inflammation plays a key role in more than just age-related diseases. Inflammation contributes to a long list of conditions that you may be dealing with right now. Like asthma, allergies, acne, eczema and other skin conditions, depression, ADHD, and mood swings.

Do we have your attention now?

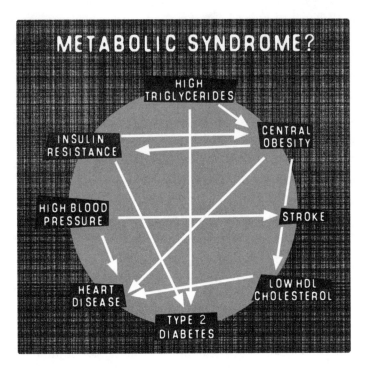

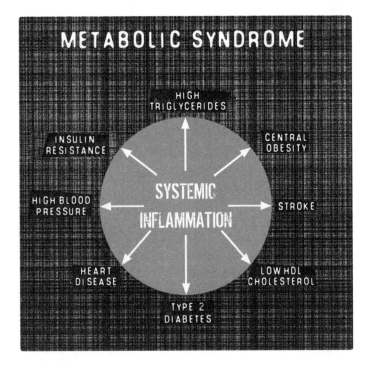

EXERCISE AND RECOVERY

Chronic systemic inflammation affects your physical fitness, whether you play a sport, are a "weekend warrior," or are just a regular gym-goer. Think of exercise as microscopic structural injury—a stressor that forces your body to adapt, making you stronger and healthier. The exercise itself isn't the most important part—you get fitter when you are *recovering* from that exercise. Giving your body enough time and resources to repair damage and build new tissue is critical to becoming stronger, faster and healthier. If you have chronic systemic inflammation, your body isn't as good at recovery and maintenance—including repairing the structural damage caused by exercise. Which makes you more likely to get injured or overtrain, and definitely means you won't be as strong or fast as you could be. Systemic inflammation ruins *everything*, doesn't it?

BUT IT'S SILENT!

At this point, you're probably wondering, "If this stuff is silent, how do I know if I have it?" That is a very good question—and we've got the answer.

First, if you are eating *any* of the foods we're about to discuss in the next section, there's a pretty good chance that you have some chronic systemic inflammation. These foods elicit inflammation both directly and indirectly, and their effects are largely universal.

If you're overweight, you are also systemically inflamed. (You don't *have* to be overweight to be inflamed, but pretty much everyone who is overweight has some inflammation.) Adipose tissue (body fat) is largely regarded by the scientific community as a separate endocrine organ, producing a number of different biologically active messengers. When fat cells are damaged by being overfilled, certain immune cells are summoned to fat tissue to help repair and clean up the damaged cells. These immune cells then secrete additional immune-reactive substances that increase inflammation in the fat itself as well as elsewhere in the body.

The more body fat you have, the more of these inflammatory compounds your fat cells can secrete. So if you're overweight, we can be pretty sure you're also somewhat inflamed. Guess what? Belly fat is *especially* active in this process, contributing to inflammation more than fat stores in other areas (like your buttocks or thighs).

More specifically, however, we believe that silent inflammation isn't so silent when you know what you're listening for. This is a comprehensive (but not exhaustive) list of conditions and diseases linked to systemic inflammation or having an inflammatory component. If you experience any of these conditions or symptoms, there's a pretty good chance you have some of that "silent" inflammation.

Related to Silent Inflammation

acid reflux/heartburn	eczema	multiple sclerosis
acne	edema	myasthenia gravis
allergies	emphysema	myositis
alopecia	endometriosis	nephritis
Alzheimer's disease	essential tremor	obesity
anemia	fibroids	osteopenia
arthritis	fibromyalgia	osteoporosis
asthma	gastroenteritis	Parkinson's disease
atherosclerosis	gingivitis	PCOS
bipolar disorder	gout	periodontal disease
bronchitis	Grave's disease	polychondritis
chronic bursitis	Hashimoto's thyroid-itis	psoriasis
cancer	heart disease	Raynaud's phenom-enon
carditis	hepatitis	rheumatoid arthritis
celiac disease	high blood pressure	sarcoidosis
chronic pain	high cholesterol	scleroderma
circulation issues	high triglycerides	seizures
cirrhosis	infertility	sinusitis
colitis	inflammatory bowel syndrome	Sjögren's syndrome
Crohn's disease	insulin resistance	spastic colon
dementia	interstitial cystitis	chronic tendonitis
depression	joint pain	trichotillomania
dermatitis	lupus	ulcerative colitis
diabetes (types 1 & 2)	Lyme disease	vasculitis
diverticulitis	migraines	vitiligo

That's a pretty long list, right?

It's what we've been saying: managing the inflammatory status of your body affects your *quality of life.*

WHAT ABOUT GENETICS?

This entire book is devoted to the idea that food plays the most important role in your pursuit of optimal health, but it's not the only factor. Lifestyle choices, exercise habits, your environment, and, of course, your genes also affect your health and predisposition for a variety of lifestyle-related diseases and conditions. But genes may play a different role than you think.

You hear folks saying, "Diabetes/high cholesterol/heart disease runs in my family!" as if to suggest that their destiny is predetermined. Most people believe that what is encoded in their DNA is unchangeable. The good news is that that couldn't be further from the truth.

Your genetic makeup certainly plays a role in everything from height to eye color to health. But even more important than the genes in your DNA sequence is which of those genes get *turned on.* A gene that isn't turned on doesn't actually *do* anything. It's the intersection of your environmental inputs and your genetics that is truly relevant to your health.

Epigenetics is the intersection of your genes and your environment.

Epigenetics is the study of gene expression—whether genes turn on or turn off, and how loudly their information is expressed. While we are all born with a certain code, we are also born with switches that tell that code what to do. Our environmental input (diet, exercise, air quality, etc.) activates those switches. Think about it this way:

Genetics loads the gun, but environment pulls the trigger.

Epigenetics is also influenced by physical and emotional stress. In fact, gene expression is impacted by how you respond to *everything* that happens in your environment, from air pollution to a move across the country to childhood trauma.

In short, you generally don't develop diabetes, high blood pressure, or heart disease simply because of a defective gene or a familial predisposition. It takes the intersection of your genes and your environment to turn on those sequences of events.

This is good news.

It means we are not doomed by our genetics.

In the case of diabetes, high blood pressure, and heart disease (among others), it means that those conditions are largely preventable.

Our gun may be loaded, but if we don't pull the trigger with a poor diet, lack of exercise, inadequate sleep, excessive stress, and other unhealthy lifestyle factors, the chance of us developing one of those diseases is dramatically reduced.

So keep reading, because this book is devoted to keeping the safety on one of the biggest potential triggers in your environment—the food you put on your plate.

THE GOOD NEWS

The good news is that, much like with your hormones and leaky gut, even after decades of poor eating habits and years of systemic inflammation, most of the health consequences are *highly reversible*. You can reduce systemic inflammation, heal from most inflammatory conditions and catch up on those repair and recovery functions your body has fallen behind on.

However, some things may not always be totally reversible.

Eventually, if systemic inflammation is left unchecked, the immune system becomes so overworked and paranoid that it creates illnesses that may, unfortunately, be irreversible. But we've found that by doing just one thing, you can drastically reduce or eliminate the *symptoms* of most of these inflammation-related diseases and conditions—and therefore significantly improve the quality of your life.

You know what we're going to tell you to do.

Change the food you put on your plate.

THE SCIENCE-Y SUMMARY

- The food you eat should promote a balanced immune system, and minimize chronic systemic inflammation.
- Chronic systemic inflammation is full-body (systemic), long-term (chronic) up-regulation of your immune system activity.
- Your immune system has two major functions—defense against threats and low-level repair and maintenance.
- Certain foods sneak past your gut's defense system, and create immune chaos.
- If certain factors, like your food choices, are overloading your immune system, it's going to be less effective at doing its main jobs, and something is going to be left undone or done poorly.
- Chronic systemic inflammation is a central risk factor for a number of lifestyle-related diseases and conditions and is at the heart of metabolic syndrome.
- Silent inflammation isn't so silent if you know what to listen for.
- Managing the inflammatory status of your body profoundly impacts your quality of life.

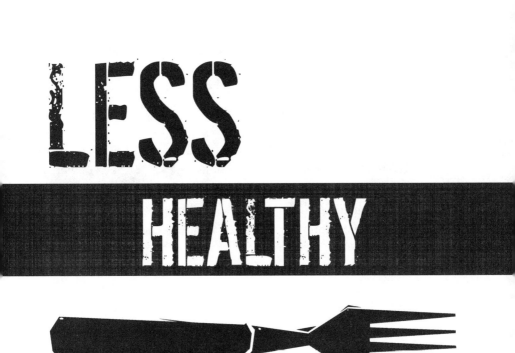

LESS HEALTHY

CHAPTER 8:
SUGAR, SWEETENERS, AND ALCOHOL

"I was diagnosed with Lyme disease in October of 2009. My symptoms were stiff neck, headache … I hurt everywhere, I was tired all the time, I could not sleep through the night because I was in so much pain! My doctor told me it could take six months of antibiotics or more to start feeling better. I thought to myself, 'I do not have six months to wait!' I found the Whole30 and thought, 'Let me try it—what do I have to lose?' Well, I had a lot to lose—like every one of my Lyme disease symptoms, and a few pounds as well! I started feeling better after day three, and I just kept feeling better—to the point at which I feel healthier now than I did before I had Lyme, as long as I stay on my dietary course!"

—Anita H., Albany, New York

Here comes the part you've all been waiting for (or dreading?). This is where we talk about all of the food groups that don't pass our four Good Food standards. We're going to use a legend to help explain why.

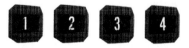

1. **These foods fail our first Good Food standard: a healthy psychological response.** These foods light up pleasure, reward, and emotional pathways in the brain, offering supernormally stimulating flavors without providing the nutrition that nature intended. These are foods-with-no-brakes, promoting overconsumption and the inability to control your cravings, habits, and behaviors.

2. **These foods fail our second Good Food standard: a healthy hormonal response.** These foods disrupt your normal hormonal balance, promoting leptin resistance, insulin resistance (and all of the negative downstream effects that follow), disrupting glucagon's energy-access function, and elevating cortisol levels.
3. **These foods fail our third Good Food standard: support a healthy gut.** These foods directly promote intestinal permeability, leading to a less-than-intact barrier that lets foreign substances get inside the body (where they do not belong). Foods that fail our third Good Food standard by default also fail the fourth.
4. **These foods fail our fourth Good Food standard: support immune function and minimize inflammation.** By creating intestinal permeability (or directly promoting chronic systemic inflammation), these foods force your immune system out of a healthy balance. This can lead to the development of systemic inflammatory symptoms or autoimmune diseases and is a central risk factor for many lifestyle-related diseases and conditions.

Before we get started, we know that there are some very fun foods in this group; foods that may form the vast majority of your daily diet; foods that may make you close this book, look up at the sky and say, "These people are *bananas.*"

Before we tell you what they are, we just want to ask you a few simple questions.

Is it *just fine* that some of the foods you eat are controlling your behaviors, making you crave things you don't really want to eat, and proving impossible to resist even when you really, truly try?

Do you *like* energy slumps, brain fogs, insidious weight gain, frequent hunger pangs, the inability to burn fat, and a metabolism that moves slower than molasses?

Can you *live* with gas, bloating, constipation, diarrhea, abdominal discomfort, fatigue, malnutrition, and food allergies?

Do you *welcome* an increase in illness, infection, aches, pains, and the signs and symptoms of innumerable diseases and conditions, some of which are irreversible?

We bet you answered every one of these questions with a resounding, "Of course not!"

So do us a favor, please?

Remember your answer to these questions as we move through this section.

At some point, you will have to weigh the fleeting pleasure of a slice of pizza, pint of beer, or frozen yogurt against one or more of these scenarios. Let's start with some of the easy ones, just to get the ball rolling.

SUGAR AND SWEETENERS

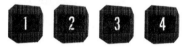

We're going to start with at least one thing we should all agree on: Sugar does not make you healthier.

Do you want to argue with that? Can *anyone* make a case that added sugar contributes positively to our health?*

What may surprise you is that both sugar and artificial sweeteners fail all four of our Good Food standards.

We think of the sweet stuff first when describing foods that provoke an unhealthy psychological response. Because the sweetness of sugar is addictive, eating an excess amount is easy. The more sugar we eat, the more we get acclimated to high levels, and the more we want.

Artificial sweeteners may be even *more* problematic because they are designed to deliver a sweetness hit that is far beyond what you could ever find in nature.

Aspartame (Equal) and stevia are 200 to 300 times sweeter than table sugar.

Sucralose (Splenda) is 600 times sweeter than table sugar.

Saccharin (Sweet'N Low) is up to 700 times sweeter than table sugar.

Remember the Vegas Strip analogy? Artificial sweeteners are the very definition of "supernormally stimulating."

---

*We doubt it. In a most unscientific experiment, we Googled "sugar is healthy" to see if we could find any support for this hypothesis. The first link that appeared was titled "Experts agree—sugar is a health destroyer." True story.

Is it any wonder we are slaves to the sweet stuff?

These artificial sweeteners provide taste and reward sensations the likes of which we (biologically) have never before experienced, burning our taste buds (and pleasure centers) out on stimuli that are simply otherworldly. It thus becomes harder and harder for us to experience the same level of pleasure and reward that we did the last time we ate them—and makes it darn near impossible to appreciate the natural flavors found in fresh foods.

Wait—we'll tell you a story.

At one of our nutrition workshops, after the section on artificial sweeteners, a lovely woman shyly raised her hand and asked, "But if I can't sweeten my strawberries with Splenda, how do I make them taste sweet?"

Bless her heart.

This phenomenon is all too common in artificial sweetener users.

REMEMBER LEPTIN? Your hormones may also have a role in this phenomenon. Research suggests that the taste organ (your tongue and taste buds) is a peripheral target for leptin. Leptin resistance (when your brain can no longer effectively sense leptin's message) may lead to an "enhanced behavioral preference for sweet substances." When you're leptin resistant, the taste of sweetness is dulled, which makes you eat more to satisfy your craving. See how that plays right into the supernormally stimulating artificial sweeteners?

Added sugar is one of the quickest and easiest foods to provoke an unhealthy hormonal response. Overconsumption of sugar-sweetened, nutrient-poor processed foods means blood sugar levels rise too high, too often, which promotes a reliance on carbohydrate for fuel. Excess carbohydrate is turned into triglycerides, which, along with chronically elevated blood sugar, contributes to leptin resistance. It also means fat isn't burned for fuel, which may lead to an accumulation of body fat. Leptin resistance promotes further overconsumption, which means fat accumulates inside cells, leading to insulin resistance, hyperglycemia, and chronically elevated insulin levels. Elevated cortisol levels promote stress-related cravings, which generally means you reach for more sweet foods with lots of added sugar.

It's a vicious cycle.

EMPTY CALORIES We'll hammer yet another nail into sugar's coffin here. From a micronutrient perspective, sugar provides virtually nothing in terms of vitamins, minerals, or phytonutrients. (No, blackstrap molasses is *not* a healthy source of iron. Since when we do look to *sugar* for iron, anyway?) All sugar provides is calories—four per gram. It's the very definition of "empty calories"—all of the energy with none of the nutrition. And that doesn't sound very sweet to us.

Sugar also messes with the healthy environment of our guts, specifically altering the delicate balance of "good" and "bad" bacteria. Unfriendly gut bacteria love refined sugars, which means your added sugar intake serves only to promote the existence of the bad guys—and can reduce the population of good guys. This condition (called dysbiosis) can lead to gas, bloating, cramps, diarrhea, constipation, and inflammatory symptoms like fatigue, body aches, headaches, and joint problems. Artificial sweeteners like Splenda may also kill off your beneficial flora, even when consumed in "normal" amounts.

Finally, sugar promotes inflammation in the body two different ways. First, concentrated sugars added to processed foods promote overconsumption, which in turn promotes inflammation via leptin and insulin resistance. In addition, sugar's effect on gut bacteria and promotion of gut dysbiosis (like when "bad" bacteria are wreaking havoc) is by definition an inflammatory condition in the gut.

NOT SO SWEET? Numerous reports have associated the use of various artificial sweeteners with various conditions, like cancer, inflammatory bowel disease, migraines, kidney disorders, autoimmune conditions, carpal tunnel syndrome, and neurotoxicity. There have not been enough long-term studies on humans to definitively confirm or deny these associations, but for us, the potential risks represent additional downsides in an already very long list—more than enough justification to avoid artificial sweeteners altogether.

Now that we've got *that* out of the way, let's talk about what we mean by "added" sugars.

First, we're *not* talking about the natural sugars found in whole foods, like fruit. Remember, we don't practice food reductionism—fruit is not sugar, fruit is *food*! There is sugar in fruit, but as we'll soon discuss, that sugar comes in a micronutrient-dense package of vitamins, minerals, phytonutrients, fiber, and water. That kind of sugar is *not* the stuff we're cautioning you against.

Added sugar is any form of sugar or sugar alternative added to foods or beverages when they are processed or prepared. It's the raw sugar you put in your coffee, the honey you add to your tea or the agave syrup that sweetens your ice cream. We don't discriminate between the source or the form, and we don't care whether it's "all natural" or "unrefined." As you'll learn in this chapter:

Sugar = Sugar = Sugar.

There are some metabolic differences between specific forms of sugar (glucose, fructose, lactose, etc.), but they all have one thing in common: a sweet taste that promotes overconsumption, and no significant nutritive value. Empty calories. Which means there is nothing special or "better" about honey, or maple syrup, or agave, or blackstrap molasses.

NOT NATURAL The same goes for artificial sweeteners. NutraSweet, Equal, Splenda, stevia—none is any more "natural" than the shoes you are wearing on your feet right now. Some are derived from nature, but after chemical processing, Splenda has more in common with pesticides than table sugar. (And stevia isn't any better. We dare you to find a stevia leaf and chew on it for a while. It ain't that sweet. At least, not until it's refined into white crystals in a laboratory somewhere.)

So in summary, sugar and artificial sweeteners fail all four of our Good Food standards and do not make you healthier. And yes, we know you're dying to ask a question right now. "But if I *am* going to eat sugar, what form of sugar is the least bad?"

Let's save the answer for after the next section.

ALCOHOL

1 **2** **3** **4**

This section is going to be short, because alcohol has no redeeming health qualities. We don't care what you've heard about red wine or agave tequila or gluten-free beer—the common denominator of all these beverages is the *alcohol*, and the *alcohol* is the primary problem. (We'll address some of the marketing claims to make booze appear to be a less-guilty pleasure later.)

Alcohol fails all four of our Good Food standards. First, in terms of a healthy psychological response, alcohol is addictive. Not just the colloquial definition of "addiction"—it's *actually* addictive in the clinical definition: promoting desire even in the face of negative consequences, tolerance to the effect of the substance, and withdrawal symptoms when use is reduced or stopped.

Regularly consuming things that are known to be clinically addictive doesn't sound super healthy to us.

But for those of us who are merely social drinkers (and not worried about addiction), alcohol still promotes an unhealthy psychological effect.

Alcohol inhibits our inhibitory mechanisms. Which means that when you are under the influence, you are more likely to make bad decisions.*

Consuming something that is going to blunt your judgment—leading to late-night splurges on pizza, ice cream, or an entire tube of cookie dough—does not facilitate your success in making good food choices. Furthermore, it takes only a small amount of alcohol to impair inhibitions and decision making—and the effects on the brain carry over until the next day. Which means that a drink or three on a Friday night may lead to a weekend's worth of poor food choices.

You may know what we're talking about.

From a hormonal perspective, alcohol consumption interferes with glucose function in the body and with the actions of regulatory hormones like insulin and glucagon. Even in well-nourished people, alcohol can dis-

---

*With food. Decisions with your food. We can't help you with those other bad decisions. That's a different book altogether.

turb blood sugar levels. Especially when combined with sugar (Jack and Coke, anyone?), alcohol increases insulin secretion, which pulls too much blood sugar out of the bloodstream, causing temporary hypoglycemia. Furthermore, alcohol can impair glucagon's normal function, leaving your blood sugar levels too low for too long—a very stressful situation for the body.

EMPTY CALORIES TIMES TWO

Ready for some math? If sugar is "empty calories," and alcohol has almost twice as many calories per gram as sugar, then isn't alcohol the *mother* of all empty calories? It's got more than enough energy to mess up your hormones, but doesn't provide a lick of valuable nutrition. Lose-lose.

Finally, as a special bonus hormonal effect, acute *and* chronic alcohol consumption have been known to inhibit testosterone production.

Ouch.

Numerous studies also show—rather conclusively, in fact—that alcohol directly promotes intestinal permeability and overgrowth of gut bacteria, contributing to a leaky gut and all of the downstream inflammatory effects. But that's not the only way alcohol affects your immune system: both acute and chronic alcohol use impair cellular immunity, leaving your immune system even less prepared to deal with inflammatory consequences. Alcohol is also pro-oxidative, meaning that it contributes to oxidation in the body: it reduces antioxidant levels by increasing free radicals, which (as we'll detail soon enough) contributes to chronic systemic inflammation.

DANCE WITH ME

Even in moderate amounts, alcohol is acutely neurotoxic. It alters the normal activity of your nervous system, may cause damage to nervous tissue, and can disrupt or even kill neurons, the cells that transmit and process signals in the brain and other parts of the nervous system. In layman's terms, it's why a few drinks makes you stumble, slur your words, and think you're a really good dancer. Other neurotoxins include mercury, lead, insecticides, formaldehyde, and biotoxins like botulism. But no one ever asks for a mercury daiquiri, now, do they? We don't think things with neurotoxic potential are a healthy choice.

Let's discuss the arguments *in favor of* certain types of alcohol—like "heart healthy" red wine. First caveat:

**These claims come from the people who manufacture
and market alcohol.**

If you sold a product that was generally deemed unhealthy in the scientific literature, wouldn't you want to find one thing about your product that might make it sound less bad? Of course you would! So if you were Mr. Red Wine Producer, you might read (or fund) some studies on the heart-healthy effects of certain antioxidants, like resveratrol,* realize your wine contains tiny amounts of this healthy compound, and start marketing your wine as "heart healthy."

We can hardly blame him. After all, Mr. Red Wine Producer isn't looking out for your health—he's looking out for his *profits* (nothing wrong with that; he's running a business, after all). Finding something healthy about his product is very, very good for business.

The problem is, it's a technicality. A fluid ounce of red wine averages 160 micrograms of resveratrol (with a wide range of variability between bottles and sources). Most research on resveratrol has been done on animals, not people—and to get the same dose of resveratrol used in the mice studies, a person would have to drink more than 60 liters (that's *80 bottles*) of red wine every day.

Seriously?

The other thing that Mr. Red Wine Producer doesn't mention is that the resveratrol in red wine actually comes from the skin of red grapes.

So ... just eat the darn grapes.

You'll get all of the potential (reported) benefits of resveratrol and none of the downsides of the alcohol. Win-win, except if you're Mr. Red Wine Producer.

The argument is the same for 100 percent agave tequila or gluten-free beer. Just because manufacturers have found a way to make their products "less bad" doesn't mean they're good for you.

Interestingly, in January 2012, a University of Connecticut researcher who worked on the health benefits of resveratrol was found to have fabricated or manipulated data in 145 separate research projects. Huh.

We are not interested in "less bad."

Our mission is to present you with *optimal*.

THE GOOD NEWS

Hear us out, now. We are *not* saying you can never eat any sugar or drink any alcohol ever again. We simply want you to make educated decisions about foods. We don't want you justifying your choices with marketing pitches or telling yourself that because it's gluten-free, low-carb, or heart-healthy, it's a perfectly fine choice.

Why go through all that self-deception, when the fact that [fill in the blank] is just plain *delicious* is a good enough reason all by itself to indulge?

We're not food robots. We like to indulge from time to time, just like the rest of you. But we're honest about our reasons, and we want you to be honest too: "This food/drink is not making me healthier, but that's OK, because it's delicious/special/culturally-relevant/emotionally-significant."

We fully support those reasons.

When it comes to less-healthy foods, understand that the less (and less often) you indulge in them, the healthier you'll be. Where you draw that line is totally up to you.

We'll talk a lot more about this later. We just wanted to mention it now, so you could stop wondering if we are trying to ruin your life.

CHAPTER 9:
SEED OILS

"I suffered my very last migraine right before I went on the Whole30 program. This change is totally amazing for me, because I've been getting migraines three to four times a year, for a week or more at a time, for the past eight years. I would be totally incapacitated—unable to do anything except just lie there in pain. Now I feel fairly confident that I can look forward to a migraine-free future. Thanks, Whole30, for changing my life!"
—Laura R.

Industrial seed oils or vegetable oils are extracted from the seeds of various plants. While these oils come from a variety of sources (peanuts, soybeans, sunflower seeds), they all share two common denominators—a high proportion of *polyunsaturated fat (PUFA)* and a large amount of *omega-6 fatty acids*. Diets high in these types of fats—specifically when derived from seed oils—have been shown to directly promote systemic inflammation, thereby violating our fourth Good Food standard.

Can we just leave it at that? Be our guest and skip the rest of the chapter if you'll take our word for it. If you'd like the background, read on.

PUFA OVERLOAD

Polyunsaturated fats (PUFA) are one of three general categories of fats. There are many different types of PUFAs, but we're going to focus on omega-6 and omega-3 fatty acids. These are both considered essential fatty acids, necessary for human health but unable to be manufactured in the body—which means that the only source of these fats is our food.

AN OMEGA-3, OMEGA-6 PRIMER

Omega-3 fatty acids have important structural and metabolic functions in the brain, influencing memory and performance, and are important for retinal health. Two types of omega-3, EPA and DHA, have also been shown to reduce inflammation and may help lower risk of chronic health conditions, such as heart disease, cancer, and arthritis. Omega-6 fatty acids are also critical for healthy brain function, metabolism, growth, and development—but if we eat too many, they can promote inflammation in the body.

We need some PUFA in our diet to be healthy—but *too much* causes problems, especially if it's too much omega-6. The trouble is, seed oils contain a lot of omega-6, and a modern diet includes a lot of seed oils, because seed oils are in *everything*.

Almost every restaurant cooks with them, whether they're fast-food joints, chain restaurants or fine-dining establishments. They're found in most processed foods as well—everything from tortilla chips to soups, salad dressings to fruit snacks. The estimated consumption of soybean oil alone in the United States increased more than a thousandfold (!) between 1909 and 1999; the National Institutes of Health estimates that soybeans, usually in the form of oil, now account for an astonishing 10 percent of total calories in the United States.

Ten percent of total calories is a lot.

These seed oils are ubiquitous because they're cheap—but they are not *healthy*.

Scientists believe our growing PUFA intake from industrial seed oils has played a significant role in the increase of inflammation-related conditions like obesity, insulin resistance, type 2 diabetes, and cancer over the past few decades. And it's quite likely that most of the diseases of modern civilization* are linked to the radical shift in the composition of fats in our foods.

*According to Dr. Joseph Hibbeln of the U.S. National Institutes of Health.

FIRST VIOLATION: OXIDATION ON THE OUTSIDE

The first concern with PUFAs in seed oils has to do with their stability when exposed to external stressors like air, light, and heat. Exposure to these stressors can cause molecules in these oils to react with oxygen in the air and form free radicals, a process called *oxidation*, or "going rancid."

FREE RADICALS Free radicals are naturally occurring, highly reactive molecules that play an essential role in many biological functions, like immunity and cellular repair. Having some in the body is good, but having too many is not. Balance is critical, because an excess of free radicals can damage cells (and your DNA). An overabundance of free radicals has been implicated in Alzheimer's disease, high blood pressure, and even cancer ... and has a severe inflammatory effect in the body.

Mother Nature gave all oily seeds a built-in defense mechanism to protect their fats from oxidation. These compounds (appropriately termed *antioxidants*) inhibit the oxidation process, delaying rancidity.* We want our dietary oils to contain these healthy antioxidants—but seed oils contain few (if any).

Industrially-produced seed oils have been refined, bleached, and deodorized—usually using nasty chemical solvents—to remove their natural flavor and aroma, making them easy to blend undetected into any food product. The trouble is, the refinement process also removes a large percentage of the health-promoting antioxidants. (Some manufacturers try to combat this by adding artificial antioxidants back into their seed oils, but numerous studies have shown that supplemented antioxidants don't work in the same protective fashion as naturally occurring antioxidants.)

Even before processing, PUFAs are the least stable kind of fat, but with their natural antioxidants largely removed, seed oils are even more vulnerable to rancidity.

We'll discuss free radicals and the benefits of dietary antioxidants in more detail when we talk about vegetables.

OILS GONE BAD These PUFA-rich seed oils are *so* vulnerable that even at room temperature and in indirect light (like the kind you find in the grocery store), oxidation occurs inside the bottle—especially as these oils are often packaged in clear plastic. That means the seed oil in your cart may be partly rancid before you even bring it home from the store!

We then *cook* with these seed oils, exposing them to yet more air, heat, and light. During the cooking process, the antioxidants that survived the refining process "sacrifice" themselves in a futile effort to prevent further oxidation. Once oxidation starts, it's hard to stop—"auto-oxidation" occurs at an increasing rate, like a free radical chain reaction.

Does eating rancid oils sound like a terrible idea to you too?

Studies show that some of these oxidized fats are transformed into toxic substances that can create damage in the liver, which means ingesting oxidized PUFAs puts your health at risk.

But that's just strike one.

SECOND VIOLATION: OXIDATION ON THE INSIDE

One of fat's jobs is to help build and maintain our cell membranes. This means that the type of fat we eat is reflected in the makeup of our cell walls. If we eat too many PUFAs, some will probably have oxidized in the bottle (and our frying pan), leading to toxic byproducts when ingested. The rest—which hasn't oxidized—is then built into our cell walls. But just as seed oils are the least stable on the shelf and in the frying pan, they are also the least stable *in the body*.

Polyunsaturated fat is the most likely type of fat to oxidize inside our bodies.

When we eat too much PUFA-rich seed oil, it makes up a larger and larger proportion of our cell membranes, which in turn makes our cells *themselves* more vulnerable. (It's like building a house with termite-ridden wood. The more termite-damaged wood you use, the more unstable the house.) The PUFAs in our cell walls can be oxidized by free radicals, creating toxic byproducts and setting off a cascade of equally destructive chain reactions. These reactions cause all sorts of damage, and provoke (you guessed it!) *systemic inflammation.*

Strike two.

THIRD VIOLATION: TOO MUCH OMEGA-6

Remember when we said seed oils are in everything, and so we eat a lot of them? It's not just about the amount of PUFA we consume—it's also about how much of that PUFA comes from omega-6 fatty acids. Seed oils contain an abundance of omega-6, while providing us with virtually no omega-3s. While some omega-6 fatty acid in our diet is essential for good health, too much throws our body's fatty acids out of balance. And if the amount of omega-6 in our bodies is disproportionately high compared with the amount of omega-3, that spells trouble—specifically, more pro-inflammatory compounds in the body, and less anti-inflammatory activity. Which is the long way of saying:

**Consuming seed oils with high levels of omega-6
promotes systemic inflammation.**

Strike three, they're out. For these three reasons, industrially-processed seed oils violate our fourth Good Food standard.

HIGH-OLEIC OILS Manufacturers are catching on to the whole omega-6 problem and are starting to modify safflower and sunflower seeds into "high oleic" versions rich in oleic acid, a form of monounsaturated fat. These modified seed oils have fat profiles similar to that of olive oil, which we say is a very healthy choice, and may be confusing to consumers trying to make smart oil choices. Don't be fooled. Unlike extra-virgin olive oil (which is always pressed without the use of high heat, solvents or extraction chemicals), most of these high-oleic oils are still highly refined—processed using unhealthy chemicals *and* heat. In addition, you can't always trust these new forms of "cold pressed" oils, as the use of the phrase is often nothing more than a marketing technique. The smartest choice is to avoid all seed oils and rely on the stable, health-promoting oils we'll outline in Chapter 15 for cooking, sauces, and dressings.

Common seed oils and vegetable oils to avoid

canola (rapeseed)	palm kernel
chia	peanut
corn	rice bran
cottonseed	safflower
flax (linseed)	sesame
grapeseed	soybean
hemp	sunflower

Even though seed oils violate only one of our four Good Food standards, that's a good enough reason for you to clean out your cupboard and throw them all away. Besides, with all the healthy alternatives we're going to give you in the next section, there's not going to be room for them—in your diet or in your pantry.

CHAPTER 10:
GRAINS AND LEGUMES

"I was diagnosed with celiac sprue in 1992, so I've been gluten-free since then. Because of the trauma to my gut, I developed other food sensitivities and environmental sensitivities as well. I learned to deal with them and be reasonably active, but I had reoccurring bouts of months of intestinal bloating and debilitating fatigue. I was trying all sorts of probiotics, digestive enzymes—nothing was helping. Then I stumbled across the Whole30. The bloating was gone in a few days and has not returned. I noticed improved energy/stamina and clearer thinking. My environmental reactions aren't as severe. For someone with celiac, this way of eating provides optimal wellness."
—Sandy H., Middleport, New York

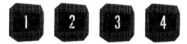

We suspect that this is one topic quite likely to spur controversy. See, our general nutritional recommendations don't include grains of any kind—no breads, cereals, pasta, rice, not even gluten-free grains or pseudo-cereals like quinoa.

No, not even *whole grains*.

We are well aware that this information may swim upstream against everything you've *ever* been told by your parents, doctors and personal trainers, by the government, and by TV advertisements. We make no apologies, however, because all the people who have been selling you whole grains for health all these years have just been plain wrong.

We understand if this makes you kind of angry—or at the very least skeptical. We want you to be skeptical! We were too. But the science, our education, and our experience have completely altered our perspective—

and we believe that by the time you get to the end of this chapter, you'll be thinking about grains differently too.

Let's talk about the trouble with grains—refined, whole, and everything in between.

SURVIVE OR THRIVE?

Most agricultural societies eat a diet that includes locally-produced grains (or legumes) as a source of cheap energy, which leads many people to say, "How can grains be so bad, if these healthy cultures have been eating them for thousands of years?" First, there are a lot of factors that play into a population's health. Sunshine, other dietary choices, exercise, and environment all contribute—so it's silly to say, for example, that traditional Asian cultures are healthy simply because they eat rice. In addition, the fact that some societies have eaten grains for thousands of years says nothing about whether grains are actually healthy. Their eating habits reflect what was available to them for *survival* in that particular place and time. But *surviving* and *thriving* are not the same thing. In today's modern world, we are interested in truly thriving, not just providing enough energy to avoid starvation—and in our culture, we can do that with optimally healthy foods that don't contain any of the downsides of grains.

Grains are seeds of plants in the grass family. This includes wheat, oats, barley, rye, millet, corn (maize), rice (including wild rice), sorghum, teff, triticale, spelt, kamut, buckwheat, amaranth, chia, and quinoa.*

The sole purpose of the seed is for reproduction of the plant. (Plants do not grow their babies just for us to eat.) When that seed matures and falls onto the ground, it needs some stored energy to get started—to germinate and grow until it produces its first leaves and can photosynthesize energy from sunlight. Grains store most of that preliminary energy in their seeds as carbohydrate.

Depending on what we do with those grains (and how we consume—or overconsume—them), all that carbohydrate *may* violate our first and second Good Food standards.

---

*Yes, we know those last few are not technically grains, but their properties are so similar (as are their health effects) that it makes sense to talk about them here.

REFINED GRAINS

Let's talk about the various components of a grain seed.

The bran is the grain's outer layer, its suit of armor. Its job is to protect the seed against outside threats, like bacteria and insects. The part of the seed that actually grows into another plant is the germ—that's where the plant's reproductive information is stored. Finally, there is the endosperm—mostly starch and some protein—which provides fuel for the seed's growth.

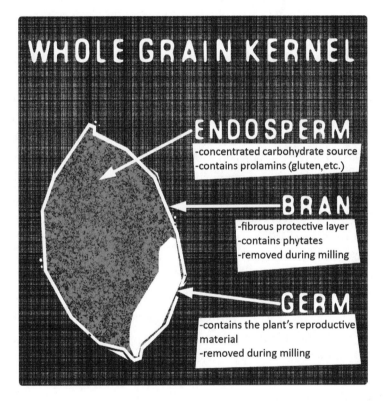

Refined grains bear little resemblance to the natural structure described above. During the refining process, the bran and the germ are removed, and so are the fiber, vitamins, and minerals present in those two layers. (Some vitamins and minerals may be added back into the product, which is then labeled "enriched," but the added nutrients don't make up for what the refining process has removed.) Milling grains in this fashion leaves us with just the endosperm.

> **Refined grains lack most of the original nutrients but still contain almost all of the calories.**

These refined grains are then made into products like white bread, instant oatmeal, snack foods, and desserts. To further increase their palatability, the water is sucked out of these products (further concentrating the calories), and then sugar, fat, and salt are added. Since there is little fiber left, these calories are also easier and quicker for us to absorb. In addition, refined grains contain no complete protein—a critical satiation factor—and little micronutrition because they are so heavily processed.

In other words, they're junk food.

The flours from refined grains form the foundation of most of the supernormally stimulating, nutrient-poor, carbohydrate-dense foods-with-no-brakes. (Remember, we don't eat these foods by themselves—they're *ingredients*.) These junk foods promote chronic overconsumption, elevated blood sugar levels, reliance on glucose for fuel, accumulation of body fat, and an increase in free fatty acids and triglycerides in the blood. And, if you *continue* to overconsume them (as is so easy to do), you can say hello to leptin resistance, insulin resistance, and all the negative downstream consequences to your health.

Which is how refined grains fail our first *and* second Good Food standards.

This should come as no surprise, as practically everyone agrees that refined grains, and the products made from white flour, do not make you healthier. But what about "heart healthy" whole grains? As you're about to see, those come with their own set of problems.

WHOLE GRAINS

For the record, whole-grain products often violate our first Good Food standard too. The words "whole grain" on a product label don't mean the product was made with 100 percent whole grain. In fact, the U.S. government has very few regulations for whole-grain labeling, and the Whole Grains Council allows the use of their Whole Grain Stamp on products containing eight grams or more of whole-grain ingredients per serving—*even if the product contains more refined grain than whole grain.* Don't let the fact that your waffles, muffins, or cookies were made with whole grains fool you. Whole-grain foods can easily qualify as foods-with-no-brakes.

WHOLE GRAINS

In whole grains, often touted as the healthy alternative to refined grains, all the natural anatomical components—the bran, germ, and starchy endosperm—are present in the same relative proportions as in the intact seed.

Because whole grains still contain fiber, they are often referred to as having a "lower glycemic index" (GI) than their refined counterparts—which is often erroneously thought of as synonymous with "healthier."

GLYCEMIC INDEX The glycemic index (GI) is a numerical scale used to quantify how fast fifty grams of carbohydrate from a particular food can raise blood glucose level. Carbohydrates that break down quickly during digestion and release glucose rapidly into the bloodstream have a higher GI; carbohydrates that break down more slowly, releasing glucose more gradually into the bloodstream, have a lower GI. The "standard" used for the GI scale—the food to which other foods are compared—is either glucose (with a score of 100) or white bread (with a score of 70 to 73).

White bread raises blood sugar very rapidly (high GI), while the starch in 100 percent whole-grain bread takes longer to break down into glucose (moderate GI). The lower GI score is largely a result of the additional fiber content of whole-grain flour, but eating a high GI food alongside other foods rich in fiber and fat will also lower the total GI of the meal.

However, the GI does not give any indication of, well, *anything else* relating to the health of these foods! It doesn't mention whether the food contains any problematic proteins, or what kind of sugars or fats it contains, or the bioavailability of the nutrients. It also doesn't tell you how much carbohydrate is contained in the food or how much insulin will be needed to manage blood glucose.

In addition, GI doesn't take into account how much of that food is typically eaten in a serving. The GI of watermelon is very high (72), but how much watermelon do you normally eat—a slice or two? The GI of peanut M&Ms® is much lower (33), but because they are supernormally stimulating and nutrient-poor, it's very easy to eat an entire bag. Which food do you think promotes better health?

The glycemic index is largely irrelevant to making Good Food choices.

But the glycemic index isn't the only thing cited in support of whole grains—proponents will point out their higher micronutrition content, too. And we'd agree—*when compared with refined grains*, whole grains are certainly more nutritious. But refined grains and whole grains aren't your only choices when it comes to carbohydrate, vitamins, minerals, and phytonutrients.

What about vegetables and fruit?

NOT SO NUTRITIOUS

The marketing from big cereal companies would have you think that cereal grains are highly nutritious—and that if you *don't* eat them, you'll miss out on all sorts of vitamins, minerals, and fiber that you can get only from grains.

That's simply not true.

Grains are not (we repeat, *not*) nutrient-dense *when compared with vegetables and fruit.*

Remember back to our prototypical healthy-hormones "good day" and our not-so-healthy-hormones "bad day" in Chapter 5? Our good day described a diet based on our Good Food standards. Our bad day represented a typical Western "healthy" diet based on whole grains and low-fat foods.

When we ran each day's meals through a nutritional-analysis system, we discovered that a diet built around "healthy" whole grains provided more than *three times* the sugar and sodium as a diet featuring vegetables and fruit.

Even better, our Good Day diet provides more dietary fiber, potassium, and magnesium, and *way* more iron, zinc, and vitamins A, B_6, B_{12}, C, D, E, and K (often in far more bioavailable forms).

Our prototypical "Good Day" vs. "Bad Day"

	Unit	Good Day	Bad Day	Difference
Calories	kcal	2,318	2,901	(20%)
Protein	g	146	115	27%
Carbohydrate	g	140	442	(68%)
Fiber	g	39	35	13%
Sugar	g	70	236	(70%)
Fat	g	142	69	106%
Sodium	mg	1,348	5,390	(75%)
Calcium	mg	779	1,451	(46%)
Potassium	mg	6,047	5,126	18%
Magnesium	mg	575	462	24%
Iron	mg	30	20	50%
Zinc	mg	24	13	85%
Vitamin A	mcg	3,132	329	852%
Vitamin C	mg	228	157	45%
Vitamin D	mcg	4	0	-
Vitamin E	mg	22	10	114%
Vitamin K	mcg	1,260	82	1435%
Vitamin B6	mg	4	3	32%
Vitamin B12	mcg	7	4	59%
Folate	mcg	935	646	45%
Beta-carotene	mcg	30,862	1,770	1644%

LIQUID CALORIES Wondering about the extra calories in our prototypical bad day? Two words: liquid calories. The coffees with skim milk and a teaspoon of sugar, the two soy lattes (one medium, one small), the 8-ounce glass of orange juice, and the 5-ounce glass of red wine contribute an extra 532 calories to the day—almost exactly making up the difference in calories between our good and bad days. Most of us don't think the liquid calories (or sugar) we're consuming "count," but when almost 20 percent of your total daily calories come in a form that's not even food ... we'd say that *counts*.

Another way that a diet high in grains leads to suboptimal nutrition is in terms of opportunity cost: if there are more whole grains on your plate, then there's probably less of some other food—like *vegetables*—on your plate. And that lowers the overall micronutrient density in your diet too. In summary:

> **There is not a single health-promoting substance
> present in grains that you can't also get
> from vegetables and fruit.**

Not a single vitamin. Not a single mineral.

Not even fiber.

Yes, the Whole Grain People will *insist* that you need your whole grains for fiber ... but have they totally forgotten that there is lots of fiber in vegetables and fruit? As you can see from the chart below, whole grains do not have a monopoly on fiber:

Dietary Fiber Content of Foods

GRAINS	Serving size	Fiber (g)
Whole-grain bread	2 slices	3.4
Oatmeal, cooked	1 cup	4.0
Rice, brown, cooked	1 cup	3.5

VEGETABLES AND FRUIT	Serving size	Fiber (g)
Broccoli, raw	1½ cups	3.5
Carrots, raw	1 cup	3.1
Cauliflower, raw	1½ cups	3.8
Green beans, cooked	1 cup	4.0
Sweet potato, cooked without skin	½ potato	3.9
Winter squash, cooked	1 cup	5.7
Apple, with skin	1 large	3.3
Banana	1	3.1
Blackberries	1 cup	7.6
Orange	1 small	3.1
Pear	1 medium	5.1
Strawberries	1 cup	3.3
Almonds	1 oz.	3.3

All of these veggies and fruits contain about as much fiber (or more!) as two slices of whole-grain bread, a cup of oatmeal, or a cup of brown rice. (We threw almonds in there just for kicks—there's fiber in nuts and seeds too!) There's no trickery here—the vegetable serving sizes are *modest* (so it's not like you have to eat a pound of broccoli to get enough fiber).

Based just on our side-by-side comparisons, it's clear that vegetables and fruit are far more nutrient-dense than even their whole-grain counterparts. We could rest our case. …

But there's even *more* to this nutrition story.

HEART-HEALTHY? But what of all the claims made by the Whole Grain People about the heart-healthiness of whole grains? Turns out those claims may be more fluff than substance, as studies show that whole grains may not prevent disease as well as you might think. According to one recent meta-analysis, there isn't any substantial evidence to back up the "heart healthy" claim beyond what poorly conducted, grain-industry-funded research has yielded. The study concluded: "Despite the consistency of effects seen in trials of whole-grain oats, the positive findings should be interpreted cautiously. Many of the trials identified were short-term, of poor quality, and had insufficient power. Most of the trials were funded by companies with commercial interests in whole grains." Enough said.

CAN YOU ACTUALLY GET TO THEM?

Grains contain a compound called phytic acid, or phytate, found mostly in the bran portion of the seed. These phytates, often referred to as "antinutrients," grab hold of minerals like calcium, iron, zinc, and magnesium found in the whole grain, creating an insoluble and undigestible complex. This means that when these nutrients get to your small intestine, they are not in a usable form—and therefore, not absorbed into the body.

Selfish anti-nutrients.

So even though those minerals are technically present in some grains, since your body can't actually make use of them, they might as well not be there at all. The takeaway? Not only are whole grains relatively nutrient-poor, but many of the minerals that are present are not actually available to you.

In other words, *eating* a nutrient is not the same as being able to *use* that nutrient.

A WORD ON PHYTATES

While other plant foods (like some vegetables) also contain phytates, the combination of relatively low concentrations plus a relatively high level of nutrients generally reduces the overall impact of the anti-nutrients. (Since there are more minerals in vegetables and not as many phytates to "bind" those minerals, a large percentage of those nutrients are still available to us.) In addition, many vegetable preparation techniques (like peeling starchy root vegetables) remove much of the phytate. Sure, if we "peeled" our whole grains (i.e., milled away the bran and germ), we'd be left with fewer phytates—but then we'd have refined grains, devoid of most of the nutrition and fiber but still containing *all* of the concentrated carbohydrate. Doesn't seem like a very good tradeoff to us.

At this point, it's tough to make the case for the regular inclusion of grains in your diet—and we haven't even talked about gluten yet.

PROBLEMATIC PROTEINS

For us, the propensity to overconsume them and their lack of nutrient density alone are enough to push grains off our plate to make room for fruits and vegetables. But there's even more to the story—which leads us to our third and fourth Good Food standards.

There are many different protein structures in grains that have been found to create transient increases in gut permeability, increasing exposure of "outside" stuff to the "inside." In addition, these proteins can improperly cross through the gut barrier, triggering an immune reaction (inflammation!).

Remember the nightclub?

These problematic proteins are, as a whole, poorly digested. In addition, some can temporarily knock out the bouncer outside your club, allowing unsavory characters to sneak inside your (formerly secure) interior. Those same components, once inside, have to be chased down and dealt with by the security guards inside (your immune cells), since they don't belong anywhere inside your body. One such class of profoundly problematic proteins belongs to a group called *prolamins*. These prolamins can damage your gut and other parts of your body through systemic inflammation.

YOU KNOW GLUTEN

While the word "prolamin" might not ring any bells, the word "gluten" should. Gluten is a protein found in the endosperm of wheat, rye, and barley, and is partly made up of prolamins. Gluten is the most infamous prolamin-containing protein because people with celiac disease have a specific intolerance to gluten.

Prolamins are especially troublesome because their particular structure makes them very difficult (often impossible) for our digestive enzymes to break down into individual amino acids.

Problem #1: These proteins are resistant to digestion.

In addition, these prolamins (including those from gluten) interact directly with some of the microscopic components of our intestinal barrier. By "interact," we mean that they trigger changes in the barrier function of the gut, temporarily opening the doors of the "club." This allows those undigested proteins to come directly into contact with immune cells *inside* the body.

**Problem #2: These proteins create localized inflamma-
tion in the gut and elsewhere if they improperly cross
the gut barrier and end up where they don't belong.**

That interaction between foreign proteins and immune cells triggers
an inflammatory response, the severity of which depends on the individual. (There is considerable person-to-person variation, though the research
on individual sensitivity is still fairly incomplete.)

One severe example of intolerance to grain proteins is found in those
with celiac disease, an autoimmune disease which occurs when genetically
susceptible individuals consume even miniscule amounts of gluten. Celiacs experience an enormous immune response in the gut and elsewhere in
the body when exposed to gluten—it's like dropping a nuclear bomb to kill
a spider.

CELIAC AND GS   *Celiac disease* (CD) is unique in that a *specific*
food component, gluten, has been identified
as the trigger in those genetically predisposed to that condition and that
the mechanism is well understood. When individuals with CD eat gluten,
the enterocytes (cells that line the small intestine) are damaged from the
"nuclear blast" of a hyper-reactive immune system. Damaged enterocytes
do not effectively absorb basic nutrients—proteins, carbohydrates, fats, vitamins, minerals, and, in some cases, water and bile salts. If CD is left un-
treated, damage to the small intestine can be chronic and even life-threatening, increasing the risk of malnutrition and immune-related disorders.
There is also a different condition called *gluten sensitivity* (GS). Those with
GS don't have the same change in intestinal permeability as celiacs (in fact,
they don't present with *any* detectable changes), but gluten still provokes a
direct activation of their immune system. This response, neither an allergy
nor an autoimmune response, can provoke similar gastrointestinal symptoms as is seen in celiacs. The research on GS is still really new, and no one
knows what percentage of the population may be affected.

Just because you don't have CD or GS doesn't mean grains are good
for you, whether they contain gluten or not. Corn and oats, for example,
contain different prolamins and other compounds that may be similarly ir-
ritating, or worse. While these protein fractions and compounds have not
yet been as well studied as gluten, it's fair to say that they have the potential

to create similar undesirable effects on your gut function and immune status.

That is how grains—even whole grains—fail our third and fourth Good Food standards.

When you regularly consume them (whether whole or refined), you expose your body to these potentially problematic proteins. This triggers localized inflammation in the gut, which (in the presence of intestinal permeability—an all-too-common condition) cascades into systemic inflammation, provoking an often silent immune response elsewhere in the body.

Or, more like *everywhere* in the body.

The inflammatory effects can show up anywhere, as anything: allergies, arthritis, asthma; autoimmune diseases like celiac, Crohn's, lupus, multiple sclerosis, and Hashimoto's thyroiditis; chronic fatigue, fibromyalgia, ulcerative colitis, diverticulitis, psoriasis, eczema, rosacea, endometriosis; these effects can even be seen *in the brain*. (Inflammatory messengers in the brain are associated with depression, anxiety, and even conditions like bipolar disorder and schizophrenia.) No two people's symptoms look the same—the inflammatory consequences are virtually *unlimited*.

Which means gluten-free is not a get-out-of-jail-free card.

Gluten-free brownies, pancakes, cookies, and breads are all the rage these days, produced primarily for celiacs. But are these products healthy—or just more marketing hype?

Many of our clients and Whole30 participants report similar reactions to non-gluten grains, leading us to believe that there are bigger problems with grains than just gluten. Gluten-free grains and non-grains like quinoa in all likelihood still contain potentially inflammatory proteins and other compounds that can provoke inflammation in the gut and elsewhere.

Finally, bread is still bread (and a pancake still a pancake), regardless of the grains with which they are made—and gluten-free grains promote the same unhealthy psychological response as their gluten-containing counterparts. In summary, "gluten free" does not necessarily represent a healthy choice.

LESS BAD   Ancient cultures reliant on grains for survival figured out ways to prepare them to mitigate some of the inflammatory and anti-nutrient downsides. Prolonged soaking, extended cooking, rinsing, sprouting, and fermenting have been shown to partly break down *some* of the phytates and *some* of the inflammatory proteins in certain grains. But note the words "partly" and "some." These preparation methods don't guarantee a safe food product in your gut. In today's modern world, we think it's an awful lot of effort to soak, rinse, sprout, and/or ferment a food just to make it somewhat less bad ... especially when vegetables and fruit provide far more nutritious benefits with none of the downsides of grains.

But wait, you're thinking, "This science isn't bomb-proof! Maybe I'm sensitive to the compounds found in grains and maybe I'm not."

You're absolutely right. And we can't answer that question for you.

But neither can you, until you've done our Whole30 program.

Remember, we can't rely solely on science to guide our recommendations, because in some cases (like the effect of proteins in non-gluten grains) data simply isn't available. But based on the research that is available, combined with the vast body of evidence we've gathered from our clients, we advise you to put the kibosh on grains, because: (a) they can be easy to overconsume and promote hormonal dysfunction, (b) they're not a good source of nutrition compared with vegetables and fruits, and (c) proteins found in all grains may very well be disruptive to the body, just as we know for *sure* that gluten can be.

We think that sounds reasonable, but to answer the question "How can I know how grains affect *me*?" we need you to do some self-experimentation.

During our Whole30 program, you'll evaluate how your body reacts, first without any grains, then with the reintroduction of grains back into your diet. Then you'll combine the science we've presented, our experience and *your own* experience to make an educated, informed decision about how often (if at all) you should eat grains.

See? We've got this all worked out for you.

LEGUMES

3 4

Next up is another plant family that has a lot in common with grains: legumes. Legumes include all types of beans, peas, lentils, and peanuts (which are not actually a "nut" at all). Like cereal grains, plants in this family have similarities in the way they behave and what chemical constituents they contain, which impacts us when we eat them.

The similarity to grains starts with the seed. Legumes are actually a plant family, but the part we eat when we consume black beans, soy, or lentils is the *seed* of the legume plant. The seeds of legumes, like the seeds from cereal grains, store a large amount of energy in the form of carbohydrate. In fact, in most legumes, the amount of carbohydrate present is double or triple that of protein.

Now, remember—we are not afraid of carbohydrate, nor do we know of anyone who has suffered metabolic catastrophe by eating too many carbohydrates from black beans! That's not to say that legumes are the healthiest choice, but the reason we exclude them is not because they contain a lot of carbohydrate. The carbohydrate content of foods *alone* is not what causes hormonal dysregulation—it starts with overconsumption.

In our experience, people generally don't chronically overconsume legumes—at least, we've never heard of anyone having an unhealthy psychological relationship with lentils. Legumes are not milled like grains often are, so legumes are essentially the equivalent of whole grains—more fiber, more water, and more nutrients than their more refined counterparts. This makes them far less likely to promote overconsumption than a refined, supernormally stimulating, nutrient-poor food.

CONTEXT MATTERS One word of caution, however: If you have chronically overconsumed supernormally stimulating, nutrient-poor processed foods and your hormones are already seriously out of balance, then continuing to overconsume carbohydrate—even from "real food" sources like legumes—*may* keep promoting an unhealthy hormonal response. Furthermore, if you take those black beans and stick them in a seven-layer dip slathered with Mexi-cheese spread and served with nacho-flavored chips, well … that's another story. As always, context matters.

Since legumes don't violate our first or second Good Food standards, does that mean they're a healthy choice?

First, legumes, like whole grains, contain considerable amounts of phytate. Remember, these phytates bind many of the minerals present in the seed, rendering them unavailable to our bodies. This makes legumes not as micronutrient-dense as you might think, in the same way that whole grains are not micronutrient-dense.

As with grains, ancient cultures that consumed legumes as a major food source had ways of mitigating some of the issues with legumes, such as rinsing, sprouting, prolonged soaking and cooking, and fermentation. However, remember that specific legumes were consumed for calories because that's what was *available*. The fact that these cultures survived on these foods does not mean that their choices were optimal, or even good— only that they had no choice. "Properly preparing" legumes using these traditional methods today is time-consuming—and frankly, it seems like a tremendous amount of work for a food that simply isn't that nutritious.

BACK TO FIBER Many people think beans are a good source of fiber, and they certainly are—but remember, so are vegetables and fruit (not to mention that the nutrients in veggies and fruit are more bioavailable). So while you *could* get a nice dose of fiber from beans, it would be like eating a Mounds bar to reap the benefits of coconut—there are far better sources of fiber that don't have the same potential downsides.

THE MAGICAL FRUIT

Because some of the short-chain carbohydrates (sugars) found in legumes aren't properly absorbed in the small intestine, they can then act as food for bacteria living in both the small and large intestines. The bacteria then "ferment" (digest) these carbohydrates (called *galactans*), which can create many unpleasant symptoms, including gas and bloating.

We suspect that you've experienced this effect.

In addition, if you have an imbalance or overgrowth of gut bacteria, large amounts of this specific type of carbohydrate may feed the "bad" bacteria, thus promoting ongoing gut dysbiosis. The significance of this concern is largely determined by the health of your gut microbiota. Given the kind of foods you used to eat and their cumulative effects on your gut bacteria, dysbiosis is, unfortunately, all too common. This is one potential outcome that would cause legumes to fail our third Good Food standard (promotes a healthy gut), and by default, our fourth (systemic inflammation, via an unhealthy gut).

FODMAPS These galactans aren't the only fermentable carbohydrate that causes gastric distress. They belong to a category called FODMAPs (fermentable oligosaccharides, disaccharides, monosaccharides, and polyols)—a collection of fermentable carbohydrates and sugar alcohols found in various foods, like grains, beans, vegetables and fruits. FODMAPs are poorly absorbed, thereby "feeding" gut bacteria and causing a host of symptoms, including dysbiosis and systemic inflammation. *Fructans* (another type of carbohydrate also in the FODMAP family), such as those found in wheat, have similar effects in the digestive tracts of sensitive individuals. The resulting gut dysbiosis is one reason that even those without celiac or gluten sensitivity still have adverse reactions to grains.

SOY FOR EVERYONE?

We'll address soy and soy products separately, as they contain unique compounds—and because, due in large part to marketing efforts, "soy" is often perceived as synonymous with "healthy."

We do not agree with that.

Soybeans are particularly good at producing seeds more protein-rich than most other legumes (and all grains). This makes them ideal for large-scale production but does *not* automatically make them a healthy food choice! You see, soybeans contain compounds called *isoflavones*, which are types of *phytoestrogens* (*phyto* meaning "plant," *estrogen* as in that female sex hormone).

These phytoestrogens are recognized by our bodies—male and female alike—as a female reproductive hormone. Got that? Our bodies recognize these phytoestrogens as *estrogen*! Some phytoestrogens act to stimulate estrogen receptors in the body, while others block the estrogen receptor. The effects of soy phytoestrogens are tissue-specific, meaning that the effect on one tissue (such as breast tissue) is totally different than on another tissue (such as uterine tissue or prostate tissue).

You may have heard that "soy is heart healthy" or that "soy reduces the risk of breast cancer," but those are radically simplified media sound bites and are not representative of the overall effect of soy phytoestrogens. The fact is, phytoestrogens may be beneficial for a very specific population (perimenopausal women, for example), but the effect on other populations is largely unknown.

SOY RX It's kind of like your doctor saying, "Hey, if you're worried about heart health, take these pills. I don't know how much you should take, or even how much 'medicine' is in each pill, but these pills are associated with heart health, so just go for it!" You would never want to take a random dose of pharmaceutical estrogens. (And for the men reading this book—do you *think* you need more estrogen?) So why would you eat a dietary source rich in similar compounds?

We think that regularly consuming a food rich in hormonally-active substances, *especially* if you do not have a specific sex-hormone imbalance, as in perimenopause (or are male and probably not estrogen-deficient), is a huge health gamble, and not one we think anyone should take. We are not ready to say that soy fails our second Good Food standard (healthy hormonal response)—but we'll keep a close watch on this subject.

PEANUTS

Peanuts are also of special concern, as they contain uniquely disruptive proteins. First, peanuts aren't tree nuts at all—botanically, they are legumes. All legumes contain protein structures that may be hazardous to humans—one type in particular is called a *lectin*. In their raw state, lectins are highly resistant to digestion and toxic to animals.

In other legumes (like black beans or kidney beans), these lectins are destroyed during the cooking process, rendering them harmless. But peanut lectins are different. They are resistant to digestion and are not destroyed by heat. When they land in your gut, they are largely intact. They can then fool your gut lining into letting them through into the body (by mimicking the structure of other proteins) and get into your bloodstream.

Once they're inside, these peanut lectins can induce an immune response. (Remember, that undigested foreign protein is totally out of place *inside* the body.) By now, you know that any abnormal activation of your immune system might negatively affect both your short- and long-term health. These dangerous proteins violate our third and fourth Good Food standards—which means that peanuts and peanut butter are banished from your plate. (We suspect that the resilience of peanut lectin is partly responsible for the rapidly growing incidence of peanut allergies.)

PB & J? Most folks don't fight us tooth and nail to keep lima beans in their diet, but peanut butter is often a different story. For those of you who love the creamy (or chunky) stuff, don't panic—we've got a substitute. Sunflower seed butter is so similar to peanut butter that your kids probably won't know the difference, and sunflower seeds don't contain the same unhealthy proteins as peanuts. All nut butters are best eaten in moderation, for reasons we'll soon discuss—but as a once-in-a-while treat, sunflower seed butter will pass your PB taste test with flying colors. (Just skip the bread and the sugar-laden J, OK?)

It's impossible to blame lectins for all the problems with legumes, since *no one* eats legumes without cooking them first, and non-peanut lectins are destroyed by high heat. It's worth noting, however, that in improperly cooked legumes (such as those cooked in a slow cooker at a lower temperature), lectins may not be completely broken down—and that could result in severe gastrointestinal distress.

MAKE YOUR OWN CASE

Admittedly, the scientific case against legumes isn't nearly as strong as the case against, say, sugar. While data suggests that certain lectins *can* be extremely detrimental, and plenty of research supports the idea that phytoestrogens in soy may adversely affect hormonal balance, researchers simply don't have enough data on all legumes to know how potentially dangerous they are.

This is where you come in.

Remember, our recommendations are based on three factors: first, the science; second, our experience and the experience of our clients; third, self-experimentation. The science suggests that consuming legumes (especially peanuts) violates our Good Food standards. Our experience certainly confirms that most folks look and feel their best when legumes are kept off their plates. But now it's time for you to step up.

You can participate in additional (small-scale) research on legumes by participating in our Whole30 program. Make *yourself* the subject of a case study to determine the effects of legumes on *you*. Eliminating legumes from your diet (at least for a trial period) will allow you to assess your own personal tolerance—and help you decide what role they should have in your daily meals.

CHAPTER 11:
DAIRY

"During and following our family's Whole30, my son Jeremiah's (type 1 diabetic) blood sugars have been completely under control ... and they never have been before. His numbers normally jump from low to high extremes without any reason—we never knew what to do about it. It's been very frustrating ... but now his numbers are perfect. I can't fully put into words how amazing this transformation has been. Thanks to the Whole30, I now know without a doubt that Jeremiah's body is working the best it can and that I am doing my job as his mom to keep it that way."
—Jacque G., New Orleans, Louisiana

The discussion of dairy* is one that interests many people and has no simple, black-and-white answers. There are many functional components of dairy that, depending on the source and the individual consuming it, can be highly problematic, generally benign, or even beneficial.

The real challenge is twofold: being honest with yourself about whether dairy is "just fine" or just the opposite, and actually finding a truly high-quality source of dairy if you are one of the people who benefit from it. Luckily, the Whole30 will help you with the first part of that challenge. In the meantime, let's talk about some of the science about dairy consumption.

While the vast majority of dairy consumed in the United States is from cows, you can also apply these concepts to sheep or goat milk.

MILK: PERFECT

Cow's milk is the perfect food ... if you are a calf. Likewise, human breast milk is the optimal food when you are an infant.

Milk is an excellent source of energy and building blocks to rapidly grow mammals that are too young to eat adult food, such as grass (cows) and a wide range of plants and animals (humans). Until a mammal's digestive system (including teeth) has completely developed and it can eat whole food, mother's milk supplies optimal nutrition.

But mother's milk is not just an inert supply of carbohydrate, protein, and fat—though it contains significant amounts of all of those macronutrients. And yes, milk also contains calcium—but what is critical to understand is that milk is so much *more* than calories and calcium!

Milk is an energy-dense hormone-delivery system.

Milk is a blend of bioactive substances that not only promote aggressive growth of a very young mammal (doubling or tripling bodyweight in a very short period of time), but also ensure the complete development of the young one's immune system. You are born with the basic framework of an immune system, but there are some missing elements which must be "supplemented" by consuming mother's milk. In this context, milk is the perfect food, and the perfect messenger.

MILK: IMPERFECT

These growth, hormonal, and immunity messages from mother's milk to newborn are biologically healthy and appropriate, *when you are a calf or an infant*. However, once weaned, calves and human infants no longer grow at such an aggressive rate, and their digestive systems and immune systems are complete. This means the growth and immunological messages from mother's milk are no longer needed, nor appropriate.

And when the biological messages *intended for a calf* are being received loud and clear by *your adult human body*, they are even *less* appropriate—and potentially downright harmful.

To demonstrate how dairy products generally fail at least one of our Good Food standards, let's talk about the already well known components of dairy (protein, carbohydrate, fat, and calcium), as well as some of the other lesser-known components.

MILK PROTEINS: CASEIN AND WHEY

Though there are dozens of dairy proteins, they can be divided into two categories—*casein* and *whey*. Casein makes up about 80 percent of total milk protein and acts as a source of amino acid building blocks that the calf can digest and turn into muscle, connective tissue, skin, hair, hormones, and enzymes and even form part of the structural matrix of bones and teeth. Calves are able to make good use of that species-specific protein supply to fuel their aggressive growth.

BUT AREN'T KIDS AND TEENAGERS GROWING TOO?

While children are still growing, they are no longer developing at the same aggressive rate as they did as infants. (Even teenage boys are not tripling their body weight in months!) Once they are weaned from breast milk, it simply doesn't make sense to keep sending children the growth, hormonal, and immune messages they needed when first born—and it's certainly inappropriate to send them biological messages intended for *newborns of a different species.* Growing kids do need adequate energy (calories!), protein, healthy fats, and micronutrients, but their age- and species-appropriate food is nutrient-dense omnivorous fare: meat, seafood, eggs, vegetables, fruit, and healthy fat sources like coconut, olives, and avocado. The bottom line: Once your toddler is weaned and eating real food, there is *no need* to supplement his or her healthy diet with cow's milk. (Not to mention that dairy consumption has been linked to a variety of medical conditions in children, including acne, asthma, juvenile myopia, insulin resistance, and type 1 diabetes.)

There are also compounds in milk that have a specific *physiological* function—proteins and "peptides" (short amino acid chains)—in the body of the intended recipient (offspring). For instance, protein sequences embedded in casein's molecular structure are released during the digestion process and send a message from mother to young.

Casein exorphins, or *casomorphins* (morphine-like substances derived from casein), are one category of these milk-derived protein fragments. Casomorphins are able to cross the gut barrier in young mammals (and in adults with increased gut permeability) and bind to opioid receptors in the enteric and central nervous systems. Casomorphins have been shown to slow down the movement of food through the gut (thanks to their morphine-like effects).

Again, let's underscore the biological context here: the presence of casomorphins in human breast milk or cow's milk is unlikely to be harmful to infants or calves (respectively), and probably serves to strengthen the bond between mother and young, improving feeding behavior and therefore improving the odds of survival of the newborn mammal. But the effects of these potently bioactive "food hormones" *from another species* on human adults remain largely unknown.*

DON'T MOVE MY CHEESE Cheese is most commonly made from concentrated casein that has been blended with enzymes that partly digest the casein molecules, liberating some of these morphine-like compounds. Is it any coincidence that a large majority of our clients and seminar attendees say that cheese is the dairy product that would be the hardest to give up? No one knows for sure whether this represents a violation of our first Good Food standard (healthy psychological response)—but we sure do find it fascinating.

Casein, especially when it comes from aged cheese, also causes a specific type of immune system reaction called a *histamine response* in many people. (So for susceptible individuals, dairy would fail our fourth Good Food standard as well.) Histamine intolerance can cause headaches, GI upset, exacerbations of asthma, and seasonal allergies.

It is unclear what percentage of the population has this response, but until you have completely removed all dairy proteins from your diet for a period of time, you won't know whether or not you are affected.

Research suggests that these peptides cannot cross an adult human's intact intestinal barrier, but if permeability is already present, the effect is unknown.

CASEIN AND GLUTEN

Casein shares some structural similarities with components of gluten. This means that gluten-sensitive individuals (including those with celiac disease) are less likely to tolerate casein-containing dairy products. Research suggests that about 50 percent of celiacs are also sensitive to milk. In genetically susceptible individuals, the incomplete breakdown of peptides with opioid activity like those from gluten or casein (in the presence of intestinal permeability) allows these fragments to enter the circulation and potentially influence neurological functioning, resulting in or exacerbating disorders such as postpartum psychosis, schizophrenia, and autism.

The other major category of milk protein is *whey*. Whey is a blend of multiple types of smaller proteins and hormones, including immunoglobulins, insulin, insulin-like growth factor 1 (IGF-1), estrogens, and other growth factors. (Remember, milk is a powerful growth promoter!) For this reason, milk is a highly *insulinogenic* food, which means that the combination of lactose plus whey dairy proteins causes the release of very large amounts of insulin when consumed.

This makes perfect sense: it all starts with biology.

The "building-storing" function of insulin is in *complete accordance* with the aggressive growth going on in those breast-feeding months. Lots of growth means lots of insulin is needed to aggressively store nutrients. But the remarkably large amount of insulin secreted in response to milk and whey protein intake is largely why dairy may fail our second Good Food standard for those with metabolic syndrome; in this population, it does not promote a healthy hormonal response.

DAIRY PROTEIN POWDERS

Marketing from some supplement companies will suggest that a large insulin response (especially after exercise) will help drive nutrients into cells to maximize recovery, but you don't need an insulin "spike" after exercise to jam nutrients into cells, because your body is more insulin sensitive immediately post-workout. In this state, nutrient uptake is elevated—meaning you can "sneak" nutrients into cells *without* large amounts of insulin. In addition, the frequent insulin spikes from regular consumption of whey protein could be harmful in a manner similar to chronic over-carbsumption and the resulting hyperinsulinism in those with metabolic syndrome. We don't believe whey protein supplements are a good choice for the majority of people (especially those who are insulin resistant and overweight), although they *may* be an easy protein source in specific circumstances for lean, insulin-sensitive, performance-driven athletes. (Casein protein supplements, while not highly insulinogenic, are poorly tolerated, and we never recommend them.) In general, opt for nutrient-dense meat, seafood, and eggs instead of nutrient-poor processed dairy proteins after exercise.

Anyone seeking to improve insulin sensitivity (or avoid becoming insulin resistant) would be best served by avoiding dairy products, including those that contain highly insulinogenic components, like sugar-sweetened yogurt or kefir, milk (regardless of fat content), whey protein powder, and, of course, ice cream. (Do we really have to tell you that ice cream is not healthy? And p.s., it's not the dairy fat that's the problem.)

Insulin is not the only potentially detrimental hormone increased by milk. Milk consumption also significantly elevates IGF-1, another powerful growth-inducer. IGF-1 promotes growth in children, but it is also associated with promotion (or indirect facilitation) of various cancers, such as breast, colon, and prostate. Of course, we're not saying that if you drink milk, you'll get cancer, but if you're at high risk, consuming substances that increase the growth of cells, including abnormal cells, seems unwise.

MILK SUGAR: LACTOSE

But there is more to this story than just the protein fractions of milk—the carbohydrate component can also pose problems. The kind of carbohydrate found in milk is called *lactose*. While there are not huge amounts present in milk (and some other dairy products have very little because of processing), lactose is an issue for a surprisingly large percentage of people. Most infants digest lactose well, but after weaning, most of us lose the ability to convert lactose into usable forms of carbohydrate (glucose and galactose).

If lactose cannot be properly digested, bloating and gastrointestinal upset may result. In addition, consuming even small amounts of lactose may contribute to an imbalance of gut bacteria, promoting dysbiosis. For those who can no longer effectively digest lactose (i.e., most of us), dairy would also fail our third Good Food standard (promotes a healthy gut).

However, lactose intolerance is not our biggest concern with dairy, given its propensity to stimulate insulin production and potential to trigger an immune system response. In fact, many people who consider themselves lactose-intolerant (by observing that dairy makes them feel poorly) may have a sensitivity to dairy *proteins* as well.

Considering the various concerns raised by the scientific evidence, we think that a cautious strategy of eliminating milk (and dairy proteins) from your diet is both intelligent and healthy. Just as with grains, when you can get all the benefits of a food from other, healthier sources, why wouldn't you?

WHAT ABOUT CALCIUM

Anytime we mention the whole "we don't do dairy" thing, we inevitably get The Question:

"What about calcium?"

The Question is generally coming from the perspective that strong, healthy bones are important and that calcium builds strong, healthy bones. We do not disagree. But despite what the pro-milk ads would lead you to believe, the whole "strong bones" thing is a lot more complicated than that. There are three fallacies when it comes to the dairy-calcium-bones triad:

1. Building strong, healthy bones depends only on calcium.
2. Your calcium *intake* is the only thing that matters.
3. Dairy is the only good source of calcium.

Let's break these down one at a time.

There's no denying that calcium is important for bone health—calcium is the substance that gives bones strength, like bricks do for a building. But bones need more than just calcium to grow and stay strong. Vitamin C, vitamin D_3 (technically a hormone), and vitamin K, along with minerals like magnesium and phosphorous, all play important roles in bone development.

Your hormones and inflammatory status also play a role in bone health—a fact that should not surprise you at this point. Chronically elevated blood sugar and cortisol levels and systemic inflammation all accelerate bone breakdown and inhibit the formation of new bone cells.

If the first fallacy is thinking that bone health is all about calcium, the second is believing that our *intake of calcium* is all that matters. If this were true, then how do you reconcile this:

The United States has one of the highest rates of osteoporosis in the world, despite having one of the highest calcium intakes.

It makes no sense ... *unless there's more to the story than how much calcium we're taking in.* And there is: It's also about how much we're able to absorb and retain.

Phytates (anti-nutrients) in grains and legumes, stress, and the aging process all inhibit calcium absorption. Acute restriction of dietary protein reduces calcium absorption and may be associated with significantly higher rates of bone loss. (Adequate protein, on the other hand, increases calcium absorption, and stimulates new bone formation.)

In addition, bone-healthy vitamin D_3 and K are both fat soluble—meaning they require some fat in order to be absorbed into the bloodstream. So a low-fat diet (like the kind we've all been advised to eat for the last twenty years) may impair your body's ability to absorb these two vitamins, which can also impair bone health.

We told you it was complicated.

THE SUPPLEMENT STORY

These factors are exactly why all the calcium supplementation we've been doing just isn't working to prevent osteoporosis and bone fractures. See, osteoporosis *isn't caused by a lack of calcium.* And studies show that calcium intake alone does not prevent fractures from bone loss. Taking calcium supplements gives you a short-term boost in bone density, but over time, your hormones (again!) will work against the extra calcium, and may even leave your bones more brittle than before. Bone-density drugs (bisphosphonates) like Fosamax and Boniva aren't much better. They deposit a long-lasting compound in the bone, giving it the *appearance* of greater density, but do not build the kind of bone matrix that actually makes bones stronger. This can result in "dense" bones that are too brittle to withstand everyday activities.

Finally, *too much* calcium is just as bad as not enough. This excess calcium generally comes from a combination of dairy *plus* calcium supplements *plus* the calcium added to a variety of products, from antacids to orange juice to cereals. Too much calcium increases the risk of developing dangerously high levels of calcium in the blood, which can result in impaired kidney function, kidney stones, and high blood pressure. Furthermore, recent studies suggest that taking calcium supplements actually *increases* the risk of a heart attack.

Of course, a "just right" calcium balance is still necessary for overall health (bone and otherwise). But it's high time we correct the "facts" promoted by years of industry-sponsored marketing and addressed the third fallacy.

Dairy is not the only good source of calcium.

You can find calcium (in bioavailable forms and significant amounts) in a wide variety of nondairy, nutrient-dense foods: vegetables (like kale, boiled spinach, collard greens, mustard greens, turnip greens, and bok choy); sea vegetables like nori; meat and seafood (like bone broth, sardines, anchovies, shrimp, oysters, and canned salmon); and nuts and seeds (like almonds, hazelnuts, and walnuts).

THE POWER OF GREEN The calcium in vegetable sources may prove *more* bioavailable (useful to the body) than the stuff you get from milk. One study compared the absorption of calcium from kale and from milk and found kale the clear winner. (Yeah, kale!) Recent studies have shown that plant-sourced calcium in particular increases bone-mineral density and reduces the risk of osteoporosis. This is probably not *just* due to the calcium content of the plant—the complement of other vitamins (such as vitamin K), minerals, and phytonutrients work synergistically to provide additional benefits to bones. Yet another reason to eat your greens.

We think we're in need of a summary here.

Your body likes balance. Remember Goldilocks? Not too little, not too much … just right. And calcium doesn't work in a vacuum, so too much calcium means your body is forced to compensate by adjusting levels of other vitamin and mineral stores, leaving you even *more* out of balance.

So how do you build strong, healthy bones without dairy and without supplements? The short answer is, just follow our guidelines! The food quality of our plan ensures a wide variety of micronutrition, includes adequate protein and fat, promotes a healthy hormonal balance and minimizes systemic inflammation.*

HEAVY STUFF For all of you overachievers, here's your bonus tip for building strong, healthy bones—pick up something heavy. Weight-bearing physical activity and strength training has long been linked to improved bone density. The compression forces of daily activity stress our bones in a healthy way. Our bones respond by building more supportive substances to structurally bear load. On the other hand, if we fail to stress our bones in this fashion (with a sedentary lifestyle or failure to use weights in our exercise routine), our bones will slowly waste away. In other words, use it or lose it.

Even if you follow all of our recommendations, however, you'll find that you're probably still not getting as much calcium as the Powers That Be insist is necessary.

Know what?

We're not that concerned.

Remember, it's not about how much calcium we're taking in. And studies support the fact that you probably don't need as much calcium as you think if the rest of your nutrition and lifestyle are supporting healthy, strong bones (and they are, if you're following our plan!).

So skip the milk, eat your greens, get some sunshine, exercise regularly, and enjoy *all* of the health benefits of a nutrient-dense, anti-inflammatory, hormone-optimizing diet—including strong, healthy bones.

BUT WHAT ABOUT...

The dairy discussion always brings up a series of questions, all of which start with, "But what about …?" Let's address some of the dairy options, and whether or not we'd classify them as healthy choices.

What about pastured dairy?

See Chapter 22 for supplementation recommendations.

Don't be confused—*pastured* is not the same as *pasteurized*. Pastured refers to the way the animal was raised (mostly outside on pasture) and the food it was fed (in the case of cows, grass). Pasteurization is a process by which milk is heated, then cooled, in an effort to delay spoilage by discouraging microbial growth.

Cows raised in a natural environment and fed a natural diet are inherently healthier. A pastured (and ideally organic) dairy product will contain a larger percentage of healthy fats like conjugated linoleic acid (CLA) and omega-3 fatty acids and a healthier essential-fatty-acid balance. In addition, pastured dairy contains larger amounts of carotenoids (a class of antioxidants) and vitamins A and E, compared with conventional dairy. Finally, pastured, full-fat dairy will not contain protein remnants from a grain-based diet, which can be a problem for people with serious grain or gluten sensitivities.

However, simply sourcing dairy from cows that roam freely only sidesteps *some* of our concerns. Pastured, organic dairy still contains the same lactose, milk proteins, growth factors and hormones as conventionally-sourced dairy, which means it's still not such a healthy option.

What about raw milk?

Proponents of raw milk will say that raw (unpasteurized) milk is a superior choice, since the pasteurization process destroys enzymes (such as lactase) that help digest some components of the milk. However, aside from those issues, *all of the other concerns still apply to raw milk.*

If you're dead set on consuming milk, raw is perhaps a "less bad" option—but if you live in the United States, you'll probably have to hunt hard for it, as selling raw milk is illegal in many states.

As for us, we can't justify working that hard for something that's *still* not optimally healthy.

What about fermented dairy?

Fermented dairy (such as yogurt or kefir) does have some advantages over regular milk. Since the bacteria in these foods have broken down a significant amount of the lactose and dairy proteins, people generally have greater tolerance for it.

The most commonly cited benefit of fermented dairy is its health-promoting bacteria, which help to maintain the balance of gut bacteria. You've probably heard of *Lactobacillus acidophilus*, one species famous for its beneficial properties, but there are dozens of other "friendlies." (These are some of the bacteria "allies" we referred to in the discussion of the nightclub in Chapter 6.)

While you can obtain some benefits from consuming these bacteria, the delivery mechanism may still prove imperfect, and individual tolerance varies greatly. Feel free to play around with unsweetened yogurt or kefir after you've done the Whole30, but make sure it's still pastured *and* organic. Conventionally-produced, sweetened, low-fat yogurt will not make you healthier, even if there is fruit on the bottom!

The good news is that yogurt is not the only place that you can find beneficial bacteria. Unpasteurized sauerkraut and kimchi, kombucha, and fermented coconut water "kefir" (as well as a probiotic supplement, if indicated) are good sources of beneficial gut bacteria without the potential downsides of most dairy.*

THE EXCEPTIONS You may have noticed that we haven't expressed any specific concerns about dairy fat. In fact, we'll talk about butter and heavy (whipping) cream in the "More Healthy" section. Surprised? Check this out—research studies that compare full-fat dairy with reduced-fat dairy demonstrate better health outcomes with full-fat dairy. This is not an endorsement of whole milk— these benefits are largely due to the health-promoting properties of dairy fat, which we encourage eating *all by itself* in the form of butter or heavy cream. For example, pastured, organic butter contains little to none of the protein fractions, growth promoters, or hormones found in milk but has many beneficial compounds including vitamin K_2, conjugated linoleic acid (CLA), and even those famous omega-3 fatty acids.

In summary, the question of whether eating dairy is healthy is complicated and depends on many factors, but we prefer to err on the side of caution. Why eat something that has so many potential downsides, especially when you can get all the nutrition your body needs from other, healthier sources?

We'll talk about these more in Chapter 22, but it's worth noting that if you have a histamine intolerance, even nondairy fermented foods may cause problems for you. Progress slowly when introducing new fermented foods into your diet.

As with our other "less healthy" foods, we recommend blending the science and our experience from the Whole30 program with some self-experimentation. Remove dairy from your diet for thirty days, so you can evaluate the effects the milk sugars and proteins are having on you. Most of our clients—especially those with acne, allergies, or asthma—experience great relief from their conditions when they stop consuming dairy, but until you try it for yourself, you'll never know for sure.

CHAPTER 12:
IT ALL ADDS UP

"I was upset and self-conscious because my vitiligo—manifesting as splotchy white 'disease-like' discolorations—was on my hands, face, breasts, and other areas. I thought I would have to pile on makeup forever and spend eternity in a light booth. Yet today, I am absolutely astonished—I have an autoimmune disease for which my doctor says there is no cure, yet I've had NO vitiligo outbreaks since the Whole30!!!! This program has paved the way for huge positive changes in my family's life. Thank you!"
—Jessica G., Vancouver, Washington

We're finished talking about all the food (and beverage) groups that we think make you less healthy. But we are not quite done.

We've discussed how these foods are problematic when eaten in isolation. They are psychologically unbalancing, hormone-imbalancing, gut-disrupting or immune-system-provoking; sometimes all four at once.

But we don't eat these foods in isolation.

We eat them all together.

We have peanut butter on whole-wheat toast, with a glass of milk.

We eat three-bean chili with sour cream and cheese.

We eat cereal with soymilk for breakfast, make sandwiches for lunch, and eat macaroni and cheese for dinner.

The effects of these foods on our bodies and our brains are cumulative.

Insulin resistance and leptin resistance don't happen overnight—it's a gradual process. The gut doesn't become chronically leaky from one meal—it often takes time for persistent permeability to develop. Chronic, systemic inflammation isn't always an observable process—it's silent, subtle, insidious.

Sometimes, as a result of your collective dietary habits and their long-term effects, your bodily systems start to break down.

Enter autoimmune disease.

WHAT IS AUTOIMMUNE DISEASE?

Under normal conditions, your immune cells won't attack cells that are "self"—your own body. In certain cases, however, immune cells get confused and attack your own body, causing the damage we know as *autoimmune disease*.

There are more than eighty known autoimmune diseases, and many more that are suspected to be autoimmune in nature. Organs and tissues frequently affected include the thyroid, pancreas, adrenal glands, red blood cells, epithelial cells (arteries and gut), the myelin sheath or neurons, skin, muscles, and joints. Autoimmune conditions, several of which we've already mentioned, include multiple sclerosis (MS), lupus, celiac disease (CD), Hashimoto's thyroiditis, Grave's disease, rheumatoid arthritis, type 1 diabetes, and pernicious anemia.

EPIGENETICS AGAIN Most autoimmune diseases are thought to develop from the interaction of an environmental factor with a specific hereditary component. It's the whole "epigenetics" thing again—you may have the gene for celiac disease, but if you are never exposed to gluten your chances of developing the disease (and suffering from the symptoms) are slim to none. Environmental factors, infectious disease, and stress all play a role in "pulling the trigger" on a genetic predisposition to autoimmune diseases … but *food* may play the most significant role of all.

IT STARTS IN YOUR GUT

Do you remember the significance of maintaining an appropriate barrier between "outside" and "inside"? And how, when that barrier is compromised, we end up with a "leaky gut"?

As a result of that increased intestinal permeability, bacteria and their toxins, undigested food, and waste may leak out of the intestines into the bloodstream.

Remember that 70 percent to 80 percent of your body's immune system is stationed in your gut.

So when this garrison of immune cells encounter stuff inside the body that doesn't belong there, they react. Strongly.

Now, maybe that "foreign invader" is just a piece of incompletely digested chicken protein, allowed to "leak" inside the body accidentally. A leaky gut forces the immune system to attack things that could be totally harmless (like a useful source of protein) if they had stayed where they belonged. But since they didn't, your immune system now identifies that chicken protein as foreign and attacks it.

This is one theory on how food allergies are born.

> **A leaky gut lets partly digested food go where it does not belong, triggering an immune response and potentially creating a reaction to an otherwise healthy food.**

It's clear that leaky gut syndrome is related to immune-mediated problems in the body. How this translates to *autoimmunity*, however, isn't as well understood. The most researched theory to date (still under exploration) involves an additional mechanism called "molecular mimicry": when something that is *foreign* looks a lot like something that is *self*.

See, parts of proteins in various foods and infectious agents resemble parts of various proteins in the body. (Remember the bad guys at the club door, wearing masks?) The theory is that when immune cells inside the body see a foreign invader that looks a lot like something that belongs to us, they may get confused and attack *us* instead of the foreign invader. This is far more likely to happen when your immune system is already overworked and stressed from dealing with all the stuff that's coming in through your food, and going where it doesn't belong.

MOLECULAR MIMICRY In celiac disease, part of the wheat protein looks a lot like a particular virus, which looks a lot like a particular gut protein. The result of such mimicry is that when this *wheat protein* is eaten, the immune system is prompted to attack the *gut*. A similar mimicry among a protein found in grains and legumes, part of the Epstein-Barr virus, and part of the collagen in joints produces rheumatoid arthritis in genetically susceptible people, as the immune system attacks the joints. For type 1 diabetes, casein (milk protein) and other viral proteins mimic proteins found in beta cells of the pancreas, leading the immune cells to attack and destroy them, and leaving the body unable to produce enough insulin to manage blood sugar.

In theory …

Leaky gut can become a confused immune system, which can become an autoimmune disease.*

The good news is that most of these cumulative effects—the unhealthy psychological effects, the metabolic dysfunction, the gut permeability, the systemic inflammation, and perhaps even the symptoms of the autoimmune condition itself—are, in most cases, *highly reversible.*

Restoring good health starts with food.

Gut bacteria probably also play a significant role in this process, but that research is still quite new.

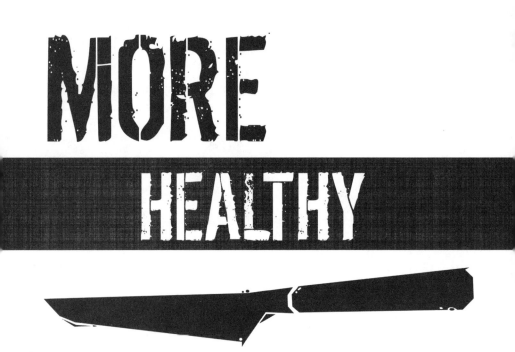

CHAPTER 13:
MEAT, SEAFOOD, AND EGGS

"My seven-year-old was diagnosed with PDD (similar to autism) at the age of four. He has always had behavior issues (screaming, tantrums, hitting his siblings, hurting himself), and I've tried everything I could to change this—including taking parenting classes, because I thought I was doing something wrong. In December 2011, my husband and I were introduced to the Whole30. Within just a few days, he was like a brand-new child! He woke up one morning with a smile on his face, was very compliant, and would even sit down and do his homework without whining and crying about it. We are so happy with the results of our whole family that we have continued to eat clean foods, and we rave about this program to anyone who will listen."
—Nicole L., Corona, California

Usually at this point, people start wondering what the heck they're supposed to eat. We assure you that there are lots of good foods on your horizon! So let's talk about the foods that meet *all four* of our Good Food standards—the foods that should be on your plate. (And it's not just that these are the only foods left over—each of these food groups also has specific properties that have positive effects on your health.)

FOLLOW ALONG You may want to download the detailed shopping list (complete with our "best choice" recommendations) from our Web site before flipping through this section. You can find it at http://whole9life.com/itstartswithfood.

Our way of eating is sometimes referred to as "radical." (That's the nice way of putting it—we hear "crazy" pretty often too.) But when you take a look at the foods we think make you more healthy, how radical is it, really?

We want you to eat meat, seafood, and eggs. You know—the stuff your great-great-grandparents ate, like beef, chicken, and salmon. You don't have to eat liver and tongue (although you can if you want to), and we are not encouraging you to be carnivores. But including some high-quality, nutrient-dense protein with each meal doesn't sound that radical to us.

We want you to balance that protein with plenty of plant matter—namely, vegetables and fruit. You don't have to "juice" or take super-green pills or replace one meal a day with a smoothie—we just want you to eat your veggies. A dietary plan that recommends that you eat a wide variety of nutritious vegetables and fruit isn't that unusual either, is it?

Finally, we're going to include healthy fats in your meals. Not fast-food-cheeseburger fat, not seed oil fat, and not fake-plastic-butterlike-foods fat, either. Healthy sources of fat to provide energy and keep your metabolism humming. Nothing too crazy there, right?

As you read through this section, close the door on all the things you *won't* be eating.

Instead, think about all the things that you *get* to eat.

Delicious, whole foods, rich in nutrition the way nature intended. Meals that satiate—leave you full, satisfied, and well nourished, not hungry, wanting, and craving. Foods that encourage a healthy relationship with food, keep your hormones in balance, make your gut healthy, and minimize inflammation.

Sounds totally sane and reasonable to us.

ANIMAL PROTEIN

The first category of foods that make you healthier includes meat, seafood, and eggs—all dense protein sources, without any of the downsides of vegetarian protein sources like kidney beans, whole grains, and tofu.*

You remember why we need adequate protein, right?

It's necessary for growth and repair of skin, hair, tendons, ligaments, and muscles; helps you recover from general activity and exercise; and is used to produce hormones, enzymes, neurotransmitters, and antibodies.

---

*We'll detail our recommendations for vegetarians or vegans in Chapter 21.

THE COMPLETE STORY Protein is made of amino acids. There are twenty-one amino acids, nine of which are "essential" (cannot be synthesized by the human body) and must be obtained from food. A *complete protein* is a protein source that contains all of the essential amino acids in useful proportions and quantities. All animal protein sources are complete, while most plant-based protein sources are incomplete.

Aside from meeting your physiological needs, protein is the most satiating of all the macronutrients. Upon digestion, complete proteins send signals to your brain that tell you to stop eating, as you are full and well nourished. Eating meals and snacks that include moderate servings of complete protein will help you avoid overconsumption, effectively stave off hunger pangs, and maintain a healthy body weight.

So what do we mean by "animal protein sources"? Here are some common examples (but not an exhaustive list).

Animal Protein Sources	Examples
Meat: Ruminants	Beef, buffalo/bison, elk, lamb, venison, moose, goat
Meat: Poultry	Chicken, duck, turkey, pheasant, ostrich, quail
Meat: Other	Pork, wild boar, rabbit
Seafood	Fish, mollusks (squid, octopus, scallops, clams, mussels, oysters), crustaceans (crab, shrimp, prawns, lobster, crayfish)
Eggs	Usually from chickens
Various: Organ meats	Liver, tongue, kidney, heart, sweetbreads, etc.
Various: Bones	Marrow, bone broths

BEAUTIFUL BROTH While bone broths are not a dense source of protein, they do provide valuable amino acids not found in large quantities in muscle meat. They are also an excellent source of vitamins and minerals, including calcium and magnesium, and digestive-tract healers like gelatin (collagen). There are several delicious bone broth recipes in Appendix A.

However, not all meat is created equal. There are two things we consider above all else when evaluating the quality of our animal protein sources.

**Here's what matters: the way the animal was raised and
the food it was fed.**

Both factors contribute significantly to the health of the animal, the quality of its meat, and ultimately your health.

NATURAL VS. INDUSTRIAL

Animals raised in a natural environment and allowed to express their normal social and biological behaviors are healthier and require fewer medical interventions. For cows, this means they're raised on pasture. For chicken and pigs, it means they've got free, unrestricted access to pasture or grazing land. Animals raised in a natural environment in a truly "organic" fashion (certified or otherwise) aren't given growth hormones, preventative antibiotics, or other potentially toxic substances and have less exposure to pesticides, fertilizers, heavy metals, and other environmental toxins.

NATURAL SCHMATURAL The term "natural" is grossly overused in food labeling and marketing. It is meant to imply that these foods are minimally processed and do not contain manufactured ingredients, but there is no legal standard. We are using the term literally, to define the environment and food supply these animals would have access to in nature.

When farmers take care to raise their animals in a natural, healthy environment, the animals are generally allowed to eat their natural diet too. This means cows and sheep (ruminants) eat grass; chickens and pigs (omnivores) forage for roots, seeds, insects, worms, leaves, and grasses; and fish eat krill, plankton, algae, and other aquatic life forms. Not only are these animals healthier, their meat is also measurably healthier (compared with the industrially-raised product), containing more vitamins, minerals, and healthy fats, and fewer environmental toxins. Since the animals are healthier, grass-fed, and pastured, they are also far less likely to transmit the harmful E. Coli bacteria through their meat.

GOOD-FOOD BUZZWORDS Not sure how to tell whether the meat you are eating was naturally raised and fed? Look for terms like *grass-finished* or *grass-fed*, *pastured*, *certified organic, hormone- and antibiotic-free,* and *wild-caught*. If you don't see them, assume that your meat, seafood, or eggs were industrially raised.

Unfortunately, the vast majority of meat, fish, and eggs sold in the United States doesn't come from health-conscious small-scale farms. Instead, a full 99 percent of our farm animals are raised and slaughtered in assembly-line fashion in mass-production operation known as "factory farming."

Factory farms don't have the green pastures and red barns most Americans imagine when they think of farms. Instead, factory farms are large industrial facilities that produce food in high volume with little to no regard for the health of the animals or the consumers.

Factory-farmed animals are denied the most basic aspects of their natural environments. They are confined in tight quarters (often indoors, crowded together in pens or cages), with no room for movement or normal behaviors and with minimal, if any, access to sunlight and fresh air.

Because of their congested and unsanitary living conditions, the animals are dosed with preventative antibiotics to ward off disease. Depending on the species, they may also be given hormones to make them grow faster. Finally, their environments and feed commonly expose them to environmental toxins like pesticides, herbicides, and heavy metals.

The animals in our profit-driven factory-farming system are fed diets designed to make them grow fast and fat—and keep feed costs down. Their feed consists primarily of industrially-produced commodity crops like corn, soybeans, and grains, and includes such unsavory "fillers" as feathers, meat from other animals, and other animal byproducts and waste, like chicken manure. (Yes, really. Chicken manure.)

Remember that old adage "You are what you eat"? We like to take that one step further, borrowing a clever turn of phrase from author Michael Pollan.

"You are what what you eat eats."

VOTE WITH YOUR DOLLAR

We cannot in good conscience support an industrialized, profit-driven, secretive "farming" system with no regard for its animals, its workers, our environment, and our health. We'd love it if all of you visited the Sustainable Table Web site (http://sustainabletable.org) or watched the documentary *Food, Inc.* and immediately abstained from supporting the factory-farming system. But we understand if that might be overwhelming for you right now, in light of the other challenging dietary changes we are promoting. Our simple hope is that you will continue to explore this issue using the resources in this book and begin to "vote with your dollar" sooner rather than later to support local, humane, ethical, and responsible farming operations.

ANIMAL PROTEIN STRATEGIES

The conditions under which factory-farmed animals are kept and the food they are fed make the meat of these animals less micronutrient-rich and more contaminated than that of their naturally raised, naturally fed counterparts. However, there are steps you can take to mitigate the negative health effects of eating industrially-produced meat.

First, buy the leanest cut possible, and trim or drain all the visible fat. Residues in factory-farmed meat (such as those from pesticides, insecticides, feed additives, hormones, and antibiotics) are often fat-soluble, which means they are stored in the animal's fatty tissues. When we consume the fat from these animals, we are also ingesting these toxins. These residues can be hazardous to humans and are dose-dependent (the more you consume, the greater the potential risk). By purchasing lean cuts of conventionally-raised meat and removing all visible fat, you can reduce your exposure to these potentially injurious substances. But allow us to make one critical point.

It's not about the fat itself.

As you'll see in a later chapter, we're not fat-phobic, and we aren't suggesting you should eat *nothing* but lean meat. We just don't like the *toxins* that come along for the ride in factory-farmed meat. However, if you're eating 100 percent grass-fed, organic meat, it's perfectly fine to eat a fatty rib-eye! The type of fat found in naturally raised and fed animals contains many healthful properties, *with none of the contaminants that result from factory farming*—and we believe that kind of fat really does make you healthier.

VITAMINS, MINERALS, MEAT Hold on—you're concerned about eating all that saturated fat, aren't you? We thought so. Remember how we cautioned you against oversimplifying the nutrients in food? Well, much as dairy isn't *just* calcium and whole grains aren't *just* fiber, red meat isn't *just* saturated fat! Many people think of meat, seafood, and eggs as protein (or as saturated-fat delivery mechanisms), but did you know that "meat" is also a dense source of micronutrients, some of which you simply *can't* effectively get from plants? All types of meat contain the most bioavailable forms of vitamin B_{12}, a nutrient essential for good health, and iron, called "heme iron." You simply can't get adequate B_{12} or this form of iron from plants—yet another reason to throw another steak on the barbie. (And, no, we haven't just ignored your concern. We'll cover saturated fat in detail soon.)

To quell some of your meat concerns, we'll also assure you that we want you to vary your animal protein sources. We don't think you should eat rib-eyes at every meal, seven days a week, even if they *are* grass-fed and organic. Different meats contain different vitamins and minerals, so the more you rotate the foods you eat, the better chance you'll have of getting the full complement of micronutrients that make you healthier. If you don't like certain types of meats, that's OK—there are still plenty of options for you.

WHAT ABOUT EGGS (AND CHOLESTEROL)?

Two of the most common questions we hear are, "Can I eat eggs every day?" and "How many eggs can I eat?"

The answers are *yes* and *a reasonable amount.*

Allow us to explain.

The concern with eggs is usually in reference to the egg yolk, and comes from health-conscious folks who worry about their cholesterol intake. Generally, they've been told that eggs are cholesterol bombs, that cholesterol in their body comes primarily from their diet, and that cholesterol is inherently "bad."

Let's clear up some cholesterol misconceptions, shall we?

CHOLESTEROL DEFINED Cholesterol is transported in the bloodstream by tagging along with structures called *lipoproteins* to form complexes of lipoproteins plus cholesterol molecules. We bet you've heard of these lipoprotein-cholesterol complexes, but you probably know them by their oversimplified abbreviations, like LDL (low-density lipoprotein) or HDL (high-density lipoprotein). When doctors talk about LDL or HDL, however, they are actually referring to the lipoprotein-cholesterol complex, which is more accurately abbreviated as LDL-C or HDL-C.

First, don't take a reductionist view here—eggs are more than *just* cholesterol. They're packed with protein (half in the white, half in the yolk), and pastured eggs provide more than a dozen essential nutrients, including vitamins A, B_{12}, D, and E, brain-healthy choline, omega-3 fatty acids, and eye-healthy lutein … all of which are found in the yolk.

That being said, one large egg yolk does have almost 200 mg of cholesterol, and conventional wisdom says that since eggs are high in cholesterol, eating eggs every day will increase your blood cholesterol, leading to heart disease and stroke.

This is one example of something that *sounds* right (eating cholesterol = higher cholesterol levels), but isn't factually accurate.

Blood-cholesterol and lipoprotein levels are controlled by far more powerful factors than the cholesterol in your diet. In fact, the vast majority of your blood cholesterol is produced by your own body: depending on your health and diet, your liver makes three to ten times more cholesterol than the amount that comes from your food. So what would make your body produce abnormally high amounts of cholesterol?

Overcarbsumption and systemic inflammation, that's what.

When, as a result of dietary and lifestyle factors, we create systemic inflammation in the body, the liver is forced to pump out more and more lipoprotein and cholesterol in an attempt to manage our inflammatory status, fend off infection, and repair damaged tissues. In addition, when we are under physical or psychological stress, cholesterol increases significantly—because cholesterol is an important precursor of cortisol. (Remember cortisol, that "stress hormone?") More stress equals more cortisol production equals more lipoprotein and cholesterol production.

So knowing that the vast majority of your total blood cholesterol comes from your own body, if your doctor says you have high cholesterol, what will have the biggest impact—eliminating three eggs a day or making changes to reduce systemic inflammation and avoid overcarbsumption, thus dramatically reducing your body's own production of cholesterol?

That's what is known as a rhetorical question.

STATIN DRUGS Many physicians will recommend statin drugs for elevated blood cholesterol levels. Statin drugs work to reduce cholesterol, but *how* do they work? They interfere with cholesterol synthesis ... and *reduce systemic inflammation!* Of course, reducing systemic inflammation is something you can do simply by changing your eating habits, thus eliminating the need to take medications with serious side effects for the rest of your life. That sounds like a better option to us too.

In addition, cholesterol is not evil—it's a necessary part of our hormonal production and cellular structure. You need cholesterol for the production of hormones like cortisol, estrogen, and testosterone, to make vitamin D, to build and repair cell walls, and to produce bile acids and salts to help you digest food. It's also critical for normal function of neurons (nerve cells), including those in the brain.

Which means our goal is not to get to zero cholesterol—in fact, cholesterol levels that are too low are quite harmful and increase your risk for a variety of disorders, including cancer, depression, stroke, and anxiety. No, the goal is to arrive at a place of appropriate cholesterol levels, with numbers that reflect a low risk for lifestyle-related diseases and conditions.

The thing is, that might still look a lot like "high cholesterol" on paper.

High cholesterol is not always an indicator of disease.
As with everything, context matters.

A diagnosis of "high cholesterol" is based on measuring the amount of total cholesterol circulating in the blood. However, measuring cholesterol and lipoprotein levels, interpreting these measurements, and drawing conclusions about their cause and effect is complicated. Some biomarkers, such as elevated total cholesterol or high LDL-C, *are* associated with increased rates of cardiovascular disease. But that doesn't mean that the cholesterol in the blood causes cardiovascular disease! In addition, while elevated total cholesterol may be an indicator of disease, it might not indicate elevated risk at all.

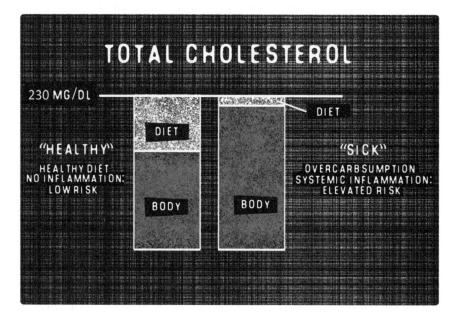

Say your total cholesterol is 230 mg/dL (230 milligrams of cholesterol per deciliter of blood). If you have no systemic inflammation, high HDL-C, and low triglycerides, you can consider yourself generally healthy and at low risk for heart disease, even though your total cholesterol is "borderline high." In this instance, some of your "high" cholesterol might come from your diet, but that is not a problem!

However, a cholesterol level of 230 accompanied by systemic inflammation, low HDL-C, and high triglycerides is a totally different story—this can happen even if you consume *no* cholesterol in your diet. In this case, high total cholesterol puts you at increased risk for heart disease and stroke.

Context matters.

Measuring just total cholesterol is kind of like watching a movie trailer—it gives you a rough idea of what's going on, but you need far more information to evaluate the whole story. A better big-picture strategy is to use cholesterol measurements in conjunction with other lab values (such as LDL particle size, triglycerides, and C-reactive protein) to paint a multi-faceted picture of your overall health.

CALCULATE YOUR RISK

So if total cholesterol by itself doesn't paint a reliable big health picture, what else can you use to estimate your risk? There are a few indicators that are relatively reliable. Low levels of triglycerides and high levels of HDL-C are generally indicators of good health, *even if your total cholesterol is high*. In addition, calculating your triglyceride-to-HDL-C ratio may be the most effective way to evaluate your risk for heart disease. Divide your triglycerides by your HDL cholesterol to arrive at your ratio. Generally speaking, the lower the ratio, the lower your risk of a heart attack. More precisely, a ratio of 2 or less is ideal, 4 is considered high, and 6 puts you square in the danger zone.

In summary, eating cholesterol-rich foods as part of a healthy, anti-inflammatory diet like this one is not problematic. If you're following our Good Food recommendations, your body won't need to overproduce cholesterol, which means it's totally safe for you to consume some in your food. We're OK with regular consumption of whole eggs—even if you're eating five or six at a time—as part of the varied, high-quality diet we're outlining here.

In fact, one 2008 study summarized: "There is no convincing evidence to link an increased intake of dietary cholesterol or eggs with coronary heart disease through raised blood cholesterol. Indeed, eggs make a nutritional contribution to a healthy diet."

Maybe we could have just said that.

PROCESSED MEATS

One last word on processed meats like bacon, sausage, deli meat, or beef jerky. While these foods are certainly convenient, they are not always the healthiest choice. Bacon and sausage often contain just as much fat as protein, and if that meat is coming from the factory-farming system, that fat contains a whole lot of potentially toxic byproducts. As with all protein, the quality of the meat and the manner in which it was processed determine how healthy the end product will be.

Some observational research suggests that processed meats are associated with higher rates of some cancers—but the how is still unknown and probably has to do with the way the animals were raised and fed (in our factory-farming system). If you are going to eat processed meats, our same quality guidelines apply. Select foods from naturally raised and fed sources (grass-fed, pastured, wild-caught, and organic), and find brands that are minimally processed with ingredients you can pronounce. And as always, make sure to vary your protein sources from day to day.

BACON While it may be liberating to think bacon is no longer off-limits, we still want you to think before you eat it. Bacon is one of those technically OK foods that may still provide enough of a flavor and texture "hit" to lead to overconsumption. If you're trying to lose weight and recover from metabolic derangement, use bacon as a condiment, rather than your main protein source. (In fact, bacon isn't really a dense source of protein for anyone.) In addition, bacon lovers *must* take the time to find a pastured, organic source. This is non-negotiable, as factory-farmed bacon is perhaps the *least healthy* cut of meat you can eat.

CHAPTER 14:
VEGETABLES AND FRUITS

"I have more allergies to more things than anyone I have ever met. In addition to nearly every form of pollen, corn, soy, and wheat, I have oral allergies to nearly all raw fruits, vegetables, and nuts. When I eat them, my mouth, head, and throat get unbearably itchy. If I continue to eat them, hello anaphylactic shock! During the Whole30, my selection of safe raw fruits and veggies expanded exponentially. I went from lettuce being the only safe thing, to eating apples, oranges, all manner of berries, carrots, peppers, hazelnuts, spinach, cabbage, and so on. After not being able to have them for years, I am downright rabid with excitement."

—Kim C., Helena, Montana

We've got some breaking news for you here—truly shocking information. Are you ready? Are you sitting down? Here goes ...

Vegetables are good for you.

That's right—vegetables really do make you healthier! First, vegetables are a nutrient-dense source of carbohydrate. Yes, we know, you don't actually *need* carbohydrate to survive, but most folks feel their best with enough carbohydrate in their diets to support brain function and activity levels. Choosing vegetables as your primary source of carbs is a great way to get all the energy you need in a micronutrient-dense package.

In addition, vegetables are distinctly anti-inflammatory. That's right, a diet rich in vegetables can actually help you battle our old arch nemesis, systemic inflammation, and reduce your risk for lifestyle-related disorders—stroke, coronary heart disease, and certain types of cancer.

Vegetables (and fruit, which we'll get to soon) are a rich source of many nutrients and active compounds. Their benefits can't be explained by a single component, like their vitamin C or fiber content. However, their anti-inflammatory properties are often attributed to the fact that vegetables provide the richest source of antioxidants, which prevent or reverse damage caused by excess free radicals.*

So how does our free radical balance get *unbalanced*?

Some free radical production is instigated by external sources, like pollution, smoking, radiation, and exposure to sunlight. Others can be created from our food, particularly when we consume certain types of fats—remember the seed oils chapter? Free radicals are also normal metabolic byproducts: they're produced when our immune system is fired up (like when we get an infection or fight off a cold), when we eat too much, or during strenuous exercise.

Remember, an overabundance of free radicals in the body can damage cells and your DNA, and are profoundly inflammatory. But we have a natural way of keeping our free radicals in balance—antioxidants. These substances both prevent free radicals from pinballing around in the body damaging healthy cells and, after the free radicals have come and gone, repair the damage they've done in our bodies.

However, when antioxidants perform these duties, they sacrifice themselves in the process (how gallant!). Therefore, even though the body produces its own antioxidants, we must continue to replenish our antioxidant stores through the food we eat—*especially* if there are variables (like illness, pollution, an aggressive exercise routine, or a less-than-healthy diet) that keep pumping more free radicals into our system.

Vegetables and fruits have the highest natural concentration of antioxidants—things we bet you've heard of, like vitamin C, vitamin E, and beta-carotene—so it makes sense that a diet rich in these noble martyrs would help us fight free radicals and reduce systemic inflammation.

But remember, food is complex, and vegetables aren't just antioxidants. You cannot attribute the benefits gained from eating certain foods to one particular nutrient, even if that nutrient is kind of a big deal. (Remember the "I eat whole grains for fiber" argument?)

People don't eat *nutrients*, they eat *food*.

---

* *Compounds from meat also add antioxidants to our arsenal and supply building blocks for our body's own antioxidant production. See? Meat does more than just provide protein!*

And like all real food, vegetables aren't just antioxidants, but an assortment of vitamins, minerals, phytonutrients, fiber, and compounds that we have yet to even identify, never mind figure out how they work in our bodies.

The good news? You don't need to understand the complexity of your vegetables to reap the benefits from eating them. Whew.

EAT YOUR VEGGIES

All this is to say: Eat your vegetables! Eat a wide variety of vegetables daily to ensure a wide range of micronutrients, and make sure you're including some of the most nutrient-dense options with each meal for maximum benefit.

Below is a list of our vegetable Top 20—the ones we recommend that you keep in regular rotation.

Eat these often!

Asparagus	Carrots	Spinach
Beets	Cauliflower	Sweet Potato
Bell Peppers	Greens (Beet, Collard, Mustard, Turnip)	Swiss Chard
Bok Choy	Kale	Tomato
Broccoli, Broccolini	Lettuce (Bibb, Boston, Butter, Red)	Watercress
Brussels Sprouts	Onions, Shallots, Leeks, Garlic	Winter Squashes
Cabbage	Rutabaga/Turnip	Zucchini/Summer Squash

We'll point out that some things you might normally spot in the produce section aren't on our Good Food list. Corn is botanically a grain, while green peas and lima beans are the seeds of legumes, so these "vegetables" are not in our general recommendations. You'll also notice white potatoes are missing too. Americans eat a lot of white potatoes—and more than a third are in the form of fries or potato chips. Keeping these familiar foods in your diet makes you more likely to return to your old, unhealthy food habits, and since there are *far* more nutrient-dense choices available, take a pass on white potatoes, please.

AREN'T THOSE LEGUMES?

However, you *will* find green beans, snow peas, and sugar-snap peas on our shopping list, despite the fact that they are botanically legumes. Confused? Let us explain. Potentially disruptive compounds are found in the *seeds* of legumes—but green beans, snow peas, and sugar-snap peas are an immature seed wrapped in a big, green plant pod. Since what you're eating is mostly pod (not seed), we don't think these three legumes have the same issues as the others. Besides … if green beans are the *worst* thing in your diet, you're doing OK.

Finally, an all-too-common refrain from clients, readers, and workshop attendees is, "But I don't *like* vegetables!" You want to know what we tell them?

We don't care.

We say it *nicely*, of course. See, it doesn't matter if you don't like vegetables, because we're all grown-ups, and sometimes, grown-ups have to do things they don't like to do. Like mow the lawn. Or pay bills. Or eat vegetables. If there were a way to be optimally healthy without vegetables, we'd tell you. Really. But there isn't, so it's now up to you to figure out a way to get them on your plate (and into your belly).

Most aversion to vegetables is a result of three factors: One, you've been eating so many sugary, salty, fatty processed foods that you simply cannot appreciate the natural flavors of fresh vegetables. But the good news is that you're not eating that stuff anymore, and taste buds are quick to adjust. In just a matter of weeks, you'll be experiencing new and delicious flavors in your healthy foods, and that will make it easier to start truly enjoying your veggies.

Two, most folks are stuck in a major vegetable rut, relying on just a few familiar choices and avoiding everything else. No wonder you're bored with your veggies! It's time to go out on a limb and try something new. Visit your local farmers' market and ask the farmers what they do with kale, kohlrabi, or leeks. Commit to trying one new vegetable a week. Buy a share in a CSA (community-supported agriculture program), ensuring seasonal variety and delicious, fresh flavors. It's time to step out of your comfort zone, because we bet you'll find vegetable options you love if you just make the effort to try something new.

Third, many of us don't like certain vegetables because of the way they were served to us as a kid. No offense to our moms, but they didn't always go out of their way to make our vegetables delicious and exciting. So … give your greens another chance. Try different cooking techniques, experiment with herbs and spices, or find a new recipe that features the vegetable. Your taste in fashion has changed in the last ten or twenty years, so why not your taste in vegetables?

ANY WAY YOU LIKE 'EM

We don't really care how you purchase and prepare your veggies (fresh, frozen, cooked, or raw)—only that you're *eating* them.* But we suggest that you make raw fermented vegetables, like sauerkraut and kimchi, a priority. They provide a rich source of nutrition and digestion-enhancing enzymes. The fermentation process also provides natural probiotics, helping the intestinal tract maintain a healthy balance of bacteria by increasing the "good guys." We recommend including these fermented veggies in your diet a few times a week. (And see Chapter 22 for details about probiotics.)

FRUIT

The next category of food we think makes you more healthy is fruit. The positive attributes of fruit, another nutrient-dense source of carbohydrate, are remarkably similar to those of vegetables, with just a few special caveats. First, the pluses.

Like vegetables, fruits are a carbohydrate source loaded with vitamins, minerals, phytonutrients, and fiber. In addition, diets rich in fruit and compounds found in fruit (like vitamin C) have been associated with a reduced risk of systemic inflammation and related conditions and diseases. (Remember, fruit is real food—a complex makeup of health-promoting substances!) In addition, fruit provides your taste buds with *natural* sweetness in a much healthier (and nutrient-packed) form than the supernormal sweetness of candy, cookies, or cake.

Those with IBD, IBS, or other digestive disorders may find raw veggies too hard on their digestive tract and should refer to Chapter 21 for more details.

VEGETABLES WIN We have one important piece of advice in this section: Don't let fruits push vegetables off your plate just because they are more fun to eat. While fruits are certainly nutrient-dense and yummy, they are not as nutritious as vegetables. In addition, if you don't particularly like fruit, you don't have to eat any! We don't know of a single micronutrient found in fruit that you can't also find in vegetables. (Translation: Veggies are mandatory; fruit is optional.)

Much as with vegetables, we'd encourage you to eat a wide variety of fruits (especially when they're in season). Refer to our chart for a list of our fruit Top 10—eat these on a regular basis to ensure you are getting the widest array of vitamins, minerals, and phytonutrients.

Best fruit choices

Apricots	Kiwi
Blackberries	Melons
Blueberries	Plums
Cherries	Strawberries
Grapefruit	Raspberries

GO ORGANIC ... SOMETIMES

You don't *have* to buy organic produce, but we do think there are major benefits to going organic. Certified organic vegetables and fruits are produced without the use of synthetic pesticides, herbicides, and chemical fertilizers, do not contain genetically-modified organisms (GMOs), and are not processed using irradiation, industrial solvents, or artificial food additives. They are generally regarded as more nutrient-dense and environmentally safe than their non-organic counterparts.

However, it's not always essential that you purchase organic produce. By shopping smart, you can effectively minimize your exposure to toxins, even if you're not buying organic.

THE DIRTY DOZEN The Environmental Working Group issues an annual "Shopper's Guide to Pesticides in Produce," detailing the "dirtiest" (most contaminated with pesticide residue) and "cleanest" (least contaminated) produce items. If you're on a tight budget, purchase organic for the dirtiest of the dirty and conventional for the rest. For items that aren't on either list, do the best you can, given the produce available and your budget. (For the full list from the Environmental Working Group, visit http://ewg.org/foodnews.)

If this approach seems too complicated, follow this general rule of thumb: If the item of produce has an inedible skin, or you're going to peel it before you eat it, it's less important to buy organic; if you can't peel it (like lettuce or grapes), consider spending the extra money for organic.

And keep in mind that not every farmer goes through the rigorous and expensive process of earning a USDA "Certified Organic" designation. Many smaller farming operations are dedicated to organic and biodynamic farming practices but can't market their products as "certified organic." When shopping at a farmers' market or your local health-food store, don't hesitate to ask how the food was grown. Labels that clearly state "pesticide-free" or "herbicide-free" are another indication that the produce was grown with environmental and health factors in mind.

HOW SWEET IT IS

Like all food, fruit is a complex combination of vitamins, minerals, phytonutrients, fiber, and many other compounds that scientists have yet to identify. Fruit also contains natural sugars (glucose and fructose) and starches in various proportions and amounts. As fruit ripens, the starch in the fleshy part of it is converted to sugar, which makes it taste sweeter.

Fructose is the sweetest of all naturally occurring carbohydrates—almost twice as sweet as sucrose. You consume fructose in a variety of sources, including table sugar (sucrose), honey, fruits, some vegetables, and in processed foods and drinks sweetened with high-fructose corn syrup.

Fructose is different from other simple sugars in the way it's processed in the body. Virtually every cell in the body can use glucose for energy, but after being absorbed from your small intestine, most fructose is sent straight to the liver, where it is metabolized and either stored as energy (liver glycogen) or converted into triglycerides (fat) and dumped into the bloodstream.

SOUND FAMILIAR? Want to know what else is processed by the liver and (when overconsumed) promotes liver damage, accumulation of fat, and other metabolic consequences? Alcohol! That's right, the ethanol in alcohol is metabolized through the liver using pathways similar to those used by fructose. Which means that those strawberry daiquiris are putting even more of a burden on your liver than you might have imagined.

The effects of a diet too high in fructose are decidedly not good and may include liver damage, inflammation, atherosclerosis, free-radical damage, and an increased risk of diabetes, high blood pressure, kidney disease, and obesity. In fact, many studies show that diets high in fructose play a key role in metabolic syndrome.

But let's be clear—eating a few servings of fruit a day (as part of an otherwise healthy diet) is not going to *create* these conditions. Nobody ever became metabolically deranged from eating fruit! The trouble comes when folks consume more fructose from processed foods than they could ever get from natural sources.

Most fructose in the American diet doesn't come from fresh fruit but from the high-fructose corn syrup (HFCS) or sucrose (a form of sugar that is 50 percent fructose) found in high concentration in soda and fruit-flavored drinks. As one example, a twenty-ounce soda contains about thirty-six grams of fructose. That's the equivalent of eating five bananas, nine cups of strawberries, or ninety cherries! Combine our soda and processed-beverage intake with our overconsumption of processed foods (many of which are also sweetened with HFCS), and you've got a recipe for massive intakes of fructose, the likes of which you could never consume from real food.

The takeaway?

You will not create metabolic issues by eating fresh fruit as part of a healthy diet.

Just because fruit tastes sweet doesn't mean it's an unhealthy choice, and just because diets high in fructose cause problems doesn't mean you

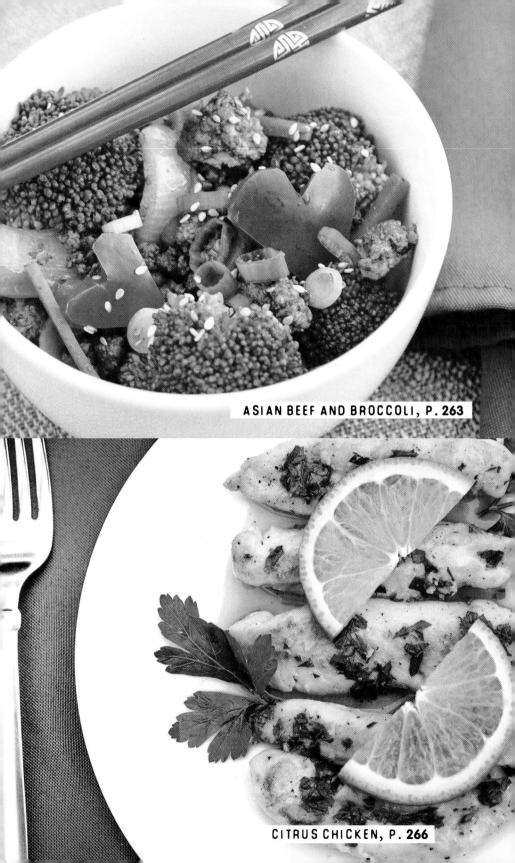

ASIAN BEEF AND BROCCOLI, P. 263

CITRUS CHICKEN, P. 266

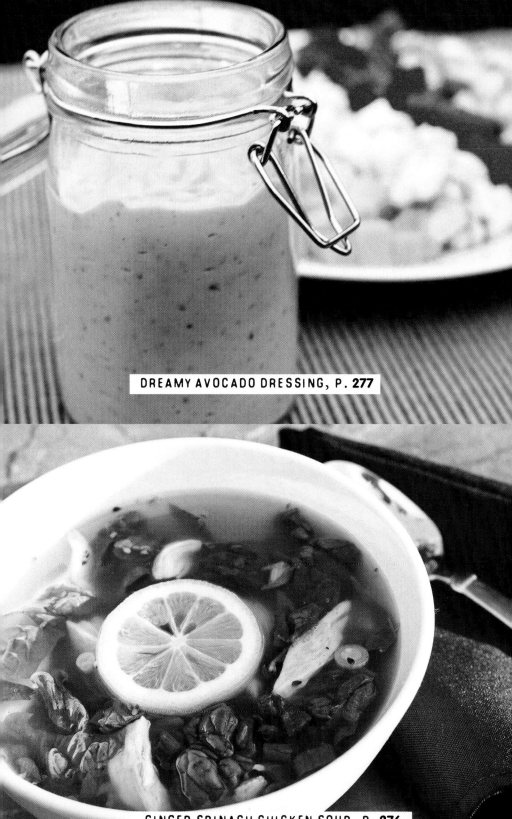

DREAMY AVOCADO DRESSING, P. 277

GINGER SPINACH CHICKEN SOUP, P. 276

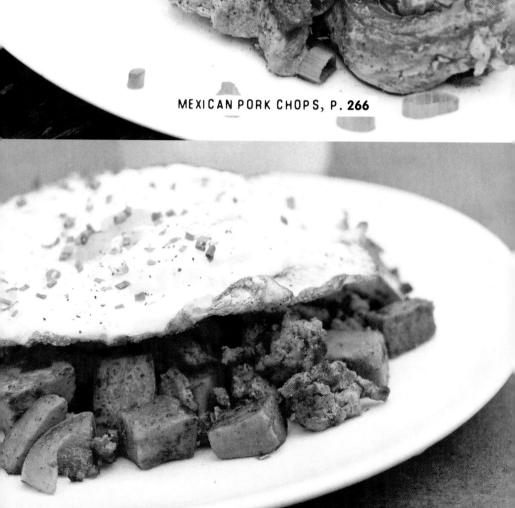

MEXICAN PORK CHOPS, P. 266

SWEET POTATO HASH, P. 263

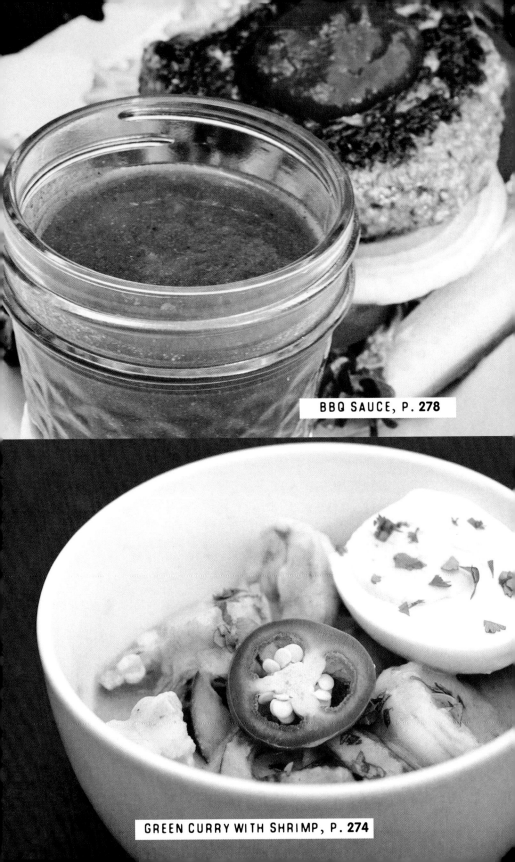

BBQ SAUCE, P. 278

GREEN CURRY WITH SHRIMP, P. 274

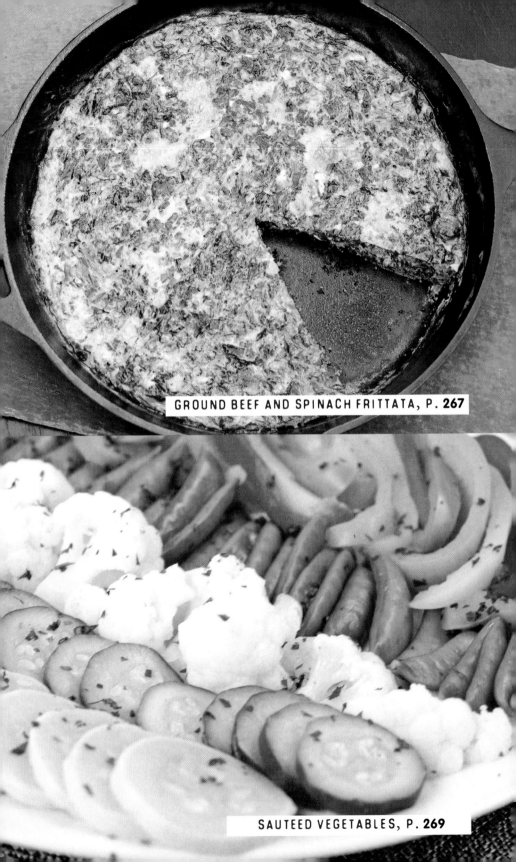

GROUND BEEF AND SPINACH FRITTATA, P. 267

SAUTEED VEGETABLES, P. 269

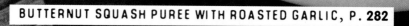

BUTTERNUT SQUASH PUREE WITH ROASTED GARLIC, P. 282

GREEN BEANS WITH FIG VINAIGRETTE, P. 282

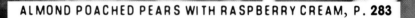

ALMOND POACHED PEARS WITH RASPBERRY CREAM, P. 283

HAZELNUT ROASTED SALMON, P. 281

NO-FUSS SALMON CAKES, P. 280

MOCHA STEAK, P. 279

should abstain from eating fruit. Remember, just as whole grains are not *just* fiber, fruit isn't *just* fructose! The naturally occurring sugars found in fruit are wrapped in a nutrient-dense package—unlike the fructose you'll find in a soft drink or breakfast pastry.

TALKING SWEET High-fructose corn syrup (HFCS) is the most common sweetener in processed foods and beverages, in large part because of how cheap it is to produce. You probably expect us to say that HFCS is the devil—but we don't think HFCS is any worse than any other form of added sweetener. Why? Because they *all* make you less healthy! Doesn't matter if it comes from corn, beets, cane, or a tree—from a psychological perspective, sugar is sugar is sugar. (Of course, not everyone agrees with this perspective—some studies do show that consuming HFCS leads to significantly more weight gain and higher triglycerides than consuming table sugar.) However, we will set the record straight on one thing: While HFCS may start out as corn, even the U.S. Food and Drug Administration says that HFCS is *not* a "natural sugar." Nice try, Corn Refiners Association.

There *is* one potential issue with fruit consumption. Because of the natural sweetness of fruit (especially in fruit juice and dried fruit, which concentrate the sugar), fruit *may* promote an unhealthy psychological response, especially in folks still battling their sugar dragons. We've seen many people use fruit to prop up their sugar cravings, telling themselves it's OK because fruit is "natural" and healthy. The scenario often looks like this:

It's 3:00 on a Thursday afternoon. You're at work, and you're hungry, cranky, and tired. You'd normally reach for a Snickers bar, a muffin, or some Oreos right about now, but you're trying to eat healthier and you know those are poor choices. So instead, you eat a dried fruit and nut bar.

There is just one problem with this situation.

Your brain doesn't know the difference.

As you learned in Chapter 4, your brain doesn't immediately differentiate between "healthy" sugar like dried fruit and "bad" sugar like a Snickers bar. The only thing your brain knows is, "I craved sugar and I got sugar."

That's right, the message you just sent to your brain is, "I craved, I satisfied that craving, and I feel better now."

Sound familiar? This is the same unhealthy pattern we described in the situation with the cookie from the downtown bakery. Except this time, your sugar of choice is "natural" and "healthy," so you don't even realize you are a slave to the same unhealthy habit ... but we do. So we'll warn you about this up front and, in later chapters, detail our recommendations for when and how to include fruit in your diet in a way that feels healthy and satisfying (but doesn't send you running for the nearest bag of candy).

DITCH THE JUICER One final word of advice: Skip the juice, even if you make it yourself. First, liquid calories aren't as satiating as real food, and as we've learned, less satiety equals eating more. Second, when you juice fruit, you're removing all of the fiber, which would normally slow the absorption of the sugar in whole fruit. More sugar in your bloodstream faster is not a good thing when you're still struggling with leptin and insulin resistance. Finally, many of the naturally occurring nutrients are lost during processing, pasteurization, and storage. Manufacturers compensate for this by adding nutrients back to the juice after the fact—but eating vitamin-enriched foods does not provide the same benefits as eating the whole, unprocessed food. Just eat the fruit.

CHAPTER 15:
THE *RIGHT* FATS

"I have always been an active, healthy girl, but in my thirties (after a bout with severe exhaustion followed by two pregnancies) I found myself a good hundred pounds over the limit. Something had to be done, as 'just eating well' was not doing my body any good. I was inspired by a close friend who had had great success doing a Whole30, and started my journey in February 2011. The first month, I lost ten pounds. And within the next two weeks, five more. In the last year, I have lost seventy pounds and over forty inches from my body. I am still a work in progress, but with the Whole30 on my side, I am making it closer to my goal every day! Thank you for changing my life."
—Heidi M., Bozeman, Montana

The last big category on our "makes you healthier" list includes many different foods with one thing in common—they're all good sources of fat.

We're discussing good fats for a number of reasons, some of which we've already talked about. First, fats are an excellent energy source. And one major goal of this dietary shift is to make your body more efficient at using fats (from your diet *and* your fat stores) for fuel. Fat is also critical to many metabolic processes, and ensuring that your diet includes adequate healthy fats means you've got the right building blocks for vital organs, cells, and hormones.

In addition, fats provide both satisfaction (via palatability) and satiety (via gut-brain hormonal pathways). A meal with a healthy amount of fat suppresses hunger longer than a meal that's primarily carbohydrate—so we don't run to the cookie jar between meals. Finally, there is another, more practical reason for including a healthy amount of fat in our meals—*calories.*

We want you to eat enough calories to maintain a healthy body weight and activity levels. But think about the way you used to eat versus the way we're recommending that you eat. You used to eat lots of calorie-dense carbohydrates (like grains, legumes, sugars, and processed foods). Now, you've replaced those with vegetables and fruit, which are comparative caloric lightweights. Which means your new diet is missing a bunch of calories—and we've got to supply them somehow.

We're not going to add more carbohydrates to the diet—you couldn't (and don't need to) eat enough veggies and fruit to fill the hole, and we're not about to resort to unhealthy food choices just for the calories.

We're not going to add more and more protein, either. We want you to eat only as much protein as you need to maintain muscle mass and support recovery from activity. (And it's not like doubling your meat consumption will double your muscle mass.) Too much protein might be just as unhealthy as not enough, so we'll outline just right protein recommendations in the next section.

So what's left?

Fat, that's what.

We're going to supply energy with good, healthy fat sources. And that's easy to do, since fat has more than twice the gram-for-gram calories as carbohydrate and protein. See—it really *is* a great source of energy!

ENERGY COMPARISON

As we mentioned in Chapter 5, our capacity to store carbohydrate in the liver and muscles is quite limited. The average person can store only enough glycogen to perform about ninety minutes of high-intensity activity. But that same person has enough energy stored as body fat to run twenty marathons! Which illustrates that fat is a much more dense and abundant source of energy in the body than carbohydrate. (That's also kind of depressing, isn't it? Sorry about that.)

DITCH THE SUGAR, FUEL WITH FAT

Fat is a dense and abundant source of energy, and with time and the right eating habits, we can create a healthy situation in which our bodies can use fat to fuel low-intensity activity (like hiking, gardening, playing with our children, or cleaning the house).

There are some major benefits to being "fat adapted," able to efficiently utilize fat as energy. First, you'll no longer need to eat every two hours to avoid the raging hunger, crankiness, or brain fog that comes with relying on glucose to fuel your energy needs. When you're fat-adapted (as in our Good Day example), you can go many hours between meals feeling and performing just fine, as your body has learned to mobilize your fat stores for energy.

In addition, once you're fat-adapted, you'll be able to start whittling away at your fat stores—something you are unable to do when your blood sugar and insulin levels are chronically elevated. (Remember, chronically elevated insulin levels impede glucagon's energy-access function!)

Finally, when you're fat-adapted, you've got the best of both worlds. Your body will still be able to run on carbohydrate for fuel when you really need it, during high-intensity activity like interval training or chasing after your runaway dog. But you'll also have an alternate energy source—fat!— for life's lower-intensity occasions (which make up the bulk of your twenty-four-hour day).*

The key to becoming fat-adapted can be explained simply enough:

Stop giving your body sugar all the time.

FAT: CONTEXT MATTERS

At this point, you've probably heard a few forward-thinking nutritionists say that *eating* fat doesn't *make* you fat. The thing is, that's not always true. A high-fat diet *in the context* of insulin resistance and leptin resistance can be profoundly damaging. Eating too much fat only adds fuel to your already out-of-control metabolic fire and provides even more energy (calories) for insulin to store. In our Bad Day scenarios, eating a high-fat diet certainly would contribute more fat to your stores. Note, however, that *dietary fat* is not the inherent problem here—it's overconsumption, your messed-up hormones, and inflammation that are at fault. The good news?

To be fair, the body always uses a mix of both carbohydrate and fat for energy. The higher the intensity, the higher proportion of that energy comes from carbohydrate. But for lower-intensity activity, your body can use a much higher proportion of fat for fuel—if you allow it to with smart food choices and a healthy hormonal balance.

When you eliminate the drive to overconsume and resultant hormonal dysfunction (via the recommendations we're making here), then eating fat *won't* make you fat.

Of course, not all fats are good fats. (Sure, we all know that … but we're also certain that our roster of "good fats" may surprise you, so stay on your toes in this section.) In addition, even some "good fats" need to be consumed in moderation, because while *some* is good, *more* isn't always better. So let's talk about good sources of each of the three different categories of fats—monounsaturated, saturated, and polyunsaturated.

TRANS FATS Do we *really* need to talk about why you shouldn't eat trans fats? These Franken-fats (often labeled as "partially hydrogenated") are not found anywhere in nature. They're common in processed foods like cookies, crackers, and potato chips, and are used to make margarine and other fake forms of butter. Ingesting industrial trans fats can double your risk of heart disease by raising your LDL cholesterol *and* depleting good HDL cholesterol. Want to hear the understatement of the century? Trans fats do not make you healthier—so throw away your margarine right now. (It's really bad for you, it tastes funky, and we're about to tell you why you *should* be eating real butter anyway.) We're serious. Go throw it out. We'll wait.

RAINBOWS, PONIES, AND SUNSHINE: MONOUNSATURATED FATS

Monounsaturated fatty acids (MUFAs), are the most popular fats in town. Their health-promoting properties are generally agreed upon, and we, your primary-care physician, the government, *and* "that doctor on TV" all believe that a diet rich in heart-healthy MUFAs do, in fact, make you healthier. (That and refined-grains-are-bad-for-you may be the *only* thing we all agree on, but we can live with that.)

Monounsaturated fats are found in a variety of plant foods and oils as well as in animal products. Studies show that eating a diet rich in MUFAs improves blood pressure and cholesterol levels, thus reducing the risk of cardiovascular disease. Research also shows that replacing other forms of fat with MUFAs may benefit insulin and blood sugar levels, which can be especially helpful if you are insulin resistant or type 2 diabetic. In addition, other compounds in foods containing high levels of monounsaturated fats (such as olive oil) may have an anti-inflammatory effect in the body, helping to keep systemic inflammation in check.

Good Sources of Monounsaturated Fats

Avocado	Macadamia nuts
Avocado Oil	Olive Oil
Hazelnuts	Olives

Avocado and guacamole are great MUFA-rich complements to a meal, and black or green olives are an often-overlooked portable source of healthy fats.

Cold-pressed (unrefined) avocado oil and extra-virgin olive oil are decent choices for cooking—not your best options, but certainly better than the seed oils you evicted from your pantry a few chapters back. The higher levels of saturated and monounsaturated fats in these oils will help protect the oil from oxidation, as will the naturally occurring antioxidants. (You may lose some healthy antioxidants in the cooking process, but if you keep the heat low and the time in the pan short, the downsides are minimal.) In addition, olive oil or any of the other MUFA-rich oils (like avocado or macadamia oil) are the perfect base for salad dressings and uncooked sauces.

If you're looking for something crunchy, macadamia and hazelnuts are the healthiest of the nuts and seeds, for reasons we'll talk about soon. Reach for these (raw or dry-roasted) when you need to add texture to a recipe or need something to grab on the go.

LIONS AND TIGERS AND SATURATED FATS, OH MY!

The next category of fats that encourage optimal health are saturated fatty acids (SFAs). Yes, you heard us right! Wrap your heads around it, folks, because this information is here to stay.

The saturated fats found in real food make you healthier.

As you'll learn in this section, saturated fat from high-quality, real-food sources is not evil incarnate—it's just misunderstood. So let's do some saturated-fat myth-busting, shall we? Don't worry, we'll start you off easy.

Sat-Fat Myth #1: Fast-food hamburgers are unhealthy because they contain so much saturated fat.

There are a *lot* of reasons that fast-food burgers are unhealthy, but it's not fair to blame the saturated fat content. We've already mentioned some of the toxic tagalongs in the fat found in industrially-produced meat, seafood, and eggs. That's not the fault of saturated fat—that's a direct result of how the animals were raised and the food they were fed. (You don't find the same unhealthy hitchhikers in grass-fed, organic burgers.) Furthermore, the industrial seed oils in which those fast-food burgers are fried contribute in a significant way to their unhealthiness.

So, yes, those fast-food burgers aren't very healthy, and it *is* because of the fat. But don't blame the saturated fat—blame the manner in which the meat was *sourced* and *prepared*. (And the gluten in the bun, and the high-fructose corn syrup in the condiments, and the monster dose of added sodium.)

Sat-Fat Myth #2: Meat = saturated fat.

As we've already explained, all foods are a complex blend of nutrients—and meat is no exception. Don't fall into the trap of food reductionism: "I don't eat red meat because it's saturated fat." In fact, animal products like tallow (beef fat) and lard (pig fat) probably contain a smaller percentage of saturated fat than you may have imagined—less than 50 percent. Even butter, which is often considered synonymous with "saturated fat," is less than two-thirds SFA! (The rest of butter is almost entirely heart-healthy monounsaturated fat, by the way.)

We like butter.

So should you.

But we digress. Point is, let's not unfairly oversimplify our fat sources—even animal fats.

Sat-Fat Myth #3: Saturated fat is artery-clogging.

This is the big one, folks. The big myth. The big lie. And we're about to expose it.

Keep an open mind, OK?

We've all heard the one about how saturated fat causes heart attacks and strokes. In fact, saturated fat is often described as "artery clogging!" But while the logic may *seem* sound (eating fat fills your arteries with fat), *the facts don't add up.*

In 2010, the *Journal of Clinical Nutrition* compiled a landmark meta-analysis of the results of 21 studies that followed more than 347,000 total participants for up to 23 years. The studies tracked dietary habits, including intake of saturated fat and the participants' incidence of heart attack and stroke. The meta-analysis found: "*There is no significant evidence for concluding that dietary saturated fat is associated with an increased risk of coronary heart disease, stroke, or cardiovascular disease.*"

Got it? This massive study-of-studies published by a highly respected scientific organization concluded that saturated fat and cholesterol do not cause heart disease or stroke.

Does that surprise you?

We thought it might.

So if saturated fat is not, in fact, "artery clogging," what is at the root of lifestyle-related diseases and conditions like heart disease and stroke? Take one guess.

Systemic inflammation.

Researchers have determined that low-grade inflammation is involved in the pathogenesis (and your risk) of many lifestyle-related diseases and conditions, such as coronary heart disease, obesity, and diabetes. (Revisit the diagram back in Chapter 7, with inflammation smack in the middle.)

Ready for a summary of what we've learned?

You don't have to be afraid of saturated fat.

LEAN MEATS Remember, we recommend eating lean cuts and trimming or draining visible fat if the meat comes from the factory-farming system *not* because of the saturated fat content, or because the fat in meat is "artery clogging." It's the *potentially toxic contaminants* inherent in the factory-farming system that we'd very much like you to avoid.

Here's the kicker, however.

Not all the saturated fat in your body starts out that way. It may not even come from fat in your diet at all. This is where we get into the myth that turns out to be true—only not in the way you think.

Was that confusing enough or what?*

Sat-Fat Myth #4: Saturated fat promotes insulin resistance and inflammation.

True.

Some forms of saturated fat (particularly the "long chain" versions) do contribute to insulin resistance and, by extension, inflammation in the body, which does increase your risk for cardiovascular disease and stroke. Palmitic acid (PA) in particular is the type of saturated fat most correlated with insulin resistance and inflammation.

But the form of saturated fat that gets all kinds of ugly in your body doesn't come from *eating saturated fat.*

The harmful kind of saturated fat comes from eating too many refined carbohydrates.

Stay with us.

Decades ago, research correlated saturated fat levels—particularly palmitic acid levels—with cardiovascular disease. (The more saturated fat people had in their bodies, the more likely they were to have a heart attack.)

As a result of that research, we were all told not to eat saturated fat because it would lead to heart attack or stroke. We were particularly warned against red meat and eggs, as they happen to be higher in saturated fat than other foods are. The premise was simple: Meat and eggs have lots of saturated fat. Saturated fat is associated with heart disease. Therefore, avoid meat and eggs.

But those recommendations were based on faulty logic.

Let's break this down, point by point.

Point #1: Identifying high levels of saturated fat, specifically palmitic acid, in folks who had cardiovascular disease does not mean that saturated fat *caused* the problems. (It's the old ice cream–shark attack correlation.)

Note, this next section presents some of the most technical material in the book. If you're up for a challenge, dive in. If not, we'll summarize the findings at the end, so you won't miss anything.

Point #2: It's impossible to eat palmitic acid all by itself. There isn't a single food out there—not even palm oil!—that contains *only* PA. Meat and eggs are high in palmitic acid, sure, but they also contain significant amounts of other fats, like oleic acid (a monounsaturated fat).

Point #3: Other fats, like oleic acid, have been found to prevent palmitic acid from inducing insulin resistance.

So what does this all mean?

Eating whole foods that *contain* PA is not the same as eating *just* PA.

Real food (like meat and eggs) contains other fats that help protect your body from too much PA. So there's basically no way to get a lot of PA into your body all by itself.

Unless …

You eat too much refined carbohydrate.

PLAN B All the way back in Chapter 5, we mentioned your body's Plan B for storing energy when the liver and muscle glycogen stores are full. In the case of full glycogen stores, the liver then turns the glucose into fat—specifically, a form of saturated fat called palmitic acid (!)—which *could* be used for energy, but is more likely (because you're a sugar-burner and not fat-adapted) to promote elevated triglycerides, leptin resistance and insulin resistance, and to be added to your fat stores.

So, when you eat too much carbohydrate, it's converted directly into PA by your liver. In which case, you *would* have a lot of PA in your system without the other protective fats—and you would have a rather large amount of saturated fat in the body *that didn't start out that way.*

And that's the behavior that *really* gives you heart disease.

**Eating whole, unprocessed foods with a rich
complement of fat and other nutrients is *not* unhealthy.
Overeating refined carbohydrates *is*.**

And it's overconsumption of refined carbohydrates that contributes to the increased "bad" cholesterol and triglycerides that are some of the risk factors for cardiovascular disease.

It's not the saturated fat in red meat or eggs at all.

EAT THESE ANIMAL FATS

So now that we've dispelled the major myths associated with SFA intake, let's talk about which foods contain these healthy saturated fats. (Say it with us: "healthy saturated fats"—the idea is quite liberating, isn't it?)

Most people think of animal products first when talking about saturated fats, so we'll start there. (But remember, even animal products like tallow, lard, and butter aren't *just* saturated fat—most are also rich sources of MUFA.)

Good Sources of Animal Fats

Clarified butter	Goat fat
Duck fat	Lard (pig fat)
Ghee	Tallow (beef fat)

Saturated fats are your healthiest choice for cooking, especially at high temperature. Saturated fats are very stable when exposed to air, heat, and light, which makes them ideal for sautéing, pan-frying, broiling, or roasting.

Another form of animal fat comes from dairy—butter. Remember, the issues we have with dairy come from its carbohydrate and protein, not its fat. In fact, we think there are some really healthy compounds in pastured, organic butter, like higher amounts of anti-inflammatory omega-3 fatty acids, CLA (conjugated linoleic acid), vitamin E, and carotenoids.

But we have one stipulation when it comes to butter—that it be *clarified*. See, butter isn't just fat. (We're like a broken record with this "food is complicated" stuff, huh?) Butter is only about 80 percent fat; the rest is water and milk solids (proteins). Those milk proteins are a butter deal-breaker in our eyes, as even tiny amounts can be disruptive to the gut if you're sensitive to dairy or have any degree of intestinal permeability.

The good news is that there's a way to remove those milk proteins: clarifying your butter.* It's a simple process by which you melt the butter at low temperature, so the fat and milk solids separate. You then filter out the

---

You can find instructions to clarify your own butter on our Web site: http://whole9life.com/butter. You can also buy richly flavored clarified butter (also known as "ghee") prepackaged in many health-food or international-food shops. We recommend Pure Indian Foods (http://pureindianfoods.com).

milk solids, leaving you with nothing but the gloriously rich, bright yellow butterfat.

Perfection.

And so much tastier than the plastic (we mean margarine) spread you used to eat.

COOKING FAT Your animal fats must be of the highest quality— grass-fed, pastured, *and* organic. Remember, the fat in factory-farmed meats is loaded with unhealthy toxins—residues from antibiotics, hormones, heavy metals, and pesticides. So the last thing you want to do is save your factory-farmed bacon fat and *cook the rest of your food in it.* Make sure you're buying or rendering your animal fats only from 100 percent grass-fed, pastured, organic sources to ensure that the rest of your food is cooked in the "cleanest" fat possible.

COCONUT: THE OTHER WHITE MEAT

There is another fantastic form of saturated fat that doesn't come from an animal—so you won't have the same concerns about sourcing. It's found in coconut and coconut products.

Coconut contains a large proportion (about 66 percent) of a very healthy form of saturated fat called "medium-chain triglycerides" (MCTs).* These MCTs have some very unique properties and are very beneficial to the body.

First, remember how we said fat is an excellent energy source? Well, these MCTs are shorter-chain fats, meaning that they are more rapidly absorbed and metabolized than their longer-chain counterparts. This means that the MCTs found in coconut products are more likely to be burned as fuel by your muscles and organs, instead of being stored as fat.

Sweet.

Studies also suggest that MCTs may help prevent atherosclerosis and cardiovascular disease, in part by reducing cholesterol levels and by imparting a slight blood-glucose-lowering effect.

Unrefined red palm oil also contains these MCTs. Palm oil has a pretty strong flavor, however, and most people don't like it as much as coconut oil.

Finally, MCTs are unique in that they do not require bile (which is made in the liver and stored in the gallbladder) for digestion. This makes them a fantastic fat source if you have impaired liver function, digestive malabsorption conditions, or have had your gallbladder removed.

Good Sources of MCTs

Coconut oil	Coconut milk (canned)
Coconut butter/manna	Coconut (meat or flakes)

Unrefined coconut oil is ideal for cooking, and most varieties don't transmit a strong coconut flavor to your food. Coconut milk (the concentrated form in a can, not the sweetened stuff in a milk-like carton) is a great substitute for milk or cream in recipes, and can be used in everything from soups and curries to "creamed" versions of your favorite vegetables. Coconut butter is a delicious snack straight from the jar, and coconut flakes or shreds can be used to coat meat or seafood for a delicious oven-baked crunch (or eaten straight from the bag as a portable source of fat).

CAUTION REQUIRED: POLYUNSATURATED FATS

The last category of fats we'll discuss are the polyunsaturated fatty acids (PUFAs). There are many different types of PUFAs, but we're going to focus on omega-3 and omega-6 fatty acids. We've already talked about these guys in reference to seed oils, but let's review:

- The omega-3 fatty acids EPA and DHA are anti-inflammatory in nature.
- More omega-6 than omega-3 promotes inflammation.
- Too much PUFA (omega-3 and omega-6) in the diet makes your cells more vulnerable to oxidation—which predisposes you to inflammation.

So you want some omega-3 in your diet to help reduce inflammation, but you don't want too much of *either* omega-3 or omega-6, lest that lead to more inflammation. It's tricky, we'll give you that—but we've got it all worked out for you in just two steps.

1. Significantly decrease the amount of omega-6 and total PUFA in your diet.
2. Eat some naturally occurring omega-3—not too much, but enough to provide some anti-inflammatory benefits.

We've already made huge inroads on that first step by eliminating all seed oils. Now, let's talk about another whole-food source of PUFAs that, if consumed in excess, could provide too much omega-6 and total PUFA in the diet: nuts and seeds.

Nuts and seeds contain a varying amount of polyunsaturated fats—anywhere from 2 percent (macadamia nuts) all the way up to 72 percent (walnuts). But please note, there is a significant difference between eating raw, minimally processed nuts and seeds and highly refined seed *oils*. Raw nuts and seeds contain a wide range of micronutrients, many of which act as antioxidants. So as long as the nuts and seeds have not been extensively heated or refined, these antioxidants should help to prevent oxidation before consumption. In addition, unlike refined seed oils, nuts and seeds contain a wide variety of health-promoting micronutrients, which studies show may work together to improve your cholesterol profile and reduce inflammation.

Of course, *some* nuts and seeds in the diet may be good, but *more* is not better. We still want to be careful not to incorporate too many of these fragile PUFAs into our cell walls, whether from whole-food sources or not.

Nuts and Seeds (and Their Corresponding Nut Butters)

Best Choices	In Moderation	Limit
Cashews	Almonds	Flax Seeds
Hazelnuts	Brazil Nuts	Pine Nuts
Macadamias	Pecans	Pumpkin Seeds
	Pistachios	Sesame Seeds
		Sunflower Seeds
		Walnuts

Let's start with your best choices—cashews, hazelnuts, and macadamias. These nuts are rich in MUFA and contain very small amounts of PUFA per serving. Nuts and seeds in the middle column have enough PUFA to be of concern, and we'd suggest eating these in moderation (no more than a few times a week).

Finally, you've got your lowest-tier nuts and seeds—the ones we'd recommend you limit in your healthy-fat rotation. More than half the fat in them comes from PUFAs, and therefore they should be eaten only occasionally, or treated like a condiment, sprinkled on salads, vegetables, or main dishes.

OMEGA-3 TECHNICALITIES

You've probably heard that flax, walnuts, chia, and hemp are good sources of omega-3 fatty acids—so why do we say they should be consumed only occasionally? The omega-3s in these sources are in a form called alpha-linolenic acid (ALA)—not the anti-inflammatory stuff (EPA and DHA). Your body *can* convert ALA to EPA and DHA, but the process is long, and can be impeded by a variety of dietary and lifestyle factors. Even if everything worked perfectly, the amount of EPA and DHA you'd get at the end is so small that it practically doesn't count. And remember, these foods all give you a *serious* dose of PUFA and omega-6 fatty acids! Getting a lot of PUFA and omega-6, and just a *tiny* amount of anti-inflammatory EPA and DHA is not a good tradeoff in our books. (We also could have just said, "Studies show that supplementation of omega-3 fatty acids from vegetable sources like flax don't decrease inflammation." That might have been simpler.)

One last thought on nuts, seeds, and especially their corresponding nut butters. Much like the natural sweetness of fruit may promote an unhealthy psychological response (and *potentially* violate our first Good Food standard), the natural fats, added salt, and perhaps added sugar found in nuts and nut butters can have the same effect.

In plain speech, people find them all too easy to overconsume.

Now, if you were to sit in front of the television and mindlessly eat a whole bag of carrots—no harm, no foul. We certainly don't encourage that kind of "auto-pilot consumption," but even an entire bag of carrots isn't going to send your metabolism spiraling out of control.

Swap those carrots for half a jar of sunflower seed butter (or almonds, or macadamia nuts), however, and we've got a serious problem. Nuts and seeds pack a far greater caloric punch than carrots, and you may just find yourself consuming almost an entire day's worth of calories before you know it. Really. Half a jar of sunflower seed butter has 1,400 calories—and a whole lot of PUFA and omega-6 to boot.

So there are a few reasons that nuts and seeds should be near the bottom of your list of healthy fat sources. They are certainly not *unhealthy*— but for the several reasons we've outlined, they're not the *most* healthy of your healthy choices. Reach for these occasionally when adding fat to meals, but choose other fats (like avocado, olives, and coconut) more often.

HEALTHY OMEGA-3 So where should you get your omega-3s? From animals raised in their natural environment and fed their natural diets. Omega-3s are found in green leaves and algae—the food that our food is supposed to eat. (Of course, we can't digest grasses—otherwise, we'd just eat them ourselves!) When grass-fed beef, pastured chicken, or wild salmon get healthy omega-3s in their diets, we get healthy EPA and DHA in ours when we eat their meat. Of course, factory-farmed animals aren't fed their natural diets, which means *they* don't get enough omega-3s, which means there isn't much EPA and DHA in their meat. So improving the quality of our meat, seafood, and eggs means we're also improving our intake of healthy omega-3 fatty acids.

FOOD QUALITY: THE FINAL WORD

Before we wrap up this section, we want to make three very important points about food quality.

Focus on meat, seafood, and eggs first.

If you can focus on the sourcing of only *one* item on your plate, we think you're better off improving the quality of your animal protein sources first—even before thinking about organic vegetables, fruits, and fats. We believe that the health of the animal has a significant effect on your health. And while we're certainly not encouraging you to ingest pesticides, in our opinion the potential downsides of industrially-raised meat, seafood, and eggs are far more harmful than the residues left on produce.

Conventional vegetables and fruit are better than no vegetables and fruits.

The potential downsides of pesticide residues don't outweigh the major health benefits from consuming vegetables and fruits. We'll reiterate: Making Good Food *choices* is the most important factor in your healthy-eating transformation. Focusing on food *sourcing* comes second, so think about it when you're able. If you can't wrap your head around organic, can't afford organic, or can't find organic in your community, that's OK. Just eat your greens!

Do the best you can with what you've got.

Thinking about how to improve the quality of your food can send you down the rabbit hole pretty darn fast. The more you learn about where your food comes from and the wide variety of health effects related to farming practices, the easier it is to become confused or disheartened. The last thing we want is for you to become so overwhelmed by all of these new concepts that you become paralyzed in your food decisions.

So, please—*don't stress about your food!* You can't ask for the full biography of every animal or plant you eat, so if the waiter says it's wild-caught or the label says "pesticide free," you have to trust that information and make the best decision you can. It's that simple—we promise.

LET'S EAT!

Congratulations! Not only have you survived the science-y stuff and our "less-healthy" information, but you've learned everything you'll need to know about choosing foods that make you healthier. So what's left? The best part—eating! Now that you've got all your foods in line, it's time to figure out how to put them all together into actual honest-to-goodness meals.

Hungry? So are we!

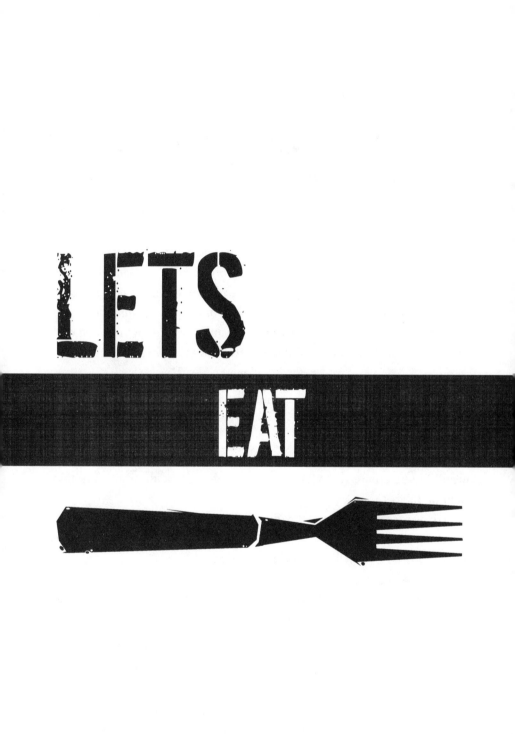

CHAPTER 16:
MEAL PLANNING MADE EASY

"I had almost every diet-related disease—breast cancer, type 2 diabetes, high blood pressure, and high cholesterol. I was also about seventy pounds overweight and almost completely sedentary. Since I started the Whole30 I have lost twenty-four pounds. I am completely off my diabetes medication and my high blood pressure medication. I had a checkup with my oncologist today, and he asked me what I was doing to look so much better. I told him about the Whole30, and he said it was wonderful that I was eating real food and doing it for health, not just to lose weight. He told me to keep it up!"
—Beth T., Richmond, Texas

It's time to put all your Good Food smarts to work building healthy meals. But before we get to the details, we're going to address one question right off the bat.

No, we are not going to tell you exactly how much to eat.

We won't give you calories, grams, ounces, blocks, or points, because you don't need us to tell you how much to eat.

Know why?

Because you've got built-in hormonal regulatory mechanisms designed to do just that. Put simply:

Your body knows how much you should be eating way better than any calculator you can find on the Internet.

The trouble is, your body's signals may have historically been *very* unreliable. Because of the foods you've been eating, and the resulting overconsumption and hormonal dysregulation, you've been getting mixed messages. Your body has been telling you to eat when you're full, that you're hungry when you're not, and sending you unsolicited cravings for foods you know don't make you healthier. And because of your metabolic status, you've never been able to trust the signals your body has been sending you. Until now.

Because when you make consistently good food choices, you can *rely* on your body to tell you what you need. Leptin's message (eat more, eat less) actually *registers* in the brain. Insulin's message (store energy) is nicely balanced by glucagon's message (release some energy). Your blood sugar levels stay within a nice, normal range, neither spiraling you into hyperactivity, nor plummeting you into crashes and cravings. And your brain is finally at peace, so you can drive right on past the bakery without blinking an eye.

Once you've been making good food choices for a while, you'll *finally* be able to trust what your body is saying. And no snazzy mathematic calculations based on your height, weight, body fat, and activity levels could possibly compete with the awesomeness of the human body.

THE MATH WORKS

We ran our meal-planning template past some really smart folks and a large test population before we unleashed it on the public. We were fortunate enough to meet one of those smart folks, Michael Hasz, MD (a spinal surgeon and longtime advocate of a Paleo diet), at one of our nutrition workshops a few years ago. He evaluated our template and ran the math for us from his perspective. As someone who has been prescribing this way of eating to his patients for ten years, his opinion carried a lot of weight. Dr. Hasz said: "While it's obviously important to have excellent food quality, you also have to be in the right neighborhood with macronutrients. I tore your meal-planning template apart, put it back together, and did all the math, and realized you have a really well organized plan. You put thought into your recommendations and your meal-planning template, and you got it right." So, you know ... just tooting our own horn a little. And making sure you know we didn't just pull this stuff out of a hat.

In addition, you won't be weighing, measuring, or tracking your calories at all. We think those are all unnatural, unsustainable, psychologically unhealthy processes that take the joy out of food and eating. Eating is an organic, natural, intrinsic behavior that we were all blessed with at birth.

Digital scales, spreadsheets, and calorie monitors have no place in our new, healthy relationship with food.

Having said that, we're not going to let you fly blind.

We'll give you some general estimates as to how much, and how often, you should be eating. But let the record reflect that our "how much" and "how often" recommendations are just a *starting point*. It's up to you to pay attention to the cues your body is giving you—hunger, energy, sleep quality, mental acuity, performance in the gym or in your sport—to tweak our plan until it's just right for you.

We can't do that for you.

Tough-love point #1:

This does require effort on your part.

You have to make sure you're eating enough, that your nutrients are plentiful, and that you're getting enough protein, fat, and carbohydrates. You'll have to figure out what to eat for lunch, how to order at a restaurant, and how often you'll need to go grocery shopping. You must teach yourself how to read labels, stay on course when you're on the road, and cope when you run into old cravings and compulsions.

We'll give you all the tools, guidelines, and resources you'll need, but the rest is up to *you*. Because getting healthy doesn't happen just because you're taking a pass on bread.

GOOD FOOD REQUIRED   In addition, this meal-planning template will work only under the condition that you are filling it with the kind of Good Food we've been talking about. We did not design our template to work with less-healthy foods: you cannot meal-template your way to optimal health if you're still eating sandwiches, pasta, and microwave dinners!

Now that we've got that out of the way, let's start with what your typical day should look like.

YOU + FOOD (THE BIG PICTURE)

- Eat meals at the table, in a relaxed fashion.
- Do not allow distractions like TV, phone, or email during mealtime.
- Chew slowly and thoroughly; don't gulp.

The first thing we want to talk about isn't how much, how often, or how many. It's just *how*. Health initiatives work only when people success-fully and sustainably change their habits. And a major focus of our healthy-eating program is changing your deeply personal relationship with food—breaking old habits and patterns and creating new associations with food and eating.

Changing those habits starts at mealtime.

Start thinking of eating as a *nourishing experience*. Don't fall victim to reductionism—our meals are not just fuel, calories, or nutrients. Our meals are so much more than just the sum of their ingredients! Our meals are our culture—the things our parents taught us and their parents taught them. They are memories and emotions, reminding us of other meals and other experiences we have shared with those we love. Mealtime is about building new traditions within our own kitchens, with our own families—and setting a good example for future generations.

But when you eat meals in your car, inhale lunch at your desk, or mind-lessly shovel in dinner while watching TV, well, you're not really fostering a relationship with your food at all. There is no cultural significance, you recall no fond memories, and you create no traditions—unless you count passing your negotiating-rush-hour-traffic-while-eating-a-Big-Mac skill down to your kids a tradition.

And the manner in which we eat our food—hurriedly, automatically, without presence of mind or consideration—plays a large role in creating our psychological and hormonal issues with food.

We don't just want you to change the food on your plate—we want you to change the way you eat it, too.

That starts with creating new mealtime habits.

First, eat as many meals as possible at the table, in as relaxed a fashion as time and company will allow. Establish a healthy-eating routine that al-lows you to appreciate your Good Food, savoring the experience. Be pres-ent, if only for a few minutes. We know most folks usually can't spend an hour at every meal, but just because your schedule is tight doesn't mean you can't relax for fifteen minutes and devote your time, energy, and senses to your food. (And for the record, your office desk is *not* a table. Take a break from the stress of work and enjoy your meal elsewhere.)

Eating slowly and in a relaxed fashion not only assists with digestion but also helps us take a much-needed break from the stressful pace of our normal lives. Tough-love point #2:

You are not *that* busy.

We know you *think* you are so busy that you can't spare fifteen minutes to sit down at the table and eat, but that is not true. You just choose to spend your time elsewhere. There is a difference.

When you do sit down to eat, do so without electronic distractions. Don't sell your experience short by eating while watching TV, sending email, or managing your calendar. If you took the time to prepare a healthy meal for yourself (and, perhaps, your family), give it the respect it deserves when it comes time to eat it. Appreciate your hard work and the final product.

If possible, share your meal with others. Conversation around a meal does not serve to distract, but rather enhances your experience. Remember, reward, memory, and emotion pathways in the brain are all interconnected. The same series of biochemical events that connected you to that downtown-bakery cookie could be used to reinforce your love and appreciation of healthy, home-cooked meals shared with the ones you love.

Taking time with your meal also means chewing your food carefully. Wolfing down food not only harms digestion because it arrives in your stomach without being properly broken down, but it doesn't give your satiety hormones a chance to send their signals, either. As you eat, receptors in the stomach are activated as it fills with food or liquid. These receptors communicate your level of fullness to the brain through various hormones (including leptin). But these signals take time to start to register in the brain—at least ten minutes. By eating too quickly, you're not giving your hormones enough time to do their job—so you eat more than you should because your brain doesn't yet know you should stop.

Now, if you're reading all this while shaking your head and saying, "In your dreams, Hartwigs," we get it. Lest you think we're envisioning some fairy tale where we all have hours upon hours every day to eat, drink, and be merry with our friends and loved ones, rest assured, we are firmly in the grip of reality. We're just asking you to make some effort here, keeping in mind our ultimate end goal: helping you change your dietary habits, and permanently instilling a new, healthy, lifelong relationship with food and eating. Your behaviors around mealtime will play a part in that change. So, please, try to meet us halfway.

And if you still feel as if this is all hippie-foodie-kumbaya mumbo jumbo, don't worry—we suppose you can still eat Good Food while driving and listening to your voicemail.

But you really should chew.

Now, on to the specifics.

DAILY GUIDELINES

- Eat three meals a day.
- Start with breakfast.
- Don't snack, if you can help it.
- Stop eating a few hours before bedtime.

First, there's nothing magical about three meals, but the concept generally works quite well from a hormonal and social perpsective. First, having a four- to five-hour break between meals gives glucagon time to do its job and mobilize some energy and keeps leptin levels normalized. In addition, most people tend to organize their work and social lives around three meals a day. Of course, if you work exceptionally long days, or have an especially active metabolism, you may end up needing four meals a day. That's OK—just make sure you allow a good chunk of time between meals to encourage the optimal hormonal response.

REDEFINING BREAKFAST

We will immediately encourage you to stop thinking about meals in traditional terms like breakfast, lunch, and dinner We just call them Meal 1, Meal 2, and Meal 3. You'll find much more freedom in building your meals around what you feel like eating, what is available at the grocery store or farmers' market, or what happens to be in your refrigerator. Plus, it will keep you from eating nothing but eggs at Meal 1. That gets boring.

As for Meal 1, don't put it off for too long, even if you're not hungry. If you're not hungry first thing in the morning, that tells us that your hormones are off. And one of the best ways to get those hormones back in line is to eat something in the morning, when it's biologically appropriate.

Ideally, eat Meal 1 within an hour of waking. It doesn't matter whether you wake at 6 a.m. for your day job or 3 p.m. for shift work—wake, then eat.* This is important.

Remember, leptin has a daily rhythm tied to your eating schedule. Which means that if you start eating too late in the day, your entire leptin pattern can be thrown off. Which means that at night, when leptin should be high, it won't be. And cortisol, correlated with leptin dysfunction, will tend to make you crave more food. Usually not the good kind, either. Which means that you'll be prowling through your pantry or freezer after dinner looking for a snack. Which leads to more hormonal disruption.

So, wake up and eat Meal 1 pretty soon afterward.

THE COFFEE CONNECTION

Our healthy eating plan can include a cup or two of coffee in the morning, with a few caveats. One, your coffee pot is not a cup. Two, if you *need* that cup of coffee first thing, it means that cortisol levels are not as healthy as they should be. Too much coffee is going to make that worse, so keep your intake down. Make sure to always drink your coffee before noon, so the caffeine doesn't interfere with sleep: do not underestimate caffeine's impact on this. And caffeine is a potent appetite suppressant, so if you're one of those people who just isn't hungry in the morning, here's your rule: You must eat Meal 1 *before* you get to enjoy your coffee. It's for your own good.

In our experience, a good Meal 1 focused on satisfying protein and fat and nutrient-dense veggies (and *not* overloaded with fruit) sets you up for less hunger, more consistent energy levels, and fewer sugar cravings, which makes it easier to make good food choices throughout your day. We're not saying you can't include *some* fruit with your first meal, but just don't make it the star of the show.

Now, each meal should be designed to hold you over until the next, eliminating your desire or need to snack. And as you become fat-adapted (a process that starts in just a few days, but can take weeks to really kick

---

If you exercise shortly after waking, your schedule will look a little different. We'll cover additional recommendations for fueling higher activity levels in Chapter 21.

in to the point that you notice the effects), your body will begin to utilize fat as fuel more readily, helping you avoid between-meal cravings, energy slumps, and brain fog.

SNACK ATTACK In general, avoid snacking between meals because it turns your eating habits into grazing, and grazing can disrupt the normal functioning of leptin, insulin, and glucagon, and may promote inadvertent overconsumption. It may take you a while to figure out the right-size meals, though, so if you find that you didn't eat enough at any given meal and need more nourishment, then we'd rather you have a snack than spend hours being cranky, tired, and hungry. Make sure your snacks are just smaller meals, and include both protein and fat—don't snack on veggies or fruit alone, as they're not very satiating all by themselves.

Finally, make your last meal the end of your daily eating cycle. If you've been doing everything right, satiety hormones *should* be at their peak in the evening, which means dinner should leave you feeling satisfied right up until bedtime. But if you're still in that transition period, or your dessert habits are firmly imprinted in your reward, pleasure, and emotion pathways, avoid the cravings as if your health depends on it.

Because it kind of does.

Eating before bed not only messes with leptin levels, but it can impede growth hormone release, which is critical for tissue regeneration and growth and repair of many cells in the body. And if that snack is sugary or rich in refined carbs, it also pushes insulin levels up, which may lead to a blood sugar crash in the middle of the night. This affects melatonin secretion, which governs our sleep patterns, and means you could wake up hungry at 2 a.m., unable to get back to sleep.

Your mom was right. Don't eat before bed.

BUILD YOUR PLATE: PROTEIN

- Create each meal around your protein source.
- Each meal should include one to two palm-size servings of protein.
- As often as possible, choose high-quality meat, seafood, and eggs.

We build each meal around protein in part because that's how we gro-cery shop, prioritizing high-quality protein sources in our budget. But there are more science-y reasons for building each meal around your high-quality animal protein source.

First, as we've learned, protein is highly satiating and helps us *stay* full until our next meal. In addition, making protein the main event ensures that we'll get enough protein over the course of our day. This is critical when you're eating only three times a day. Skipping protein at one meal means you'll have to overload at your other meals to keep intake adequate, which can be difficult. Finally, eating protein with each and every meal helps to stabilize blood sugar levels (via glucagon) in the absence of large amounts of insulin-promoting foods.

Which, of course, you don't eat anymore. Good for you!

Now, we know you have questions about this, because "palm-size" is still too general for most people. So we'll give you some additional guide-lines, but also caution you not to get too caught up in analyzing your por-tions. The *exact* portion size doesn't really matter, because you'll be adjust-ing it based on the signals your body sends you.

The bulk (thickest part) of your protein source should be roughly the same size as the palm of your hand. If you've got some thinner parts hang-ing over (like with salmon, or a chicken breast), don't sweat it.

For whole eggs, a meal-size portion is the number of eggs you can hold in one hand. This is usually between three and five. (If Dallas is *very* hungry, he can hold six.) And to all of you ladies who would respond to our breakfast inquiry by demurely responding, "Oh, I had my egg this morning," we have one thing to say.

We don't care how petite you are, we *know* you can hold more than one egg.

Adequate protein is the key to this whole plan. And if there's one meal at which you can afford to overindulge, it's breakfast. So err on the side of generous, please. Also, yes, you're eating the whole egg. We've already talked about this. Plus, half the protein is in the yolk, so it's darn hard to get enough protein if you're eating only the whites.

For deli meat, stack slices to approximately the thickness of your palm. For oddly-shaped protein (tuna fish, shrimp, scallops, etc.) simply do your best to estimate a palm-size portion. Again, don't sweat the exact portion size. We don't want to see anyone playing shrimp-Tetris on his palm. That is wholly unnecessary, and kind of gross.

Now, our guidelines say "one to two palm-size servings." So how do you know whether you're a one-palm or two-palm kind of person? Go by your *size* and your *activity levels*.

If you're big, try two palms. If you're small, try one palm. (If you don't know whether you're big or small, we can't help you.)

If you're very active, either with your job (construction worker, landscaper, firefighter) or with your sport or exercise routine, try two palms. If you're less active, try one palm.

Also, for the record, these are not your only options. You've also got 1.25 palms, 1.5 palms, 1.942 palms, and every possibility in between.

This should not be overwhelming. You all have palms. Choose your protein, look at your meat, look at your palm, call it good.

TOO MUCH PROTEIN?

Some of you may be thinking, "Is this much protein bad for my kidneys?" The answer is no—for three reasons. First, as long as your kidneys are functioning normally, even a high level of dietary protein (25 percent of total calories) won't cause problems. Studies show that your kidneys can easily adapt to accommodate the elimination of the waste products from protein metabolism—and that adaptation is not at all harmful. Second, our plan isn't to turn you into a carnivore. Our recommended protein portions are just right—enough to support activity levels, recovery, and build muscle mass but not excessive by any means. Third, even if we *did* recommend stuffing your face with meat at every meal, you probably wouldn't be able to. Remember, dense protein sources (from real food) are satiating, which means they're *really* hard to overeat. Processed protein shakes and other forms of "liquid food," however, are another matter. Bodybuilders use those to gain weight, since you can chug large amounts of liquid protein faster than your brain can register that you're full. But we're not bodybuilders trying to gain weight at all costs, are we?

BUILD YOUR PLATE: VEGETABLES

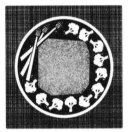

- Fill the rest of your plate with vegetables.

Um, that's it. We could pretty much end this section right here. Put your protein on the plate, and fill the rest with vegetables. How easy is that?

Of course, you have some questions.

First, we do mean *fill* your plate. Because seven leaves of spinach don't really provide you with the carbohydrate or the micronutrients you need to be healthy. And don't try arranging the meat on your plate so it takes up as much space as possible, either. (What are you, twelve?) Don't worry, by the time we're done, you'll like certain vegetables so much that you'll gladly make room for them. Really.

That having been said, we're not the Veggie Police, insisting that you eat your weight in leafy greens every day. And we also know that some days you won't even *have* a plate—like if you're eating a bowl of curry or stew, in which the veggies are already mixed right into the meal. We're just encouraging you to do your best to eat a healthy amount of vegetables with each of your three meals. That's all—just do your best.

To help with variety, we like to include at least two vegetables with each meal—sometimes more. An entire plate full of green beans can feel pretty boring, and including a variety of veggies per meal helps to maximize nutrients too.

SPICE IT UP! This is one area where you'll benefit tremendously from keeping a large assortment of herbs and spices on hand. You can change the flavor of a dish in a snap, just by varying your seasonings. (We'll give you plenty of examples in our Meal Map.) Think cumin, cayenne, basil, cilantro, oregano, curry powder, garlic, and onion … even salt! Most of the salt in an unhealthy diet comes from processed foods—which we are no longer eating. So feel free to add a few shakes to your meals, alternating between iodized table salt (often the only source of valuable iodine in our diet) and sea salt. Just be sure to read your labels—you may be surprised at how many seasoning and spice mixtures add sugar, fillers, and other not-so-healthy ingredients.

Finally, there are vegetables that are both nutrient-dense and carbohydrate-dense. You don't have to be afraid of sweet potato, beets, butternut squash, acorn squash, parsnips, or pumpkin just because they contain carbohydrates. We assure you, no one ever made herself diabetic by overeating beets or pumpkin.* In fact, if you're healthy and active, you'll need to make a point of eating some of these carb-dense vegetables on a regular basis to support your activity levels.

If you're overweight and insulin resistant, you don't want to fill your whole plate with mashed sweet potato, because your metabolism isn't good at managing energy. In this case, include the more carb-dense veggies in smaller portions and fill in the rest with leafy greens or other fibrous vegetables.

---

*We don't have a scientific study to support this statement, but we're pretty sure it's true.

BUILD YOUR PLATE: FRUIT

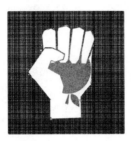

- Start with one to two servings of fruit a day.
- A serving is about the size of a fist.

Feel free to add some fruit either with your meals or immediately after. Remember, fruit should not take the place of vegetables during meals!
However, adding fruit to meals, or enjoying a sweet treat after a meal, is a
great way to take advantage of nature's nutritious sweetness.

We do have some caveats with fruit, however, going back to that healthy
psychological response and your hormones. These caveats can mostly be
described in two words:

Fruit. Smoothie.

We know that *sounds* really healthy. Unfortunately, waking up in the
morning and blending large amounts of fruit into a breakfast smoothie is
not a good idea, for a few reasons.

First, liquid foods, while convenient, don't promote the same satiety
response as eating real food. Which means your fruit smoothie isn't as satiating as the eggs, spinach, and avocado you'd have to chew and swallow. A
smoothie is likely to fill you up short-term, but leave you hungry between
meals, *especially* if you drink it all by itself. In addition, eating mostly fruit
in the morning means you'll have to make up for the missed nutrients and
calories from protein and fat in your other meals, leaving you stuffed if you
manage to jam it all in, or generally underfed if you simply can't eat that
much in one sitting.

In addition, it's better to eat smaller servings of fruit throughout the
day than a large amount in one sitting. Remember, fructose (one of the
sugars found in fruit) must be processed by your liver. Large amounts of
fruit in one sitting can put a burden on your liver, especially if you're still

working through insulin resistance or obesity. Research has shown that people who are insulin resistant and obese are more sensitive to fructose, so large amounts in one sitting is a very bad idea for that population—but that doesn't make it a great idea for the rest of us, either.

Finally, from our perspective, when clients eat a bunch of sugar first thing in the morning, they are far more likely to experience volatile energy swings, sugar cravings, and abnormal levels of hunger throughout the rest of their day. So think about Meal 1 as setting the tone for the rest of your day, both physically and psychologically. If the first thing you taste when you wake up is sugar, it may be hard to shake that taste, and any subsequent cravings. But if your first meal is a nutritious and satiating combination of protein, healthy fats, and vegetables (with perhaps a little fruit thrown in for flavor), you start your day off with steady, long-lasting energy, nutrients, and the feeling of satisfaction and fullness that comes from a complete meal.

That sounds way smarter to us too.

Now, we're not saying you can't have any fruit at breakfast. We're just saying don't drink it, and don't eat it all by itself. One of our favorite breakfast creations is an egg scramble with poached peaches, spinach, fresh basil, and chopped pecans—a dense protein, some healthy fat from the cooking oil and pecans, and just the right amount of natural sweetness from the peaches. Fruit and eggs are a surprisingly delicious combination.

Just don't forget your veggies.

Finally, as we've already mentioned, if you find yourself reaching for fruit after every single meal, satisfying those leftover cravings for dessert, you may want to stop and think. Remember, addressing your *habits* is the most important factor in making sustainable healthy eating changes—and dessert just might be one of those habits you'd be better off shaking.

SLAY THE SUGAR DRAGON

So what do you eat when you find yourself battling the sugar dragon? Anything *but* the sweet stuff. As Dallas likes to say, you can't battle the sugar dragon outright—the only way to slay it is to *starve* it. So conscientiously avoid the fruit, nut butters, Larabars or anything else that may prop up your sugar cravings. If you are legitimately hungry, reach for protein and fat, as they are both satisfying and calorie-dense enough to see you through until your next meal. And instead of reaching for fruit after a meal, try a cup of herbal tea instead. Rooibus (pronounced "ROY-boos") blends, a Hartwig favorite, are naturally decaffeinated and rich in flavor, and may just help you break your after-dinner sweet-treat habit in a way that is satisfying and healthy.

One last thing—in nature, fruit is highly seasonal, available only for short periods of time during the year. If you want to go with the seasonal flow, as Mother Nature intended, we're good with that. If you find yourself reaching for more fruit in summer, when it's local, fresh, and delicious, that's OK! Enjoy nature's deliciousness while you can. But this also means that you shouldn't eat much in the winter, when most fruit is out of season.

BUILD YOUR PLATE: HEALTHY FATS

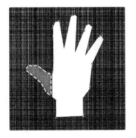 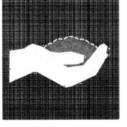 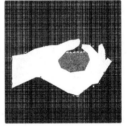

- Choose one or more fat sources per meal.
- Add fats in the following recommended quantities, per person, *per meal.*

All oils: (olive oil, coconut oil, etc.): one to two thumb-size portions.*
All butters: (coconut butter, nut butters, clarified butter, and ghee): one to two thumb-size portions.
Olives: one to two open (heaping) handfuls.
Coconut (meat/flakes): one to two open (heaping) handfuls.
Nuts and seeds: up to one closed handful.
Avocado: half to one avocado.
Coconut milk: between ¼ - ½ of a (14 oz.) can

We'll give you an actual measurement here, because "thumbs" don't always translate for those who are challenged with spatial relations (like Melissa). One or two thumbs is about a tablespoon or two.

This is the one area of our meal plan where people need the most comforting—or tough love. See, up until this point, you've probably been a little fat-phobic. (We can't blame you, given the misinformation you've been getting.) And now, here come these crazy Hartwigs, encouraging you to eat an *entire avocado* in a single sitting.

We understand if that sounds a little scary … but we've already talked about this.

In the context of a healthy diet that doesn't promote overconsumption or hormonal dysregulation, dietary fat isn't going to make you fat. And remember, we need to make sure you're eating enough fat to both cover your caloric requirements and promote satiety between meals. But it's not like we're saying *everyone* needs to eat an entire avocado with every meal. We've given you a range, because some people are big and some are little, some are very active and others less so, some people need to put on weight and some need to lose.

We're pretty sure you know which you are.

So, if you're little, not that active, and need to lose weight, choose fat from the lower end of our recommended quantities. If you're Dallas (205 pounds, very active, with the metabolism of a teenage boy), you'll probably eat more than we're starting you off with, because your context requires the extra calories for energy.

REAL-LIFE COOKING In reality, you'll probably end up incorporating more than one of these fat sources in every meal. Most people cook with oil and may want to add another source of fat for texture, flavor, or crunch. No problem! Just choose the smaller quantity from the ranges, and you won't end up consuming too much fat at any given meal.

Which reminds us to tell you that fat is probably going to be the meal-planning factor you experiment with the most, depending on your current health condition, your size, and your goals. Here is the basic rule for experimentation:

**Feel free to add *more* than our recommended quantities,
but never add *less*.**

If you're Dallas, and your body is telling you to eat more at each meal than we've suggested, that's totally fine. If you're smaller, less active, or still struggling with metabolic derangement, then stick with the quantities at the lower end of our spectrum, but do not cut your fat intake below the low end of our range, *even if you're trying to lose weight.*

Trust me, we've got safe, healthy, sustainable weight loss built right into our model, because we know that is a major goal for the majority of you. So don't try to outsmart the system in an effort to lose weight faster, as your efforts may backfire. Remember, it's not about fat grams or calories; it's about *hormones.* Your delicate hormone balance will be thrown off if you're chronically underfeeding yourself—plus you'll be hungry all the time, and your energy levels will take a dive, and you'll be cranky because you're tired and hungry. So stick to the lower end of our spectrum if you want, but resist the urge to cut your fat intake even more. Because as crazy as it sounds, you now know that eating less could be counterproductive to your weight-loss efforts.

YOUR MILEAGE MAY VARY

Eventually, we want to hand our plan over to you to make adjustments as needed, but this probably isn't going to happen right away. You've historically not been able to rely on the signals your body has been sending you, because of psychological factors and hormonal disruptions. This isn't going to change overnight—and that's OK. It generally takes a few weeks (or, in some cases, months) of consistently eating Good Food before this system starts to find its level.

For the first several weeks, use our meal plan as your baseline. We still want you to regularly check in with yourself, to evaluate how you think you feel: Hungry? Not hungry? Tired? Cranky? But we'll ask you to filter the messages your body is trying to send you, because it probably won't be telling you the truth just yet. Experience has shown us that most people with an imbalanced hunger mechanism fall into one of two camps: *hungry all the time,* or *not really hungry at all.*

If you're hungry all the time, you are either legitimately not eating enough or your brain is telling you that you're hungry when you're actually just *craving.* In the first instance, try making each meal a little bigger than the last and see if that quells your hunger. If it does—that's your new baseline. If not, there's more than just hunger going on.

CRAVINGS VS. HUNGER

It can be easy to confuse cravings for actual hunger, but we've got a quick-and-easy approach to differentiating between the two. Simply ask yourself, "Am I hungry enough to eat steamed fish and broccoli?" If the answer is no, then you're not *really* hungry; you've just got a craving. So go for a walk, phone a friend, or drink a glass of water and ride it out. If the answer is yes, then you're definitely hungry—so eat something!

Some of you will fall into the other camp—you're simply not going to be hungry for the first few weeks. It's partly because of the hormonal recalibration, and partly because you're now eating meals that are sending honest-to-goodness satiety signals to your brain.

If you simply never feel like eating, common sense should tell you it's not normal. In this case, you will have to temporarily override the signals your body is sending you, or risk further hormonal disruption because of chronic lack of nutrition. Our basic three meals a day are the minimum requirement for your caloric needs, so make sure you're at least getting those. Consider adding some activity to your day too—a brisk walk, weight training, or an exercise class should fire up your appetite. Within a few weeks, your hormones and hunger mechanism should self-regulate, and you'll be able to start listening to your body for real.

Generally a few weeks after changing your diet, you'll be ready to take the wheel of your own meal plan. This is perhaps the most critical step in our entire program, so when you're ready, start adjusting your own plate based on the signals your body is sending you.

We've given you the tools. It'll be time for you to take off the training wheels. And here are three reasons that we trust you'll do a stellar job of managing your food intake.

1. **You have been developing a new relationship with food:** spending time with your meals, chewing thoroughly, enjoying each bite, and paying attention.
2. **You have been filling your plate with Good Food:** food that isn't going to mess with your mind, *or* your hormones.

Therefore …

3. You will be able to trust the messages your body is sending you.

For perhaps the first time in your life, you can rely on your own body to tell you what it needs. Hallelujah! Because you're making good food choices *and* engaging with your food in a new way, you know that if you feel hungry, you're actually hungry (and not just having a craving or suffering from hypoglycemia). So what do you do? You eat something!

When you're full, you know you're *actually* full, because you've given your food enough time to send the right signal to your brain, and your hormones are working the way they're supposed to, to regulate your appetite. So what do you do? You stop eating!

And if you're hungry or brain-foggy between meals, your energy is flagging or your performance in the gym or playing sports is starting to slip, then you can surmise that you're not eating enough. So what do you do? You start making each meal a little bit bigger!

See? You're *brilliant* at this already!

So here's how it works.

Plan your first meal using your best judgment and our guidelines. Eat slowly, chew thoroughly, relax while digesting. Then, evaluate fifteen to twenty minutes later. Are you still hungry? If you are, eat more—particularly, more protein and more fat. Then evaluate your hunger levels, energy levels, and general mood in the hours before your next meal. Are you ravenously hungry an hour before dinnertime? Did your energy fade? Were you cranky, foggy, tired? If so, then your next meal needs to be bigger right from the start.

Make small changes—you don't have to double your portions just because you noticed you're a little hungry between meals. Try adding more protein and more fat, and see if that helps. If it does, that's your new personalized template. If it doesn't, then add some more fat—the great equalizer. Continue to add fat in small quantities until you hit that sweet spot—enough food to support activity levels, energy, and appetite, but not so much that you start getting flabby or putting on weight.

Finally, your own personal template will change over time. As your activity level changes and you lose weight or put on muscle mass, your nutritional needs will change too. So it's always important to pay attention to those signals, and not to rely on today's "perfect" template to fuel you a year from now.

So there you have it—you are now an expert meal planner! Congratulations.

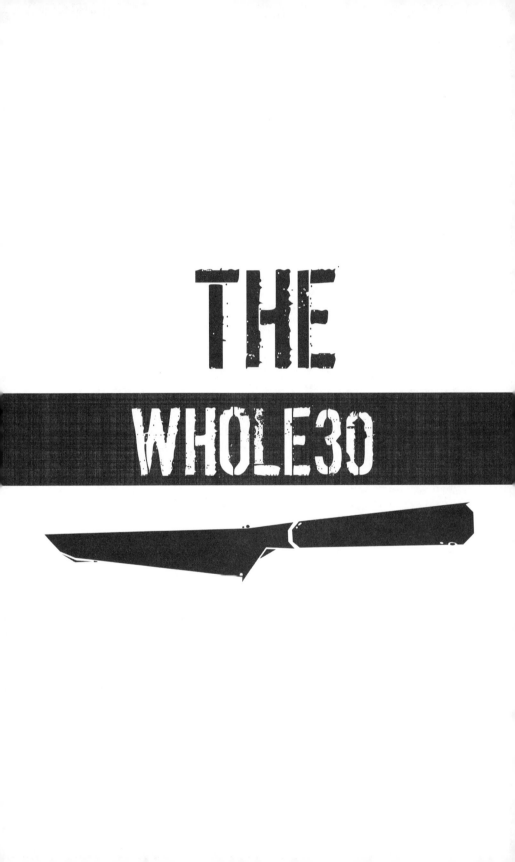

CHAPTER 17:
PREFACE TO THE PROGRAM

"Before I tell you what the Whole30 is, I would like to share my thoughts on what the Whole 30 is not. The Whole30 is not a diet. It is not a twenty-two-day program with eight cheat days (weekends) built in. It is not 30 days of restriction, to be followed by 335 days of gluttony. Here is what the Whole30 is. It is life-changing. It is the path to healing your insides. It is about eating real food and learning that what you put into your body actually matters. It is a test of the level of respect you have for this one body you were given. Simply put, if you follow it the way it was written, it works. If you don't, it doesn't. My only regret is that I waited so long to do it."
—*Tara O., Edwardsburg, Michigan*

Up until now, you've been somewhat passive in this relationship. We've been yapping our heads off, you've been patiently listening, and the flow has been mostly unidirectional. You've absorbed information from us, sure, but you haven't really rolled up your sleeves and jumped into the conversation.

In the last chapter, we asked you to start contributing. We gave you our meal-planning template and encouraged you to start making some of your own decisions by customizing the size and contents of your meals. (Good work there.) But now, our relationship is at a turning point. We think you are ready to truly take charge of your own health, and your own nutrition program. We can't do that for you. Frankly, we don't *want* to do that for you.

We're big fans of that whole "teach you how to fish" thing.

See, we've done as much as we can to educate you about foods that we believe are making you less healthy, and those that we think contribute to your health in a positive way. But at this point, it's all just theory—pretty solid theory, based on reputable science and our own extensive experience, but theory nonetheless. The thing is, *you* are not represented in any of the scientific experiments we've referenced. And unfortunately, we've probably never met you, which means you *personally* are not a part of our experience, either.

Now, we can still make an educated guess as to what your optimal diet should look like going forward. And if you're OK with us dictating what you can and can't eat for the rest of your life, you can go ahead and skip this chapter. But we suspect that you're not OK with that. We suspect that you'd like to know, definitively, how the foods you've been eating—particularly, the ones we've described as less healthy—are actually affecting your health. We suspect that you'd like to decide for yourself if including these less-than-healthy foods in your diet is worth it. We suspect that you'd prefer to make educated, informed decisions about your own diet for the rest of your life.

We don't blame you. We want that for you too. But it means that you're going to have to step up now. You're ready. It's time.

NO CHEATS. NO SLIPS. NO EXCUSES.

We'll be honest—the Whole30 is strict. It demands a full thirty days, and requires that you *radically* alter your daily diet for the duration. The rules are clear, and do not allow for substitutions or exceptions. Believe us, if there were another way—a gentler way—to get the same degree of success, we'd put it out there. But the science and our experience show that "baby steps" and "moderation" simply aren't effective at changing your habits long-term.

Despite what you may believe, habit research shows that dramatic changes are actually *easier* for us to manage, both physically and psychologically. Conscious decisions are made in the frontal lobe of the brain, and require active attention. But habits—automatic behaviors—take place in other parts of the brain, including the basal ganglia, and require much less cognitive effort.

SIGNAL, PLEASE Remember when you learned to drive a car? In the beginning, you had to think about *everything*—which pedal was the gas, which lever was the turn signal, and what to do when the light turned yellow. But now, you drive practically on autopilot, without exerting effort thinking about your pedals, the steering wheel, or your signals. The act of driving has progressed from a series of conscious decisions to a habitual set of behaviors—you don't have to *think* about it, it's just what you *do*.

Behaviors (like dietary choices) that start out as effort can eventually become habit, as easy to maintain as it is to drive a car. But that requires consistency in your decision-making process, and dedication to making good choices until they become relatively effortless.

Making small changes or "baby-stepping" the process keeps every decision in the frontal lobe of your brain, in "effort" territory. Simply limiting added sugar ("I'm going to have only one sweet treat per day") leads to incessant battles of willpower, continued cravings, and small sugar hits, which keep your brain focused on sugar. When faced with the offer of a cookie, your decision-making process is extensive, and painful: "Should I eat it? Is this what I want for my one treat? Maybe just today I'll have two treats. ..." But by committing to eliminate *all* added sugar, you've taken it out of the equation and made that decision more automatic, which makes it easier to continue that behavior until it becomes a habit. When faced with the same cookie offer, your decision-making process is easy: "Thanks, but I'm not eating sweets today."

In addition, the *only* way this program will work is if you give it the full thirty days—no cheats, slips, or special-occasion foods or drinks. This isn't us playing tough, or trying to make the Whole30 "hard-core." The thirty-day no-cheat policy is based on science and our experience.

First, just a *tiny* amount—in the case of folks with celiac disease, as little as ten milligrams (or about one-five-hundredth of a teaspoon)—of the inflammatory compounds found in off-plan foods may break the healing cycle. One bite of pizza, one splash of milk in your coffee, one brownie corner from your friend's plate within the thirty-day period could short-circuit your "reset" button, forcing you to start the entire process over from day one. And we're pretty sure that half a slice of pizza on day twenty-three isn't going to be worth starting over!

CAT MATH   Think of it like this: You're allergic to cats, and you own ten of them. One day, fed up with your allergies, you decide to get rid of *nine* of your cats. Will you feel better? Maybe a bit—maybe not so stuffy, itchy, or headachy. But will your allergies go away entirely? Not a chance, because you're still living with a cat! Removing only some commonly problematic foods from your diet is like getting rid of nine of your cats—with even a little bit remaining in your diet, you can't hope to be free of the negative effects it may be having.

In addition, most folks are trying to overcome ten, twenty, thirty years of less-than-healthy eating habits. Common sense should tell you that you cannot reasonably expect to make major improvements in your health with just a week or two of good, clean eating. Some research has shown that effectively establishing a new habit takes, on average, about two months— but may take as many as eight!

We based our program on the idea that thirty days is the minimum amount of time necessary to solidify a new habit. And in our experience, a full thirty days of our program is essential to give you a taste of "the magic"—that's why we call it the *Whole30*. Many Whole30 participants report that their most significant transformations take place in the final few days of the program. Still others require a Whole45 or a Whole60 to firmly root their new habits, banish stubborn cravings, and allow their bodies extra time to heal. In any event, your health isn't going to radically improve in *less* than 30 days—so we'll start there.

Another tough-love point:

It's only thirty days.

It's for the only body you will ever have in this lifetime.

And you have no idea how powerful this program can be.

After only thirty days, you'll know how those foods you *used* to eat work in *your* body—how they affect your energy levels, sleep, mood, and physical performance. You'll know how your food choices were affecting your skin, your hair, your joints, and your digestive tract. You'll learn how your diet played into your disease, medical condition, or hard-to-define collection of symptoms. In just thirty days, you will see for yourself, first-hand, how these things we've been talking about—an unhealthy psychological response, hormonal disruption, gut permeability, systemic inflammation—have been affecting *you*. And then you'll *know* whether these foods truly make you less healthy, which will then give you the power to decide what you're going to do about it.

It's time to step up and do what's right for you, and for your body, for the long-term.

It's time for your Whole30.

WHAT IS THE WHOLE30?

The Whole30 is our unique program designed to change your life in thirty days. Think of it as a short-term nutritional reset, designed to help you restore a healthy metabolism, heal your digestive tract, calm systemic inflammation, and put an end to unhealthy cravings, habits, and relationships with food. The premise is simple.

Certain food groups (like sugar, grains, dairy, and legumes) are probably having a negative impact on your health and fitness *without you even realizing it*. Are your energy levels inconsistent or nonexistent? Do you have aches and pains that can't be explained by overuse or injury? Is it almost impossible for you to lose weight no matter how hard you try? Do you have an undesirable health condition (like skin disruptions, digestive trouble, chronic pain, or infertility) that medication hasn't alleviated? As you now know, these ailments are directly impacted by the foods you eat— *even the "healthy" stuff.*

WHAT IS NORMAL?

But wouldn't you *know* if these foods were making you less healthy? Not necessarily. Say you're allergic to a tree outside your bedroom window. Every morning, you wake up with itchy eyes, a runny nose, and a slight headache. But those symptoms eventually start to become your "norm." You no longer notice the headache, runny nose, or itchy eyes, because that's just your experience *every single day*. Then one day you go on vacation somewhere where there are none of those trees. The first morning you wake up, you're clear-headed, your eyes are bright, and you couldn't summon a sniffle if you tried to. You feel fantastic—and you become acutely aware of how terrible you used to feel. That's kind of like what we're trying to do for you here—remove all potential triggers, so you can be truly, honestly aware of what your life would be like without them.

So how do you know if (and how) these foods are affecting you?

Remove them from your diet completely.

Cut out all of the mind-messing, hormonally disruptive, gut-damaging, inflammatory food groups for an entire month. Let your body recover from whatever effects those foods may have been having on you. Break old cravings, compulsions, and unhealthy relationships with food. Push the "reset" button on your metabolism and systemic inflammation. Learn *once and for all* how the foods you've been eating are actually affecting your day-to-day life and your long-term health.

The most important reason to commit to thirty days?

It can change your life.

We cannot possibly put enough emphasis on this simple fact—the next thirty days can CHANGE YOUR LIFE. It can change the way you think about food, it can change your tastes, it can change your habits and your cravings. It can permanently change the relationship you have with food *... for the rest of your life.* We know this because we did it, and tens of thousands of people have done it, and it changed our lives and their lives in a remarkable and surprising fashion.

Our program has two phases: elimination and reintroduction.

CHAPTER 18:
THE WHOLE30:
PROCESS OF ELIMINATION

"I have been a lifelong acute asthmatic. Hundreds of ER visits, hospitalizations, and so forth. It was around week two of my Whole30 when my miracle happened. I went out for a warm-up run—something I dread every day, and something I have never been able to do. But it was during this run where there was suddenly a feeling like I had the legs (and lungs) of a gazelle. I had never felt this in thirty-three years. So much so that I voluntarily went on another run ... and another. Since the Whole30, I have been unmedicated for the first time in my life. I would normally have to take four or five control medications and use my inhaler multiple times a day. It is something miraculous to feel life as you have never known it."
—Andrea B., Minneapolis, Minnesota

THE WHOLE30® PROGRAM: ELIMINATION

Follow these guidelines for the entirety of your program. No cheats, no slips, no excuses.

YES: Eat foods that make you more healthy – meat, seafood and eggs, lots of vegetables, some fruit, and plenty of healthy fats.

NO: Do not consume any added sugar, alcohol, grains, legumes or dairy.

NO: Do not attempt to recreate junk foods or desserts by using "approved" ingredients.

NO: Do not step on the scale for the entirety of your program.

**YES: Eat foods that make you healthier—meat,
seafood, eggs, lots of vegetables, some fruit,
and plenty of healthy fats.**

Eat foods with pronounceable ingredients, or, better yet, no ingredients listed at all because they are whole and unprocessed. It's what we've already talked about—the things that should be on your plate, using the same meal planning recommendations we've just covered.

**NO: Do not consume any of the following foods or
beverages for the duration of your Whole30 program.**

- **Added sugar of any kind, real or artificial.** No table sugar, maple syrup, honey, agave nectar, Splenda, Equal, NutraSweet, xylitol, stevia, etc. Read your labels, because food manufacturers sneak sugar into products in ways you might not recognize or even imagine.
- **Alcohol.** In any form, not even for cooking. (And it should go without saying, but **no tobacco products** of any sort, either.)
- **Grains.** This includes (but is not limited to) wheat, rye, barley, oats, corn, rice, millet, bulgur, sorghum, amaranth, buckwheat, sprouted grains, and quinoa. This also includes all the forms in which wheat, corn, and rice are added to our foods: bran, germ, starch, and so on. Again, read your labels.
- **Legumes.** This includes beans of all kinds (black, red, pinto, navy, white, kidney, lima, fava, etc.), peas, chickpeas, lentils, and peanuts. No peanut butter, either. This also includes all forms of soy—soy sauce, miso, tofu, tempeh, edamame—and all the ways soy is sneaked into foods (like lecithin).
- **Dairy.** This includes cow's, goat's, or sheep's milk products such as cream, cheese (hard or soft), kefir, yogurt (even Greek), and sour cream, *with the exception of clarified butter and ghee.* (Keep reading for details.)
- **White potatoes.** If we are trying to change your habits, it's best to leave white, red, purple, Yukon gold, and fingerling potatoes off your plate. There's a world of new veggies waiting for you to make room for them!

DO YOU STILL SMOKE?

If you still smoke, you might be thinking, "There is no way I can quit smoking and make these dietary changes all at the same time." And you might be right. If you feel like all of these changes are too overwhelming, then we'd encourage you to focus on getting rid of your tobacco habit first, and then come back to the Whole30. That's not to say you can't make some dietary improvements while you quit—many smokers report that taking better care of their health with diet and exercise makes it easier to stop smoking. But if you just can't manage it all, the cigarettes *should* be your top priority. On the other hand, if you've been looking for a program to help you quit, the Whole30 may just be your ticket. Many former smokers have told us they used the Whole30 in part as a smoking-cessation program, and that eliminating sugar and other psychologically unhealthy foods at the same time made the process that much easier. Either way, we encourage you to seek help for your nicotine addiction, prioritize ditching the smokes, and take on the Whole30 as soon as you are ready.

NO: Do not try to recreate junk foods or desserts with "approved" ingredients.

This is a very important rule, mostly because we know you're already thinking about how you can take the foods you used to eat and make them compliant with approved ingredients. "There *must* be a way to make Whole30-approved pizza/pancakes/brownies/ice cream. …" And a quick Internet search will bring up thousands of "Paleo" treat temptations.

Most people make this mistake during their first Whole30. But we know from experience that one of the fastest ways to negate the potential benefits of your program is to try to shove your old, unhealthy diet into a shiny, new Whole30 mold. Pizza, pancakes, brownies or ice cream are still junk food, even if they're made from "healthier" ingredients. They're still pushing more nutrient-dense foods off your plate. And their flavor, texture and taste aren't generally as good as the "real thing," which means they aren't as rewarding—which makes you crave them even more. When it comes to the psychological hold certain foods have over us, the whole (muffin) is *far* more than just the sum of its parts (ingredients).

Do you really want to spend the entirety of your Whole30 focusing on all the stuff you *can't* have, and eating the same kinds of foods you've been eating all along? If you come out of the program under the shadow of the same habits, patterns, and food choices you had when you started, what are your chances for long-term, life-changing success? After all, those very same habits, patterns, and food choices are what got you into trouble in the first place!

Use the Whole30 to change your habits, alter your patterns, break unhealthy cravings, and create a new, healthy relationship with food. Starve the sugar dragon once and for all! You won't be sorry, as those new habits and patterns will stay with you for the rest of your life.

NO: Do not step on the scale or take any body measurements for the duration of the program.

This one may be the hardest rule of all and requires another dose of tough love.

We don't care if you lose weight during your Whole30.

We know *you* care, though, and we *do* care about you. So, please, hear us out.

The Whole30 isn't just another weight-loss diet. The program is designed to jump-start *optimal health for the rest of your life.* We tell people to get off the scale altogether for the first thirty days because scale weight tells you almost nothing about your overall *health*—and is one of the fastest ways to lose motivation, even if you thought you were making great progress in other areas. ("I only lost half a pound today—this program isn't working at all!")

Scale weight fluctuates. It doesn't reflect improvements in your health. And it's one of the parties holding you hostage to your unhealthy relationship with food. So give yourself a long-overdue, well-deserved break from your preoccupation with body weight. You deserve it.

However, because we know weight loss is important to you—and because we get that there's a connection between a more pleasing physique and motivation to maintain your new, healthy habits—we're going to let you in on a secret: Our nutrition plan will improve your overall health, and that is almost always reflected in an improvement in body composition. Which means that if you focus on eating better, sleeping better, and making yourself *healthier* … your shape will have no choice but to shift. Yes, automatically. But it doesn't work the other way around.

You can achieve short-term weight loss by taking some drastic steps (like eating a super low calorie diet plus doing two hours of cardio a day), but that's not going to make you healthier, nor is it sustainable long term. So trust us, and be patient. We'll get you there the healthy way—the *right* way—and you'll be able to maintain the new, improved you for the rest of your life.

OUR SURVEY In a 2011 survey of more than 1,000 Whole30 participants, 95 percent reported having lost weight and/or improved their body composition. The majority lost between six and fifteen pounds in just thirty days. So, there you go—proof that weight loss is built right into the program, *without your having to think about it.*

The Whole30 is about so much more than *just* weight loss, and if you focus on the small picture, like body composition, you'll miss out on the big picture—the dramatic and lifelong benefits the plan has to offer. But simply by doing the Whole30, you'll probably lose weight anyway. So why waste brain cells obsessing about something you don't need to obsess about?*

THE FINE PRINT

These items, even though they don't all necessarily meet the strictest criteria for the Whole30, are allowed. Including them should not have a negative impact on your results.

YES: Feel free to include these foods as part of your varied healthy-eating plan.

- **Clarified butter and ghee.** Clarified butter and ghee are the only dairy products allowed. Plain old butter is *not*, as it contains milk proteins.
- **Fruit juice as a sweetener.** Some products use orange or apple juice as a sweetener. We have to draw the line somewhere, so we're OK with a small amount of fruit juice as an *added* ingredient.

---

*We do, however, encourage you to document your "before" and "after" selves: weigh yourself or take body measurements as well as photos, so you will have proof positive of your success.

- **Certain legumes.** Specifically, green beans, sugar snap peas, and snow peas.
- **Vinegar.** Most varieties of vinegar, including white, balsamic, apple cider, red wine, and rice, are allowed. But vinegars with added sugar or sulfites, and malt vinegar (which generally contains gluten), are not.
- **Processed foods.** Minimally processed foods like canned coconut milk, applesauce, tomato sauce, chicken broth, or canned olives are all acceptable—but avoid anything with **MSG**, **sulfites**, or **carrageenan**: these additives all have potentially nasty side effects.

WHY THESE THREE?

While we'd prefer that none of your foods contain additives, we're singling out MSG, sulfites, and carrageenan for very good reasons. Monosodium glutamate (MSG), a common flavor enhancer in many processed foods, is known to have neurotoxic effects and is also linked to obesity by promoting leptin resistance. In fact, MSG is used to induce obesity in lab rats! Sulfites occur naturally in many foods and beverages and are a byproduct of fermentation, so they are found in most wines, as well as balsamic and red wine vinegars. They are also added to processed foods to increase shelf life, preserve color, and inhibit microbial growth. Sulfites can cause significant dermatological, pulmonary, gastrointestinal, and cardiovascular symptoms in sensitive people. Carrageenan is a concentrated seaweed extract used to thicken processed foods and is found in everything from deli meat to yogurt to chocolate. Carrageenan is inflammatory if it gets into the body, which could happen if you have increased gut permeability. (Carrageenan is actually used to *create* inflammation in lab animals.) Furthermore, in the digestive process, carrageenan may be broken down into components that can cross even a healthy gut barrier.

READY TO START?

Now that you have the elements of the plan, you need to know how to implement them. It's simple, actually.

Start now. Today. This minute.

Block out thirty days on your calendar. Clean out your pantry. Plan a week's worth of meals with the help of our Meal Map in Appendix A. Take our shopping list to your local grocery store, health-food store, or farmers' market and stock up on ingredients for all the yummy meals you'll be making. And then ... go. Just start! Don't put this off, not for one more day. If you give yourself excuses to delay, you may never begin.

Do it now.

Your only job for the next thirty days will be to focus on making good food choices. You won't need to weigh or measure, you won't need to count calories, you won't need to stress about whether you're doing it "perfectly." Just figure out how to stick to the Whole30 regardless of the circumstances, in the face of any amount of stress, for the next thirty days.

Your only job? Eat. Good. Food.

WHAT TO EXPECT

We won't lie—things will probably get worse before they get better. Here's a general template for what to expect, based on the feedback we've received from thousands of Whole30 participants.

Days 1 to 7: The first week will be tough as your body heals and adjusts to this new way of eating and your brain wraps itself around going without all its habitual sweet tastes and sugar-driven energy spikes. In addition, the reward, pleasure, and emotional connections to supernormally stimulating, nutrient-poor foods will take a *lot* longer to overcome, so the cravings can be intense. In fact, many Whole30 participants have reported craving-driven dreams about off-plan foods—some so intensely real, they wake up feeling *guilty*. Talk about an unhealthy psychological response!

Since you've removed many of the dense carbohydrates from your diet (like sugars, grains, and legumes), your body can no longer rely on those sugars as a primary energy source. That often leads to "withdrawal" symptoms like headaches, lethargy, and crankiness—the "carb flu"—as your body adjusts to its new fuel source. Ease off your physical activity this week—don't take part in any big races or events, and don't expect to set any personal bests in the gym. Your body is desperately trying to recalibrate during this first critical week, so give it the time, space, and rest it needs to do so.

You may see a significant change in your body as you shed excess water weight and the incumbent bloating. Don't get too excited: This probably doesn't represent much true fat loss—it's just your body's way of letting go of some of the physical effects of your old way of eating.

Days 8 to 14: Most people report that their "carb flu" symptoms are gone by the very end of the second week. During this week, most people report falling asleep faster, sleeping better, and more consistent energy levels. At this point, your body is already more efficient at using fat (dietary and body fat) as fuel. Once your metabolism has become "fat adapted," you'll notice that your energy levels are much more stable than they ever were with processed foods and an incessant influx of sugar.

However, although you are starting to feel better, the healing process takes much longer than a week or two. Digestive distress is common and may take a few months to completely resolve. The inflammation-causing foods you've been eating have been like sandpaper in your digestive tract for all the years you've been eating them. Remove *all* of them, and your digestive tract starts to heal—but the healing process *can* be unpleasant. Constipation or diarrhea, cramps, bloating, gas, and general discomfort are common, and are all a normal part of the process, as your intestinal lining starts to repair itself, some gut bacteria die off, and the extra-thick protective layer of mucosal lining starts to slough off.

If you've dramatically increased your fruit and vegetable intake, that could also be playing a role in your digestive distress. Try eating more cooked vegetables than raw and having more frequent, smaller servings of fruit throughout the day, as opposed to one or two larger serving. In addition, if you're relying too heavily on nuts and seeds, you may find digestive relief from swapping those out for fats like avocado, coconut, and olive oil.

We know this part isn't fun, but ride it out. It gets better quickly, we promise, and once your digestive tract has healed, it will be happier—and healthier—than it has been in years.

Days 15 to 30: Much of what happens during the second half of your Whole30 depends on your health history and habits. You may notice improvement in ailments—skin clearing up, allergies diminishing, joints no longer aching. Most people are sleeping well and are energetic and attentive throughout their day. Your gym or sports performance may take an upturn, and you may find that your mental focus and physical coordination are better. And you'll probably notice that your clothes are fitting differently by this point, too.

Your taste buds should also be waking up right about now, allowing you to truly appreciate the flavors found in the fresh foods you're eating. But you may also be getting a little bored with your food if you relied on the same basic "go-to" meals for the first two weeks. Time to revisit our Meal Map and try something new!

During this time, you also may start thinking, "I'm really feeling better now—two weeks is probably enough." We call this the "bright, shiny toy" mentality—the novelty of the program has worn off, but you're still two weeks away from completion. Time to snap to attention—don't get lazy or let your guard down! Now is the perfect time to experiment with new foods, new spices and herbs, and more exotic dishes—and draft a few strategies to combat the sugar dragon when it unexpectedly roars back to life in your brain. (And, we're sorry to say, it probably will.)

Even if you haven't achieved all the results you'd hoped to by the twenty-ninth day, hang on: you cannot reasonably expect to completely reverse decades of poor eating habits in just thirty days. At some point, we promise … the magic *will* happen. In the meantime, be patient, don't ease up on your hard-won discipline, and focus on all the things that *have* improved in your life since starting the Whole30—that should supply all the motivation you need to keep up the good work. But we'll caution you now …

There is no magic number.

You don't have to abandon your efforts just because you've done your thirty days. If after a month, your tastes have yet to change, if you're still craving all your "old" foods, if you're still a slave to the sugar dragon, or if you haven't noticed a significant improvement in a particular factor that was important to you at the beginning of this program … please consider sticking with the Whole30 for a little while longer. You've already put in thirty long, hard days of reconditioning your body and your brain. And we bet that if you're feeling a little frustrated right now, it's because you're trying to counteract the effects of twenty or thirty *years* of less-than-stellar eating habits. That damage doesn't miraculously come undone in a month.

STICK WITH IT For some, a Whole45 or even a Whole60 is necessary to get the job done, and we believe that the results you are hoping for *will* appear, if you can be patient for just a little bit longer. Your body is slowly reverting to a healthy hunger cycle and metabolism, and to having a happy (intact) gut, reduced systemic inflammation, and a balanced immune system. And as this happens, you *will* notice a reduction in cravings, a shift in body composition, an improvement in energy, and a reduction in symptoms—but it takes longer for some people than for others.

So stick with it, for as long as it takes. You owe it to yourself, and you owe it to your body. But let's also address one really important point right here.

This is not *just* about your body. This is also about resetting your *brain*.

If there is one thing we've learned from our clients' Whole30 experiences and our own, it's this: Food is emotional. It's comfort, it's celebration, it's punishment, and it's reward. Food is often the *only* thing people come together over. It's used to establish common ground, form a bond, smooth over rough personal interactions. And you cannot take that aspect out of this equation.

So if you're still feeling the same way about food after your initial thirty days, if that relationship is *still* too dysfunctional to feel healthy ... hang in a little longer. Allow your body *and your mind* to catch up to this new way of eating, this new way of being. This thirty-day program is the kindest thing you've done for your body in a long time, and your brain simply may not know what to do with that. Be patient, embrace the intention and spirit of the program, and allow those new habits, patterns, relationships, and tastes to change right along with the changes you are seeing with your body.

IT'S FOR YOUR OWN GOOD

Now ... for those of you who are thinking about taking on this life-changing challenge but aren't sure you can actually pull it off, cheat-free, for a full thirty days, for those of you who really *want* to do this, but just need a little extra motivation—here comes the famous Whole30 tough love in a few talking points.

- **It is *not* hard.** Please don't tell us this program is hard. Quitting heroin is hard. Beating cancer is hard. Birthing a baby is hard. Drinking your coffee black. Is. Not. Hard. You have no excuse not to complete the program as written. It's only thirty days, and it's for the most important health cause on earth—the only physical body you will ever have in this lifetime.

- **Don't even consider the possibility of a "slip."** Unless you physically trip and your face lands in a box of doughnuts, there is no such thing as a "slip." You make a *choice* to eat something unhealthy. It is always a *choice*. So don't talk as if you had an accident. Own it. Commit to the program 100 percent for the full thirty days. Don't give yourself an excuse to fail before you have even started.

- **You never, ever, ever *have* to eat anything you don't want to eat.** You're all big boys and girls. Toughen up. Learn to say no (or make your mom proud and say, "No, thank you"). Learn to stick up for yourself. Just because it's your sister's birthday, or your best friend's wedding, or your company picnic does not mean you *have* to eat *anything*. It's *always* a choice, and we would hope that you stopped succumbing to peer pressure in seventh grade.

- **You can do this.** You've come too far to back out now. You want to do this. You *need* to do this. And we know that you *can* do this. So stop thinking, and start *doing*. Right now, this very minute, tell someone that you are starting the Whole30. Tell your spouse, tell your best friend, post it on our Facebook page, and prove to yourself that you are *committed* to your health.

There—that wasn't so bad, was it?

And before you know it, you'll be done with the first part of your program. Hooray! So go do your Whole30 (or Whole45, or Whole60 …), and then come back here when you're ready for the next phase. (Or for all of you overachievers, keep on reading and get a sneak preview.)

CHAPTER 19:
THE WHOLE30: REINTRODUCTION

"This program has shown results that I didn't think were possible. I recognized that I had severe difficulties dealing with food cravings and knowing when to stop eating. Daily I asked myself, 'How can I get these urges under control? Why do I feel like I need these bad foods?' The Whole30 is the answer. I haven't felt the deep desire to binge since I've submerged myself into this program. I don't feel like I have to struggle to make decisions when trying to decide what to eat. It's as simple as knowing that what I have been eating is beneficial to me, and that is how I will continue to nourish myself."
—Aubrey H., Manassas, Virginia

THE WHOLE30® PROGRAM: REINTRODUCTION

Follow this sample reintroduction schedule when your program is over. Keep the rest of your diet Whole30-compliant during this period.

DAY 1: Reintroduce and evaluate dairy products.

DAY 4: Reintroduce and evaluate gluten-containing grains.

DAY 7: Reintroduce and evaluate non-gluten grains.

DAY 10: Reintroduce and evaluate legumes.

You've eliminated added sugars, alcohol, grains, legumes, and dairy from your diet for an entire month. But every once in a while, maybe you'd still like to drink a beer, have some ice cream, slather a piece of toast with peanut butter and jelly.

We are completely on board with that. (Does that surprise you? We're healthy, not automatons.)

But let's use the efforts you've made during your program as a springboard for approaching this intelligently. Yes, you'll have to be patient here, too—don't waste the last thirty (or more) days! You've spent valuable time cleaning out your system and allowing your body to heal. But if you run right out the day you've completed your program and binge on pancakes, pizza, ice cream, and beer, when you feel like junk that night (yes, you *will* feel like junk), how will you know what to blame for which symptoms? Was it the dairy that bloated your belly, or maybe the grains? Were you headachy because of the sugar, the booze, or both? And where did those pimples come from—the soy, the dairy, or the sugar? What a waste. You've spent so much time and effort ... and missed a critical opportunity to learn from your experience.

Here's what we'd like you to do instead: introduce "less healthy" foods back into your diet *one group at a time*, while keeping the rest of your diet as Whole30-clean as possible. Think about it like a scientific trial, in which your Whole30 is the "control" and the one food group you are trying to evaluate is the "experimental group." Sure, you'll get some added sugar in many of your "experimental" foods, but the key is not combining *food groups* in any one testing day.

DON'T MISS IT? We shouldn't have to say it, but if you don't miss a particular food or drink that you know makes you less healthy, don't bother reintroducing it. If you made it through the entire Whole30 without longing for cheddar cheese or martinis or black beans one tiny bit, then why bother "testing" it? Only reintroduce those foods that you suspect you'll really *want* to include in your diet once in a while, and consider the rest history.

REINTRODUCTION, SCIENCE-Y STYLE

Here is a sample ten-day reintroduction schedule. Feel free to alter the food groups and particular food choices to suit your needs.

Day 1: Evaluate dairy, *while keeping the rest of your diet Whole30-compliant.* Have yogurt in the morning, some cheese in the afternoon, and ice cream after dinner. Evaluate how you feel that day, and the next day, and perhaps even the day after that. Stomach feel like you're about to birth an alien? Suddenly feeling all congested and headachy? Skin break out in the next day or two? You may need to limit your dairy consumption to very small quantities or only certain items (yogurt, but not ice cream) during "off plan" meals, or you may decide that the aftereffects mean that all dairy is simply never worth it.

Day 4: Evaluate gluten-containing grains, *while keeping the rest of your diet Whole30-compliant.* Gluten is such nasty stuff that we want to break it out from the other grains, so you can evaluate it all by itself. Over the course of your day, eat a whole-wheat bagel, a side of pasta, and a dinner roll. See how you feel that day, and the next day, and so on. Evaluate your experience and decide how often and how much to incorporate gluten grains into your regular diet—if at all. (We recommend not at all.)

Day 7: Evaluate non-gluten grains, *while keeping the rest of your diet Whole30-compliant.* Eat a serving of white rice, some corn tortilla chips, and a slice of gluten-free bread. See how you feel that day, and the next day, and so on. Pay attention to your reactions and decide how, how often, and how much to incorporate grains into your regular diet—if at all.

Day 10: Evaluate legumes, *while keeping the rest of your diet Whole30-compliant.* Try some peanut butter, a bowl of lentil soup, some tofu, and a side of black beans. See how you feel that day, and the next day, and so on. Evaluate your experience and decide how, how often, and how much to incorporate legumes into your regular diet—if at all.

THAT COVERT YOGURT   One word of caution here. Just because that slice of toast or glass of milk didn't leave you clutching your stomach doesn't mean it isn't causing physiological (and psychological) damage. Cravings, hormonal disruption, intestinal permeability, and inflammation are, as we said earlier, often silent, hiding behind the scenes. People who don't notice any obvious effects from one or two exposures to a certain food may start to notice the results catching up with them after a few days or a week. In addition, you may be tempted to downplay the effects of a certain food, simply because you really like it. The point is, you need to evaluate your own experiences carefully and honestly when making decisions about which foods to reintroduce post-Whole30.

This invaluable information, and the self-awareness you gain as the result of your own hard work, is a big part of the Whole30 program, and a huge influence on how you eat going forward. In a very short period of time, you've learned how the foods that we've been saying make you less healthy actually affect *you*, personally. You've completed your scientific experiment, and now it's time to take that knowledge with you, and create new, lifelong healthy eating habits.

We are not telling you where to draw your own individual "worth it" line. Maybe ice cream *really* makes your stomach hurt, but you *really* love ice cream, so you decide it's worth it for you. That is entirely your call. But don't you at least appreciate knowing what the repercussions of that ice cream will be, so you don't indulge in a bowl before a tough workout or while out on a date? Draw your own line, and arrive at your own conclusions—and use your Whole30 experience to add some smart context to those decisions.

Easier said than done, you're thinking?

That's exactly why the next section is devoted to transitioning your Whole30 experience into sustainable, healthy habits. Because that's what this is all about: it's not about a short-term fix or a temporary solution, but about creating lifelong behaviors designed to always move you in the direction of "more healthy."

Sounds too good to be true?

It's not.

In fact, you're already well on your way.

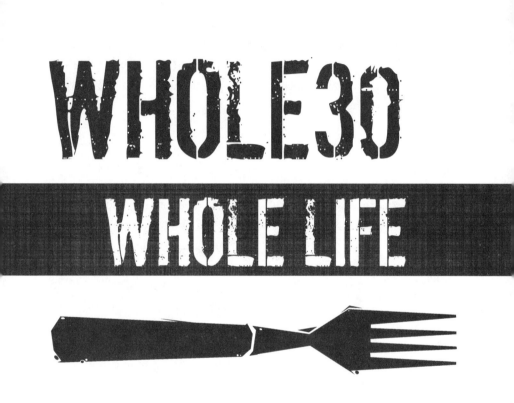

CHAPTER 20:
STRATEGIES FOR LONG-TERM SUCCESS

"The Whole30 has set me free of so many things. Now I can look at my plate as I am creating my dinner and know when enough is enough so after my meal I am neither hungry nor uncomfortably full. I have, for the first time in my life, learned how to listen to my body. I can list all of the 'classic' bonuses of the Whole30 with an emphatic yes. I am sleeping better. I am feeling better. My intestines are behaving the way they should for the first time ever. My skin is clear. I have lost weight, and my clothes fit better. I have kicked the sugar demon to the curb and am coping with stress without eating the entire kitchen, packaging and all. But even with that entire list, if I could only tell someone one benefit of my Whole30 experience, my answer would be a single word: freedom."

—Laura C., Mullingar, Co. Westmeath, Ireland

You've finished your Whole30, and you're probably feeling pretty good. You've worked hard to change your habits, and you're finding it easier to turn down foods you used to find "irresistible," thanks in part to a reduction (or elimination) of cravings. But you may also be a little bit nervous about what's to come. Here is one universal truth:

It's much harder to make Good Food choices out there in the "real world."

The rules of the Whole30 program are very specific, and completely non-negotiable. They remove some of the stress from making your own food choices, take all the guesswork out of our expectations, and give you a clear goal. ("Start eating healthy" is a far more difficult challenge to wrap your head around than "Eat no added sugar, alcohol, grains, legumes, or dairy in any form whatsoever for thirty days.") The program also gives you an easy fall-back when faced with social or peer pressures—a built-in excuse for why you don't want that piece of cake or glass of wine. Blame us. We can handle it.

The rules of the Whole30 function much like training wheels on a bike, giving you all the support you need while allowing you to *complete* the program under the power of your own pedal strokes. But what happens when your thirty days are up? All the comforts of our rules, your built-in excuses, your clear objectives disappear with the end of your Whole30. Which leaves you with the *desire* to continue to eat healthfully, but no clear plan to make that happen.

So, let's create a plan. We'll outline our best suggestions for transitioning your Whole30 program into lifelong, sustainable habits—and then *you* can customize the plan to suit your lifestyle and goals.

IT'S NOT THE WHOLE365

Remember, the Whole30 is just a *springboard* into a lifetime of healthy eating habits. We don't expect (or want) you to stay on the program forever, or eat according to our rules all the time! Think of the Whole30 as a tool, allowing you to build new, sustainable habits that will be with you for the rest of your life.

IT'S A MARATHON, NOT A SPRINT

Here's what most of you Whole30'ers can expect when your first program is over. You may wait a few days before eating anything off-plan, nervous about taking that first step. Eventually, though, you'll reintroduce some less-healthy foods. Most likely, these foods won't taste as good as you remember, and perhaps they won't make you feel as good as you felt during your Whole30—which makes it pretty easy to set them aside and return to your Whole30-ish eating habits.

But slowly, eventually, inevitably, poor choices will start to creep back in. Vacations, stressful situations, family events, and celebrations are common catalysts for the backslide into old habits, although perhaps the backslide starts with a glass of wine or bowl of ice cream on a random Tuesday night. It might take a month, or two, or three … but we predict that eventually you will wake up and realize that (a) you've somehow slipped back into mediocre eating habits, (b) you don't feel so fantastic anymore, and (c) it's really time to clean things up again.

When you get to this place, hear us clearly:

This does *not* mean you've failed your post-Whole30 test.

Habits are hard to break, pressures are hard to resist, and the temptation of delicious, less-healthy foods are everywhere. In the real world, it's easy to have a relapse—it happens to everyone, including us. And it will, at some point, happen to you.

CHEAT DAYS This is why we are not fans of scheduled "cheat meals"—and even worse, "cheat days." When you purposefully *plan* to make poor food choices, you are literally setting yourself up to fail! Plus, you are more likely to eat something you don't really want, just because you've told yourself you *can*. In addition, devoting an entire day to poor food choices (allowing yourself to binge on all the super-normally stimulating, processed, nutrient-poor foods you want) wreaks havoc for days to come. Your sugar cravings, GI tract, energy levels, and mental health will take far less of a "hit" if you eat healthy, slip in your less-healthy choice, then go right back to eating healthy foods (versus an entire day of Carb-a-Palooza).

This process of restoring your health (and then some) is just that—a *process*. While the Whole30 was a fantastic jumping-off point, and will form the foundation of your healthy eating habits for the rest of your life, remember that it's a marathon, not a sprint. You cannot expect yourself to be a "perfect eater" today, or tomorrow, or probably ever. In fact, we don't generally think that's a good goal to strive for. And it's unreasonable to expect a lifetime of habits, patterns, and relationships with food to completely change in a mere month.

Which means that your lifelong healthy-eating journey will take you, well, the rest of your life. And that's OK. Because much like your Whole30, this healthy-eating thing gets easier with time and practice.

MAKE CONSCIOUS DECISIONS

Instead of preplanning your "nutritional off-roading," we recommend a more flexible, intuitive approach. The basis of your everyday meals should look a lot like our "more healthy" recommendations, focused on high-quality meat, seafood, and eggs; vegetables, fruit, and healthy fats.

If you are happy with your food, feeling great and lovin' life, there is no reason whatsoever to stray from this template.

The idea that dietary "cheats" are necessary to "shock the body" and "jump-start your metabolism" is total malarkey. Binging on pizza, pasta, cake, and cookies has absolutely *zero* positive impact on your health, and may have serious consequences, depending on the food and your context. However, there *are* a few reasons to eat foods that are less healthy.

First, there are culturally significant or family-related events in which food and drink play a major role. A wedding, a special vacation, or your family's Christmas dinner may involve foods that don't make you physically healthier but have important emotional significance. In addition, there are valid psychological reasons for eating less-healthy foods. You crave a special food from your childhood. Your brain rebels against the rigidity of "can have" and "can't have." You get the urge to "test" a food group again, because you're not yet *totally* convinced that those foods make you feel as terrible as you remember.

But perhaps the most compelling reason to go off-roading with your food from time to time is:

Because they are delicious.

Sometimes, the fact that a food or drink is *so delicious* is a good enough reason to indulge. So, how do you work these choices into your everyday life?

On a case-by-case basis, making conscious, deliberate, informed decisions.

Keep eating your healthy foods until you bump into something that you believe might be worth it. Maybe it's the homemade cookies Mom bakes, your favorite pomegranate martini on a dinner date, or that decadent-looking dessert in the bakery window.

THAT AIN'T SPECIAL One thing we'll tell you right now—the box of doughnuts (or the open bag of pretzels, or the bag of M&Ms) sitting on the break-room counter *is not special*. You're a grown-up. You earn your own money. And if you want doughnuts, pretzels, or a bag of M&Ms, you can walk right into any supermarket or convenience store and *buy them*. These foods are not special. They're not homemade, or a once-a-year treat, and we're pretty sure they don't evoke fond childhood memories of sitting around the dining room table while Mom pulls things out of the oven. Now, if a chocolate-glazed doughnut is your favorite food in the whole world, that may be a different story. But don't indulge in something that's less healthy just because it's *around*. That's not a good enough reason in our book.

Once you've identified something you think might be worth it, ask yourself a series of questions to help you decide if it's *really* worth it. Do I have a *specific desire* for this particular food, or am I just emotional, hungry, or craving? Is it going to be incredibly special, significant, or delicious? Is it going to mess me up—negatively affect how I feel or the quality of my life?

This process might seem tedious or unnecessary. After all, you've been choosing your own food for a long time now—surely, you are capable of deciding what you want to eat or drink, right?

Not so fast.

Isn't that kind of automatic "decision making" what got you into trouble in the first place? Because of the *kinds* of foods and drinks we often indulge with (supernormally stimulating, nutrient-poor, calorie-dense, and highly processed), it's all too easy to let your reward, pleasure, and emotional pathways do the talking. And if you allow that to happen, you often find that cookie, martini, or breakfast pastry half gone before you even realize it. So please, stop and think critically at this point. It may make the difference between reinforcing your new, healthy habit and taking one step backward into an old one.

If you decide the food or drink really is worth it, congratulations! You can move on to the next step—*enjoying it*.

NEED MORE HELP? If you're a visual learner, or need more help deciding whether that less-healthy food is *really* worth it, we've created a handy flow chart just for you! Download our free "Guide to Nutritional Off-Roading" at http://whole9life.com/it-startswithfood.

EAT SMART

The first thing we'd like to suggest is, don't use the word "cheat" to describe your less-healthy indulgences. We want you to be able to make *guilt-free* choices to indulge in less-healthy foods from time to time, but "cheating" has a negative connotation. (And really, there *is* no guilt—only consequences.) We don't believe those negative associations have any place in your new, healthy relationship with food, so going forward, we'll call them "treats" instead.

The second tip: Eat only as much as you need to satisfy your craving. If you've been dreaming about your favorite treat—say, homemade chocolate-chip cookies—and you decide today is the day, then by all means, bust out the cookie sheet and make some. But remember:

**You don't have to eat the whole tray
just because it's there.**

How will you know how much is enough? Because you are going to *savor those cookies*. It's a terrible thing to mindlessly eat a plate of homemade cookies while watching TV. That is a shameful waste of a delicious food. So when you finally pull that hot tray of cookies out of the oven, put one on a plate and spend *time* with it.

**Light some candles, put on some soft music, and get
downright *romantic* with your cookie.**

Take small bites. Chew thoroughly. Savor the flavor, smell, and texture. Make it last. Share the experience with a friend or your family, or simply enjoy the quiet time. Since we indulge partly to provide mental satisfaction, squeeze as much satisfaction as possible out of what you are eating.

With this approach, you should have plenty of time to notice that your craving has been satisfied, and that satisfaction has been achieved. So when it has, *stop eating*. Maybe that's half a cookie. Maybe it's four cookies. It doesn't matter, as long as you are mindful of the process every step of the way.

THE SLIPPERY SLOPE

If you're following this general prescription, your overall diet should be consistently moving you in the direction of "more healthy," with just enough "treats" to make the plan feel sustainable and satisfying. Please note, however:

Where you draw that line is entirely up to you.

One person's "healthy and balanced" may be another person's "I really need to clean things up!" In addition, where you draw the line, and which foods you crave, will most likely change as the years go on. Sure, we'll go out on a limb and say that 99 percent of the time "treat" equals processed or sugary food or drink. But with time and the reinforcement of your new habits, tastes, and awareness, your perception of what constitutes a treat *will* evolve.

THE 80/20 RULE Resist the urge to classify your overall diet in numerical terms—"I eat 90 percent healthy" or "I follow the 80/20 rule." First, it's a bit like scheduling a cheat day— you're practically setting yourself up to eat less-healthy foods a set percentage of the time. But more important, what does that number even *mean*? If you're "80/20," does that mean that one out of every five foods on your plate is less healthy? Or that every fifth meal is a highly processed sugar-fat-and-salt bomb? In addition, the food that makes up that 20 percent is of critical importance. If those "off plan" foods are peas, hummus, and corn tortillas, that's totally different than off-plan cookies, pizza, and dirty martinis. Long story short: Keep this process *intuitive* and *fluid*. Don't paint yourself into a corner with meaningless numbers or percentages!

Now at some point, we're betting that even with careful analysis of the "worth it" factor and the deliberate manner in which you enjoy and savor your treats, your overall diet will eventually start to slide from more healthy to less healthy. You may be a few weeks into the process of daily treats, overconsumption, and automatic eating before you even realize that you're spending more time in less-healthy territory than you mean to. Maybe you notice that you've gained a few pounds, you're not waking up as easily, or your energy levels aren't as consistently high. Maybe you're experiencing allergies, asthma, migraines, acne, aches and pains, or other symptoms of conditions that you *thought* you'd gotten rid of.

And at this point, you're likely to be discouraged. After all, you've been here before, haven't you, every time you've tried a new diet? You do well for a while, lose some weight, feel better. But then, usually sooner rather than later, you're back to your old habits and patterns, and it's as if nothing changed. But in this case, we want you to remember one very important fact:

This is not that scenario.

You are no longer on a diet. In fact, you will never have to "diet" again! You have used the Whole30 to change your habits, gain awareness, and establish a new, healthy relationship with food. This is your *lifestyle* now— and though things might not be as good as they could be at this very moment, please do not panic.

Because this time, you've got all the tools you need to get yourself right back on track.

Whole30 (or Whole7, or Whole14) to the rescue!

All you have to do to regain that awareness, reset those good habits, and remind yourself how amazing clean eating makes you look, feel, and live is to jump right back on the Whole30. And while you can if you want to, you don't always have to do the program in full! There's no reason that you can't follow Whole30 rules for a weekend, a week, two weeks … just long enough for your body and your brain to remember how good you feel, how delicious healthy food tastes, and how much you enjoy this way of eating. Once you're back on solid ground, kick off your training wheels and head right back out into the real world, with your newly reinforced knowledge, habits, and awareness keeping you as safe as a bike helmet.

See? Easy!

In addition, one of the best parts of our program is that each of your Whole30s builds on the last one. This means that as you stay connected with our program, your periods of slipping back into bad habits will grow shorter and less frequent, and your clean-eating adventures will grow longer in duration (and easier). And of course, should some special occasion, vacation, or stressful event knock you right off your bike, the Whole30 will always be there to help you get right back on.

JOIN OUR COMMUNITY One of the most helpful factors in staying on track during your Whole30 and beyond is having a support network—people who believe in this approach, who have "been there, done that" and who can provide motivation, inspiration, encouragement, and accountability for one another. If you don't have a local community to reach out to, join ours! We host Whole30 programs monthly and have a thriving, supportive community on our Web site (http://forum.whole9life.com) and Facebook page (http://facebook.com/whole9).

FRIENDS AND FAMILY

Seeking (and obtaining) support from family and friends is another important part of your good-health transformation. Some may offer support unconditionally, others may start paying attention once they notice the changes in your appearance, mood, attitude, and health. But we feel it's fair to warn you—despite the fact that you're taking healthy, sustainable steps to improve your quality of life, you may encounter negative reactions, too.

"All that fat can't be good for you."

"It's just another fad diet."

"It's so restrictive—you can't eat anything!"

We're sorry, but you'll probably hear all this and more, regardless of the life-changing results you achieve through the program and your hard work.

It can be tough enough to stick to your guns, let alone have to defend yourself against the onslaught of negativity-doubt-criticism from family, friends, and coworkers. So here are some of our best tips for dealing with the naysayers in a way that won't get you divorced, defriended, or fired.

Lead by quiet example.

This one is first for a reason, and it's your most powerful ally. *Your Whole30 results will speak for themselves.* And in the months to follow, when your energy is high, your skin is glowing, your aches and pains are gone, and you've shed some fat or built some muscle, people will notice, and they will ask you what you've been doing. It's hard to doubt the method when the proof of its value is staring them in the face, so let your experience shine through, and answer questions if asked—but don't waste your breath proselytizing. Just be a living example of what the Whole30 could do for them.

A HORSE AND HIS WATER This is perhaps the hardest lesson to learn. Chances are, you feel *amazing* right now. You want to shout from the rooftops about this plan you've discovered and the results you've experienced. And, if you have friends and family members who could use a little help with their health, it's all too tempting to start preaching the Good Food word. Just remember, you can lead them to water ... but your friends and family may not be ready to take a drink. Be patient—when they're ready, they'll come to you.

Pick your battles.

You can make people feel bad about their food choices *just* by rolling up to the table. The way you eat may remind people that they aren't eating the way they should, or might want to. So they'll be on the defensive the minute the waiter sets your salmon and veggies down next to their macaroni and cheese or BLT with fries.

But beware—now is *not* the time to point out the dangers of grains, or comment on the correlations between diet soda and obesity. Keep your lunch to yourself, and encourage others to do the same by ignoring snide remarks or attacks on your "weird diet." If someone is truly interested, have the conversation away from the crowd (and the food), when you can speak privately and not be interrupted by the criticism of others.

Educate yourself.

You know you'll have to deal with questions, comments, and challenges from time to time, so you'd better be prepared. If we asked you right now, "Why aren't you eating grains?" how many of you would have an answer on the tips of your tongues? Your answer could range from the fact that grain proteins are potentially inflammatory to the fact that when you gave up bread your stomach lost its bloat—anything from scientific data to personal experience. The point is, you'd *better* have an answer, and it can't just be, "Because Dallas and Melissa said so." (Although we do like that answer.)

So, do your homework. Be able to explain why you don't eat certain foods. Memorize our Web address. Prepare some remarks based on your own experience. Just don't show up empty-handed, because if you do, you'll lose any chance you may have had to get the other party to buy in. And if that other party is your mom, who shops for all the family's food; your husband, who cooks all the food; or your roommate, who pays for half the food, you really can't afford to lose that chance.

On that note, however …

Refer to "scientific evidence" cautiously.

We're not saying you shouldn't research and cite the conclusions of scientific studies. What we *are* saying, however, is that for every science-y article you find that talks about, say, how dairy can create hormonal disruption … there are a hundred *just* as science-y articles that will say the exact opposite.

Our recommendation? Unless you're totally up to speed with scientific references and able to smartly refute the opposing side on the fly, don't let the scientific research be the only leg you choose to stand on. Lead by example, the first line of defense, and cite *real* people who have had *real* results. Which brings us to our final point …

When outnumbered, fall back.

You may very well find yourself stuck in a battle that you just can't win. It's a family dinner, and you're being hammered with questions, skepticism, and outright criticism. So take a deep breath, smile, and simply fall back. In the end, the only person's health and wellness you are responsible for is *yours*. And while it may pain you to witness the unhealthy behaviors of your friends and family, they are, ultimately, responsible for their own lives, and their own choices.

So rather than spark a bitter feud and ruin a family gathering, swallow your ego and your frustration and simply say, "Well, this is actually working really well for me right now, but I do appreciate your thoughts. Now let's get back to enjoying this delicious meal!" Sometimes, that's all you can do … and that's OK. Refer back to our first point: If people are open to change, *they* will eventually come to *you*, and you'll get the opportunity to help them change their lives too.

A FAMILY AFFAIR You may at some point find yourself faced with a dilemma—eating something less healthy that you really don't want to eat, or hurting someone's feelings by refusing. Handle these situations delicately. First, if the food in question is seriously going to affect your health, then you have to speak up. Your loved ones don't want to make you sick, so if they simply didn't realize that you don't tolerate dairy well, explain (without getting too graphic) and politely decline the dish. If it's just a matter of preference—you don't want the dessert, but your mom made it special for the occasion—then it's best to go with the flow. Accept a small piece, eat just enough to participate in the celebration, and deal with the consequences—which will be nowhere near as serious as turning down the triple-layer chocolate cake your mom spent the afternoon making just for you.

Finally, there are some "special populations" that could benefit from the program by modifying our general recommendations to accommodate their medical conditions, lifestyle, or nutritional needs. Let's talk about those now.

CHAPTER 21:
FINE-TUNING FOR SPECIAL POPULATIONS

"I was diagnosed with my first autoimmune disease at 19—autoimmune hepatitis. Then seven years later, I was diagnosed with lupus. I had a rash on the face, mouth sores, fatigue, hair falling out, swollen, painful joints, shortness of breath. Then, my kidneys started to fail, and I was diagnosed with lupus-induced swelling of the brain. I started chemo treatments, reached remission, then came out of remission in 2010. Nothing worked—I was heading toward dialysis and more chemo. During all of these years, I gained weight from the steroids, and my legs were was so full of water my skin would crack. This is when my cousin told me about the Whole30, and how it helped her arthritis. In the first week, my pulse fell from 98 to 78. It only took the Whole30 seven days to get the water out of my legs! I could see and feel the inflammation leaving my body. My BP is now 120/80, and my blood sugar is more regular. I feel great, I have energy to make it through the day and then some, and most importantly, I'm pain-free. Your program has changed my life—if not saved it."

—Heather B., Stevens Point, Wisconsin

While we believe that our dietary recommendations, and our Whole30 program, would benefit everyone, there is no one-size-fits-all nutritional plan. There are those with specific medical conditions, lifestyles, or activity levels who may require the modification of our general guidelines to achieve optimal results.

If you fall into one of these categories, feel free to make the adjustments that we're going to recommend during your Whole30 program and beyond.*

Please note, we are not doctors, and cannot "prescribe" a treatment, dietary or otherwise, for your particular medical condition. We always recommend speaking with your health-care provider before undertaking any new nutritional protocol.

DIABETES

This program is *ideal* for managing blood sugar and insulin levels, and for preventing (and even reversing!) type 2 diabetes. We have seen first-hand the effects of our Whole30 program and healthy-eating guidelines on those with both type 1 and type 2 diabetes, and the scientific literature also supports our protocol.

However, diabetics must work very closely with their doctors to ensure that the powerful effects of these dietary changes are monitored and medications are properly adjusted. We have seen dramatic results in as little as one week, with one client being able to cut his oral medication in *half*. Radical improvements, in just seven days—which means that you'll need to speak with your doctor *before* making changes in your diet, so that together you can decide how to monitor and adjust your medications.

In addition, those with type 1 diabetes will need to make changes far more gradually than the Whole30 program calls for. Start with *small* modifications to meals, gradually substituting your "less healthy" foods for high-quality meats, vegetables, fruits, and fats. Working with your doctor, adjust your insulin dose and/or oral medication as necessary to accommodate these new foods, until you've successfully replaced all the less-healthy foods on your plate with more-healthy choices.

AUTOIMMUNE DISEASE

Our protocol is ideal for normalizing an overactive immune system, reducing systemic inflammation, and minimizing (or eliminating) symptoms related to an autoimmune disease. There are some additional caveats with respect to our autoimmune guidelines, however, as certain foods that are generally "safe" for many people may provoke inflammation in those with an autoimmune disease. Since your margin of error is that much smaller, you may want to consider removing these additional items from your daily diet.

- **Eggs (whole eggs and egg whites):** Egg whites contain proteins that can adversely stimulate the immune system—a contributing factor in autoimmune diseases. We recommend that those suffering from autoimmune diseases avoid eggs for at least ninety days, to evaluate sensitivity.

- **Nightshades:** Nightshades are a group of plants that contain compounds that promote gut irritability, inflammation, and joint pain or and stiffness in sensitive individuals. Nightshades include white potatoes, tomatoes, sweet and hot peppers, eggplant, tomatillos, tamarios, pepinos, and spices like cayenne, chili powder, curry powder, paprika, pepper sauce, pimento, and crushed red pepper flakes. We recommend avoiding nightshades for at least ninety days, to evaluate sensitivity.
- **Dairy (including heavy cream, clarified butter, and ghee):** Milk solids (proteins), even the trace amounts found in ghee, can be problematic if you have an autoimmune disease. For this reason, you should avoid all dairy products during your Whole30, and potentially indefinitely.
- **Nuts and Seeds:** Nuts and seeds contain compounds that may be inflammatory in those with an autoimmune condition. Consider other sources of dietary fat per our recommendations.
- **NSAIDs:** Nonsteroidal anti-inflammatory drugs like aspirin, ibuprofen (Advil, Motrin), naproxen (Aleve), and Celebrex disrupt the lining of the gut, leading to intestinal permeability, a contributing factor in autoimmune disease. For pain relief, Tylenol (which is not an NSAID) is a better choice—or ask your doctor about other pain-control strategies.

IBS AND IBD

Medical professionals agree that our general recommendations and Whole30 program are safe, healthy, and effective for those with IBS (irritable bowel syndrome), IBD (inflammatory bowel disease) and similar digestive disorders. However, having a serious digestive disorder does require you to follow some protocols specific to your type of inflammation. These modifications should make your transition easier.

In addition, those with IBD (Crohn's disease or ulcerative colitis) should also adopt our autoimmune protocol, especially with respect to eggs and nightshades. Only after you have seen symptomatic improvement and, ideally, improvement in inflammatory lab markers, would we recommend reintroducing these foods, starting with eggs first, and then night-shades.

- **Vegetables:** Eat plenty of fiber-rich vegetables, but make sure they are cooked thoroughly, as this makes their fiber content way less likely to cause problems. We also recommend that you prepare veggies by first chopping them into small pieces, which makes it easier to guarantee thorough cooking, or to add them to soups or stew.
- **Fruit:** Be cautious with fruit consumption, as there are strong links between fructose malabsorption and IBS. Make sure you peel all fruit, avoid what you can't peel (like grapes and cherries), and eat your fruit as ripe as possible. You should also avoid fruits that have seeds and a rough exterior (like berries). Although no one knows why for sure, many IBS sufferers report increased symptoms after consuming citrus fruits, so we recommend avoiding those as well. Finally, dried fruits and fruit juices pack too much sugar into a small package for folks with serious GI disturbances.
- **Nuts and Seeds:** Avoid all nuts and seeds. They can be profoundly inflammatory in the intestinal tract, mostly because of their physical structure. (They can "scrape" the intestinal lining, causing discomfort when inflammation is already present.) This includes nut butters, even the "creamy" kind.
- **Coffee:** Avoid coffee—even decaffeinated. Coffee is a powerful GI-tract irritant, and even decaffeinated coffee can trigger abdominal spasms and diarrhea in IBS/IBD patients. In addition, caffeinated coffee is a double-whammy, as caffeine speeds up every system in the body (including the colon), which can lead to diarrhea, followed by constipation. Coffee can also increase stomach acid, which can contribute to inflammation in the GI tract.
- **Water:** Drink plenty of water throughout the day, but *not* with your meal, as it can inhibit proper digestion by diluting stomach acid and digestive enzymes.
- **Fish Oil:** Consider taking a high-quality fish oil. (See Chapter 22 for details.) Fish oil supplements containing omega-3 fatty acids have been proven a complementary or alternative treatment for IBD.

Finally, understand that your digestion may get *worse* before it gets *better*. As your GI tract starts to heal, your mucosal layer will adjust, unhealthy gut bacteria will start to die off, healthy bacteria will begin to repopulate, and the intestinal lining will start to rebuild itself, plugging gaps and filling in holes. This can lead to gas, bloating, diarrhea, or constipation. In conditions such as IBD and IBS, it's not uncommon for digestive issues to continue for three to six months after making such radical dietary changes—but it is a *necessary* first step in restoring normal, healthy gut integrity.

ADDITIONAL FACTORS Note, there are other food groups that may potentially be inflammatory or digestively disruptive— like FODMAPs (see page 119), high-oxalate foods, or high-histamine foods. If you've been following the Whole30 and these special protocols for sixty to ninety days and are still experiencing digestive issues or other autoimmune-related symptoms, consider working with a qualified nutritionist or functional-medicine practitioner to help you arrive at an ongoing protocol that will work for your particular condition and symptoms. A food journal can also help you identify potentially "healthy" foods that may be triggering unpleasant symptoms. Write down all the foods in your meals and snacks for a week, and note the severity and type of symptoms you experience after each to try to pinpoint the culprit(s).

FOOD ALLERGIES

This may seem like a no-brainer, but we get plenty of questions from people asking if they can follow our plan if they are allergic to eggs, seafood, nuts, or avocado.

The answer is, yes, of course! Just don't eat the foods you are allergic to.

If you suspect that you have an allergy or intolerance to any one food, please don't test your limits during your Whole30 program.

You want to *completely eliminate* your exposure to any potentially inflammatory compound during your Whole30, so avoid that food or food group. None of the foods on our shopping list are mandatory—and there are plenty of healthy options in each category (protein, vegetable, good fat), so it should be easy for you to make appropriate choices.

In addition, your "allergy" to certain foods may not be a *true* allergy—it may just be an intolerance or sensitivity, in which case, it *may* be reversible. Many have reported the reduction or elimination of food "allergies" after successful completion of their Whole30. Perhaps by eliminating intestinal permeability and restoring normal gut flora and fauna, your body's immune system will relax enough to permit the reintroduction of certain foods.

However, this process requires at least six months of absolutely *no* exposure to the problematic food, and may not be safe or feasible for those with long-standing, life-threatening allergies. Work closely with your doctor and test this cautiously, please.

VEGETARIANS AND VEGANS

These particular lifestyle choices do present more of a challenge to our nutritional recommendations and Whole30 program. While our diet is not exclusively carnivorous, we do recommend the inclusion of animal protein for optimal health. However, it is still possible to reap many of the benefits of our healthy-eating plan while still honoring your ethical or religious obligations.

HEALTH-CONSCIOUS If your primary reason for becoming vegetarian or vegan was for health, we certainly hope we have made you reconsider! We don't believe you can enjoy optimal health without eating animal protein (dairy doesn't count), and we think we've provided a well-reasoned, well-sourced argument to back up our position. So if this is where you are coming from, give our plan a try! Go back to eating high-quality animal protein for thirty days (while implementing the rest of our recommendations) as a self-experiment. We'd be shocked if your health did not dramatically improve!

If you'll eat some animal products (eggs, fish, etc.), then we recommend getting the bulk of your protein from these sources and supplementing with plant-based sources as little as possible. If your concerns are largely ethical—animal welfare, sustainability, your local economy, or global economic factors—know that there *are* ways to responsibly, ethically source meat, seafood, and eggs and supporting those efforts sends a strong message (financial and otherwise) to the large corporations invested in factory farming. We believe it is important to create an alternative food-supply system, but that cannot be done without the support of committed consumers.

If dairy is a viable source of protein, we recommend putting pastured, organic, fermented sources like yogurt or kefir at the top of your list. You could also use whey protein powder from grass-fed, organic sources, which would provide the protein you need with fewer downsides than other dairy products, including all forms of milk and cheese.

If you don't eat any animal products, or if you find you still need to supplement your diet with plant-based protein sources, your best choices are minimally-processed, fermented soy products like tempeh or natto, or organic edamame (soybeans). You can also include nonfermented soy (like extra-firm tofu) and various legumes in rotation, making sure to soak them for twelve to twenty-four hours, rinse, and boil them for at least fifteen minutes to reduce the anti-nutrient and inflammatory compounds. A hemp- or pea-protein powder is also an option for you.

Avoid all grains and grain products, including seitan (which is made from wheat gluten) and pseudo-cereals like quinoa, as the downsides are too numerous. In addition, vegans will need to eat more carbohydrate and fat, to cover the missing calories from their relatively low protein diet.

VEGETARIAN SHOPPING LIST

You can download a free copy of our shopping list for vegetarians and vegans on our Web site (http://whole9life.com/itstartswithfood). In addition, refer to Appendix B for responsibly-sourced animal and vegetarian protein.

ACTIVE INDIVIDUALS

If you exercise regularly or play a sport, you'll need to support that activity with extra nutrition and calories. Remember, your energy stores function like gas in your car. The more you drive, the quicker you'll use up the gas in your tank.

Lower-intensity activity, like casual cycling, walking, hiking, or golf, burns more fat than carbohydrate, so you may not need to load up on starch on a daily basis. However, if you participate in high-intensity activity (like CrossFit, P90X, sprinting, or basketball) or longer-duration activities, like running or biking, you will probably need to include more carbohydrate than the average (less-active) person in your daily meals to maintain adequate glycogen stores. Throw in some carb-dense veggies like sweet potato, butternut squash, acorn squash, beets, pumpkin, or parsnips, and perhaps bump up your protein and fat and/or add an extra meal.

WHAT IS HIGH INTENSITY?

"High intensity" means the exercise is brief and you are close to an "all-out" effort. Often, it's based on the rate of perceived exertion (RPE), how hard you *think* you're working. You could also use heart rate to determine the level of your intensity, especially if you're new to this of kind of training. If you are working above 75 percent of your max heart rate (conversation is impossible, save for short phrases or one-word bursts), that's generally considered high-intensity effort. From our perspective, high-intensity training generally lasts less than ten or fifteen minutes—any longer, and you simply cannot continue to sustain near-maximal output. However, some exercise programs include workouts that last longer than that and expect participants to work as hard as possible the entire time. For the purposes of this discussion, we'll call these training sessions "high intensity" too.

In addition, for those participating in either high-intensity or longer-duration activity, you'll need to support your training session or athletic event with proper nutrition to help you fuel and recover.

- **Pre-Workout:** Your pre-workout "snack" is *not* fuel for your workout! You've got tens of thousands of calories stored in your body—plenty to support your activity. Your pre-workout food simply sends a signal to your body to prepare it for the activity that is coming. Eat fifteen to seventy-five minutes before your workout, choosing foods that are easily digestible and palatable—the timing is highly variable and depends on what your gastrointestinal tract can tolerate before physical activity. Focus on protein and fat and avoid lots of fruit or carb-dense vegetables. Remember, elevated insulin levels undermine glucagon's energy-access function—and you need your energy stores during a training scssion. A pre-workout snack might be: two hard-boiled eggs, some deli turkey and a small handful of macadamia nuts, or a few strips of beef jerky. If you exercise first thing in the morning, a little something is better than nothing, so do the best you can.

- **Post-Workout:** Your post-workout meal is a special "bonus meal" designed to help you start the recovery process faster and more effectively. After you train, your muscles and connective tissue need protein, and your glycogen stores *may* need replenishing. Eat your post-workout meal as soon as possible—ideally, within fifteen to thirty minutes of training. Bring it to the gym or competition site! Have a meal-size serving of an easily digestible protein and add carbohydrate in the form of starchy vegetables based on your activity level and health status. Fruit is not your best choice here. Fructose-rich fruit will preferentially replenish *liver* glycogen, but your *muscles* did all the hard work. A good post-workout meal might be: chicken breast and sweet potato, salmon and butternut squash, or egg whites mixed into mashed pumpkin. Eat a normal meal sixty to ninety minutes after your post-workout meal.

All high-intensity exercisers need protein post-workout, but whether to include carbohydrate depends on the type of activity and metabolic status. If you are lean, muscular, healthy (insulin sensitive), and performance-oriented, you have a totally different context than someone who is overweight, metabolically deranged, and trying to get back on track with his health. For that reason, we recommend following our "post-workout carb curve," which accounts for both your particular health status and the type and duration of activity.

- **Duration:** On the left side of the chart, find the number that corresponds to the total duration of the high-intensity portion of your exercise session. If you were at the gym for an hour, but spent only twelve minutes actually working hard, then 12 is your number.
- **Health Status:** Identify where your current state of health lies along the spectrum at the bottom of the chart. It's subjective, but it's just a conceptual guideline.

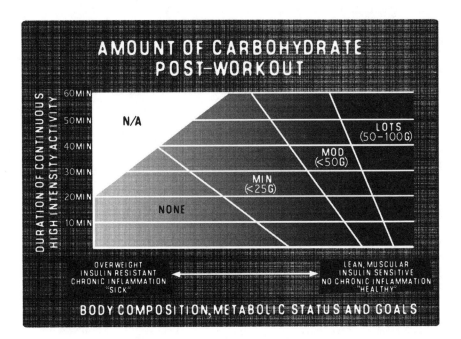

- **Post-Workout Carb Intake**: Use those two coordinates to plot the point that determines the approximate amount of carbohydrate you should consume after each high-intensity training session.

If your health status is toward the left end of the continuum, perhaps just starting to exercise and eat healthier, restoring your *health* takes priority over fueling your athletic performance. In that case, we don't think you need carbohydrate post-workout, regardless of the duration of your high-intensity activity. You have thousands of calories stored in your body already, and adding a bunch of carbs in any one sitting isn't the smartest hormonal strategy when you're already insulin resistant. Therefore, your post-workout meal should include *only* protein.

THE X FACTOR   Notice how there's a big "N/A" area on our chart? That's because we don't think it's appropriate for overweight, insulin-resistant, inflamed folks to work out hard for longer than twenty minutes straight. Adding more stress to an already over-stressed system is counterproductive to improving health. So keep your workouts either long in duration *or* high in intensity—but not both. As always, context matters.

If you are closer to the lean, healthy, performance-oriented end of the spectrum, you'll need to start replenishing calories (and glycogen stores) after even short-duration activity to maintain performance levels and muscle mass. Follow our recommendations and include both protein and varying levels of carbohydrate in your post-workout window.

PREGNANT AND BREASTFEEDING WOMEN

If you are pregnant or breast-feeding, you know how important Mom's nutrition is to her baby's health and development, and we believe that the diet that's healthiest for *you* is also going to be the healthiest for your baby. The more nutrition Mom receives from her diet, the more she is able to pass along to the little one—and there is no diet more nutritious than one that focuses on healthy protein and fat, vegetables, and fruits.

ASK THE DOCTOR Dr. Michele Blackwell, OB-GYN, has done our Whole30 program herself and recommends it to her pregnant and breast-feeding patients. Dr. Blackwell says, "I wholeheartedly recommend the Whole30 plan to my patients to optimize a woman's health during pregnancy and lactation. The nutrient-dense foods recommended provide ample vitamins and minerals without the need for the standard prenatal supplement. Eating in this manner will also help regulate blood sugars, alleviating hypoglycemic spells common in pregnancy."

However, you'll want to make some minor tweaks to your healthy-eating plan, as your nutritional needs (and those of your baby) are different during these special times. Recommendations for pregnancy include:

- **Protein:** A very high protein diet isn't the healthiest thing for your baby, and may contribute to low birth weight, poor feeding, and other longer-term effects. Pregnant women should limit protein consumption to *no more than* 20 percent of total calories. (Nature usually helps us out here—many women report an aversion to, or loss of appetite for, protein during pregnancy.)

- **Total Calories:** While pregnant, it's critical for you to consume enough calories. Make sure you are incorporating more starchy vegetables and healthy fats into your diet to make sure you're not underfeeding yourself or your baby. Sipping on a can of coconut milk throughout the day is a easy way to add calories.

- **Omega-3 Fatty Acids:** EPA and especially DHA provide excellent benefits for your baby's neurological and early visual development, and may reduce the risk of pregnancy complications like preeclampsia, gestational diabetes, postpartum depression, and pre-term delivery. We recommend shooting for 300 mg of DHA per day while you are pregnant (but do not exceed a total of 1 gram of EPA and DHA combined).

- **Prenatal Vitamins:** The problem with most prenatal vitamins is that they contain too many potentially harmful nutrients (like iron and folic acid) and not enough of what a pregnant woman really needs (like vitamins D_3 and K_2). It's best to meet as many of your nutritional needs as possible with food, even while pregnant. That said, the recommended amounts of certain nutrients, like folate, vitamin K_2, and vitamin D, during pregnancy may be difficult to obtain solely through diet. For this reason, taking a prenatal vitamin with the appropriate nutrients in the right dosages and forms may be a good insurance policy. You want at least 1,000 IUs of vitamin D_3, 500 mcg of vitamin K_2 (MK-4 form), and 800 mcg of folate (not folic acid). A good choice is Nutrient 950 with vitamin K from Pure Encapsulations.

While breast-feeding, the same protein restrictions are not necessary. However, breast-feeding mothers need to make sure their hydration and caloric intake are adequate for ongoing lactation. Most women's appetites are stimulated when they breast-feed, and increasing fat intake is the best way to keep up the calories. Keep coconut milk or individual packets of coconut butter on hand, or snack on olives or avocado—and make sure you always have a bottle of water on standby.

Omega-3 supplementation is just as important while breast-feeding as it is during pregnancy. Continue taking the same daily dose of EPA and DHA while you are lactating.

KIDS

Once again, we believe that the diet that is healthiest for us grown-ups is also healthiest for growing children. There isn't a single nutrient in cereals, biscuits, or formulas that can't also be found in healthy meats, vegetables, and fruits!

For infants, breast milk is the perfect food. The scientific literature supports the health benefits of breast milk, reporting that infants who are breast-fed have lower rates of respiratory illness and ear infections as babies, and lower rates of type 1 diabetes, asthma, and allergies as adults. Better yet, babies who are breast-fed longer grow up to have higher IQs than those who are breast-fed for fewer months. Because of the numerous advantages breast milk provides for an infant's development, we encourage mothers to breast-feed for longer than twelve months, if possible.

Once your infant is weaned, there is no need to supplement his or her real-food diet with cow's milk! Once a cow starts eating grass, it does not return to suckle—that's simply not natural, biologically appropriate behavior. And while cow's milk perfectly supports the needs of a rapidly growing calf, your baby has different nutritional requirements.

Since your kids are working so hard to grow into adults (though we can't imagine why they want to do that), they need plenty of calories to support growth, activity, and normal cognitive development. But eating well isn't *just* about getting adequate protein, fat, and carbohydrates—*micronutrients* also contribute significantly to our health, and that of our children. One significant reason that fresh, unprocessed foods like meat, vegetables, fruit, and good fats are so healthy is that these foods supply generous amounts of vitamins, minerals, and phytonutrients—the stuff that directly benefits your child's health. Choosing foods that supply adequate calories and copious amounts of micronutrition is the "best-case scenario" for growing kids, from toddlers to teenagers.

Your child's diet should comprise nutrient-dense foods that require minimal preparation—beef, chicken, and fish; sweet potato, carrots, and spinach; blueberries, cantaloupe, and plums; avocado, olives, and coconut milk.

Sound familiar?

It should!

As we've mentioned once or twice, eating Good Food confers a *host* of benefits on us adults, including effortless weight management, decreasing systemic inflammation, optimizing hormonal levels, and reducing the risk for a number of lifestyle-related diseases and conditions. And kids are just adults-in-the-making, right? This same food promotes *their* healthy immune function, supports activity and growth, and contributes a wide variety of micronutrients that have been shown to decrease risk of (and improve) conditions such as asthma, allergies, ADHD, and various autoimmune diseases.

On the opposite end of the spectrum, much in the way foods like sugar, grains, legumes, and dairy negatively affect *our* health, they also have a negative impact our children's health—perhaps even more so, as their immature immune system and GI tract can be even more vulnerable than ours. Even in the youngest of us, typical "kid foods" like milk, yogurt, cereal, peanut butter, and bread can promote systemic inflammation, create immune system dysfunction, and increase the risk of diseases like type 1 diabetes.

Lots of parents we've talked to say, "But my kids don't like vegetables ..." or, "But my son *loves* his sugary breakfast cereals." This is where we often get into trouble, asking, "Does your toddler do his own grocery shopping?" Admittedly, we don't know how difficult it is to try to take away a child's Golden Grahams—although we can imagine, knowing how hard it is for our adult Whole30 participants to change *their* eating habits. But until your children are buying their own food with their own money, you as the parent are the single largest supplier of your child's nutritional needs. And we believe it's just as critical to your children's long-term success to feed them healthy food as it is to make sure they don't drop out of school after the third grade.

Admittedly, getting kids to love Good Food is easier said than done, especially if they're accustomed to sweeter, more processed foods. But we think that there are few parental duties more noble than loving your children wholeheartedly, and feeding them as best you can.

Even if you have to fight them on it.

Even if they go to bed hungry for a night or two.

Even if you have to resort to the old standbys:

It's for your own good. Because I said so.

CHAPTER 22:
SUPPLEMENT YOUR HEALTHY DIET

"I've had rheumatoid arthritis since childhood. As a waitress, I used to get to the end of the day, and my feet, knees, and hips would hurt so much. My joints were always swollen and stiff, and I've tried numerous medications that failed to provide relief. After consulting with Dallas and Melissa, I changed my diet and started taking a high-quality fish oil to help get my inflammation in check. After my Whole30, I was completely pain-free for the first time since diagnosis. My joint stiffness and swelling were gone, I was able to go off my medication, and I no longer hurt after a long day on my feet. And I've been able to maintain my pain-free status as long as I stay compliant with my program."

—Amber H., Kelowna, British Columbia, Canada

While the idea of getting all of your necessary micronutrition from real food, water, and your environment sounds lovely, it's not always feasible. We're not 100 percent perfect eaters, and our food and environment don't always supply us with the nutrition we need—even if we're eating Good Food on a regular basis.

In some cases, supplementing with natural compounds already found in the healthy foods we eat, and in our natural environments, can help us shore up our already excellent nutrition. But hear us clearly:

You cannot supplement your way out of a poor diet.

Vitamins and other supplements may *promise* to supply the missing nutrients we're not getting from our food or our environment—but that's a promise yet to be fulfilled. Nutrients delivered by foods taken directly from their natural environment (like vegetables, fruit, and meat) contain phytonutrients and enzymes that are not—and in some cases *cannot be*—

included in any supplement. And remember, these micronutrients work synergistically with other compounds *in your total diet* to provide their health-promoting benefits.

PROMISES, PROMISES It's no wonder studies show that vitamin and mineral supplements don't work the same way as the vitamins and minerals found in your food. For example, vitamin C from real food helps prevent many types of cancer and cardiovascular disease, but vitamin C from a bottle doesn't seem to have the same protective effects. And a diet high in antioxidant-rich vegetables and fruits is associated with a lower risk for many chronic diseases, but there isn't much evidence to support the use of antioxidant supplements to prevent disease.

Our takeaway is this: Supplements can never replicate the awesome effects of eating real food. However, that doesn't mean supplements can't support an otherwise healthy diet. There is plenty of evidence to suggest that certain supplements (like fish oil or vitamin D_3) have benefits in the context of a healthy lifestyle that includes eating Good Food. Think about it this way:

Dietary supplements are a *supplementation* to, not a *substitution* for, a balanced, nutrient-dense diet.

So what are our supplement all-stars? Our (short) list follows. These are substances already present in a healthy diet and environment that show clear benefit in the research. Now, we're not saying you *have* to take these supplements, nor are we saying you should. We are simply discussing compounds that we believe have health-promoting properties and may be able to support your already healthy diet.*

FISH OIL

You only need to do a quick Web search to discover the benefits of fish oil, because there is a *wealth* of scientific literature on this subject. The omega-3 fatty acids, particularly the long-chain forms found in fish oil

---

*And it goes without saying—check with your doctor before taking any new supplements.

(EPA and DHA), have been well-documented to have health-promoting effects, including improvement in blood chemistry and a reduced risk for a number of lifestyle-related diseases and conditions. EPA and DHA are natural anti-inflammatory agents, and as such play a role in brain and heart health; protection from cancer, Alzheimer's, and depression; improvement of skin conditions like psoriasis and acne; fetal brain development; inflammatory bowel disorders; and arthritis, to name a few.

FATTY-ACID FLASHBACK Remember, EPA and DHA are specific types of polyunsaturated omega-3 fatty acids. Your body cannot produce them—you must get them from food or supplements. EPA and DHA are found in high-quality (grass-finished, pastured, wild-caught) meat, seafood, and eggs and in fish oil supplements.

Reducing the amount of omega-6 fatty acids in your diet; eating high-quality meat, seafood, and eggs to maximize omega-3 intake; and supplementing with a high-quality fish oil all help to reduce systemic inflammation and the wide range of downstream effects. However, remember that in the case of all polyunsaturated fats, some is good, but more is not better. We don't want to overdo our fish oil intake, as too much PUFA in the diet (even the healthy kind) may promote oxidation and inflammation in the body.

If you're eating lots of grass-finished meat and wild-caught, cold-water fish (like salmon or mackerel), you may not need to supplement with fish oil at all. However, if your meat quality isn't perfect, or if you frequently dine out or travel (and are exposed to omega-6-rich seed oils in restaurant cooking), you may want to consider a daily dose of fish oil.

General recommendations: 2 to 4 grams of EPA + DHA daily.*

Look for a concentrated omega-3-rich fish oil with lots of EPA and DHA per pill or teaspoon. (Skip the omega-3-6-9 blends—most people get more than enough omega-6 from their diets as it is.) We like Stronger Faster Healthier's liquid fish oil (http://strongerfasterhealthier.com) for a

---

For more information on fish oil supplementation, visit http://whole9life.com/fish-oil-faq.

few reasons. First, it's highly concentrated, with almost three grams of total EPA and DHA in just one teaspoon. Second, the ingredients are 100 percent natural—no sugar or unhealthy additives. Most important, it tastes pretty darn good for fish oil. See, the fish oil that sits in your fridge isn't actually anti-inflammatory. You actually have to *take* it. So five flavors of fish oil that actually taste good (and not at all fishy) make it far more likely that the "taking" part will happen.

CONTRAINDICATIONS One word of caution: Fish oil can affect blood clotting by inhibiting clotting factors and platelet aggregation. If you have a bleeding tendency, are on anticoagulant medications (like Coumadin), or are about to have surgery, talk to your physician about whether you should take fish oil.

In addition, because EPA and DHA are rather unstable when exposed to air, heat, and light, don't ever heat your fish oil! It's OK to add the lemon-flavored one to a cold salad dressing, but don't drizzle it over hot food or store it in warm places—in fact, we recommend storing it in the fridge, just to be safe.

VITAMIN D$_3$

This vitamin-that's-really-a-hormone should be no stranger at this point—we've mentioned the benefits of D$_3$ for everything from immune support to bone health. While vitamin D$_3$ is found in many foods (like meat and eggs), sun exposure is the biggest natural source of our vitamin D stores.

Skin cells are able to synthesize vitamin D$_3$ when the sun's UV-B rays hit the skin. If you're fair skinned, spending just ten minutes in the summertime sun (sunscreen-free, with arms and legs exposed) can produce about 10,000 IUs of the vitamin.

However, dark-skinned individuals and the elderly produce less vitamin D$_3$, and those who live in the Northern Hemisphere may not be able to produce enough vitamin D in the winter, as the sun may not get high enough in the sky for its UV-B rays to penetrate the atmosphere. Which means that many of us are walking around chronically deficient in vitamin

D_3 and at higher risk for conditions like osteoporosis, heart disease, and certain types of cancer.

Luckily, supplementation with vitamin D_3 is quite effective at replenishing and maintaining stores in the body. Of course, some is good, but more is not better. While you can't overdose on D_3 if you're getting it from the sun, some research suggests that supplementing with more than 10,000 IUs a day may be toxic.

**General recommendations: Up to 5,000 IUs daily,
depending on your geographical location and sun
exposure.**

Since D_3 is fat soluble, we recommend taking it first thing in the morning, with your fat-rich breakfast. Look for olive oil-based or "dry" D_3, not the stuff in soybean or corn oil. Yes, even with supplements, you need to read your labels!

MAGNESIUM

Magnesium is the fourth most abundant mineral in the body (but we bet you didn't know that, because its big brother, calcium, gets way more attention). About 50 percent of your body's magnesium is found in bone, the other half predominantly in tissues and organs.

Magnesium is critical to bone health but also plays a major role in muscle and nerve function, heart rhythm, immunity, regulation of blood sugar, and blood pressure. And from our own experience, we have found magnesium to be of great help for those who are having trouble obtaining restful sleep. In fact, we often call magnesium the "magic white powder," as it helps us fall asleep so easily!

Magnesium is found in many foods, including leafy greens (spinach, Swiss chard, mustard greens, and turnip greens), other vegetables and fruits, and several types of nuts and seeds. However, according to several studies and the World Health Organization, a substantial number of people in the United States are magnesium deficient. The processing of food and higher percentage of "junk food" in our diets have been contributing factors. Furthermore, many blame the depletion of our soil because of long-term industrial-farming practices, excessive use of fertilizers, changes in varieties of plants grown, and loss of microorganisms in the soil—if our soil doesn't contain as much magnesium as it used to, the plants we grow in that soil won't either.

Magnesium supplements come in many forms. A citrate form is generally well tolerated and easy for the body to absorb. Citrate can be taken in capsules, but we prefer a powder like unsweetened Natural Calm.

General recommendations: 1 to 3 teaspoons (200-600 mg) dissolved thoroughly in water shortly before bed every evening.

You can also get your mag the old-fashioned way—in an Epsom salt bath. Throw two cups of the salts in warm bath water and soak away—some of the magnesium in the salts will be absorbed by your skin.

TOO MUCH MAG One word of caution: Too much magnesium will have a laxative effect. This may be great for those suffering from constipation—a regular dose of magnesium may help alleviate that digestive issue—but for those of you who want to supplement without the extra bathroom "help," start your dose off small and gradually work your way up. You can always split your supplementation up into smaller doses throughout the day, or switch to an ionic or topical form of magnesium, if the citrate form is not well tolerated.

DIGESTIVE ENZYMES

Enzymes are proteins found in food (but mostly manufactured by your own body) that facilitate chemical reactions. These enzymes—and good mealtime habits, like the kind we describe in our meal-planning template—are critical for proper digestion.

Ideally, you'd all be eating whole, unprocessed foods, taking time to chew your food thoroughly to make it easier for your small intestine to absorb the nutrients. However, processing, cooking, gulping down meals, and drinking fluids while eating reduce the number of enzymes that make their way into the digestive tract—and may make it hard for your body to actually "use" (digest and absorb) the nutrients in the food you are eating.

Broad-spectrum digestive enzymes containing HCl and pepsin help your body break down fats, carbohydrates, and protein and maximize the amount of nutrition you are able to absorb. We like NOW Foods Super Enzymes, but any brand that contains HC1 and pepsin (and, ideally, papain and bromelain as well) would work.

General recommendations:
1 to 4 capsules with each meal.

Take a bite of food, the digestive enzyme(s), then the rest of your food If you feel any sort of "heat" in your stomach after taking your enzymes, back off by one of more pills per meal, as necessary.

PROBIOTICS

Remember way back in Chapter 6, when we talked about our "friendlies," those health-promoting gut bacteria? Our alliance with them is largely what helps regulate our delicately balanced immune activity, digest our food, absorb micronutrients, manufacture vitamins, and generally take up space that would otherwise be snapped up by pathogenic bacteria.

Balanced gut bacteria is the key here—the right kinds, in the right amounts. But many factors can cause our gut's bacterial population to become unbalanced—and that spells trouble.

Bacterial infections, the use of antibiotics, stress, alcohol, and specific dietary factors can disrupt the delicate balance of beneficial bacteria in our gut. If left unchecked, gut dysbiosis can contribute to a number of health conditions, including diabetes, obesity, cancers, and autoimmune disorders.

However, before you go running out to the store to stock up on (often expensive) probiotic supplements or buy out your local health-food market's sauerkraut supply, a word of caution.

There are about 500 different species of bacteria living in your gut.

Without knowing how much of which kind you have (and which ones you're missing), how will you know what kind of supplement to buy, and how much to take?

We're not big fans of willy-nilly supplementation with live bacteria. Remember, *balance* is key—and too many of *any* one kind could be problematic.

General recommendations: Don't dump a bunch of
probiotics into a disordered system without guidance or
testing.

So, if you suspect that your bacterial allies aren't so well organized, start by reaching out to your doctor or nutritionist for some testing. If you can't do the lab work, then you can still take steps to restore a healthy balance of bacteria with naturally fermented foods and drinks—an excellent choice for regular consumption.

However, *start slow* with raw (unpasteurized) sauerkraut, kimchi, kombucha beverages, or coconut-based kefirs. Overdoing fermented foods can also provoke some pretty ugly symptoms in people who have dysbiosis. This may mean as little as one tablespoon of "live cultures" from real food a day, working up to a higher "dose" as your gut adjusts to the infusion of new friends.

Another great helper for gut health and healing are bone broths—but you have to make your own, as the stuff in the store doesn't have nearly the same nutrition as homemade broths. Slow-cooking the bones extracts vital nutrients that are seldom consumed in our regular diets, including gelatin, glucosamine, and important amino acids that form the building blocks of a healthy, balanced digestive system.

Use our recipe in Appendix A, choosing bones from pastured, organic animals whenever possible. Start with a cup of bone broth a day, but feel free to increase your intake to a cup with each meal.

MULTI-VITAMINS

In response to the question, "Should I take a multi-vitamin," we generally answer with one word.

Meh.

We're pretty agnostic on the subject of "multi-vitamins"—supplements that include a wide range and variety of vitamins, minerals, and micronutrients. On one hand, we know that the nutrients we get from real food interact in complex and beautiful ways in our bodies, providing us with a level of health that supplements simply cannot match. On the other hand, it's idealistic to think that we can get perfect nutrition just from the foods we eat and our environment. After all, we don't always eat perfectly, and our modern world (the soil, the water, the seeds themselves) may not provide us with as much nutrition from our foods as it used to.

However, the micronutrients found in multivitamins are nowhere near as bioavailable as those found in real food, and some of the synthesized forms of vitamins contained in multivitamin supplements may actually be harmful.

General recommendations: May not hurt but probably won't help, either.

If taking a broad-spectrum multi-vitamin makes you feel good, go right ahead. But we certainly don't think it's a *necessary* addition to your already healthy diet and lifestyle.

FINAL THOUGHTS

While your initial introduction to our Good Food philosophy may be over, our journey together is just beginning! Improving your health and quality of life is a gradual, evolutionary process. Our Whole30 program is a great way to jump-start your healthy-eating transformation, but you will continue to develop your new, healthy-eating habits and relationships with food for the rest of your life. And we promise, working your new food selections and habits into a sustainable, satisfying lifestyle gets easier with practice.

Still, you'll probably want a little help, support, and guidance along the way, and we are more than happy to oblige. Our Web site (http://whole9life.com) is a wealth of resources, including an active forum where readers can post questions, connect with others, and share their experiences with like-minded people at various stages of their healthy-eating journeys. We encourage you to visit, participate, and become a part of our growing community.

Of course, while we believe your journey to optimal health *starts* with food, there are other factors that also play important roles. Health and fitness is multifactorial, and while nutrition is always the foundation, we also believe that you cannot focus on just one aspect of health at the exclusion of others. Sleep, exercise habits, and stress also factor into your personal health equation.

If your health is still suboptimal after many months (or years) of healthy eating per our recommendations, consider looking deeper into non-nutritional factors. At our seminars we often say, "Don't look for a nutrition solution to a lifestyle problem." So at some point, we encourage you to expand your scope of focus beyond food and start making positive, sustainable changes in other areas of your life too.

We have enjoyed sharing our stories and our message with you. Now we encourage you to do the same. Please visit our Web site or our Facebook page and tell us how the Whole30 and *It Starts With Food* has changed your life.

We wish you the best in health.

APPENDIX A

THE MEAL MAP

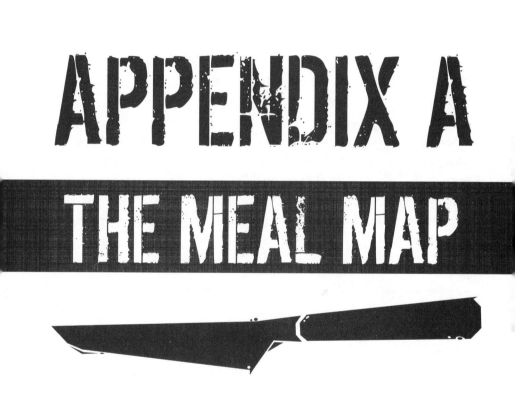

APPENDIX A:
THE MEAL MAP

"I've battled to control my reactive hypoglycemia for what seems like forever, even as a young child. I attempted to manage it by eating small meals throughout the day and followed the suggestion to try regularly timed, conventional 'round meals' when the constant snacking did not help. As a result of my uncontrolled and overaggressive insulin response, there were many times when I would wake up with paralyzing night sweats and heart palpitations. Since doing my first Whole30, I've been able to manage my blood sugar more easily than I ever have before, and I no longer have to think about food with fear. Whole30 has helped me to eat in normal intervals without having to constantly snack, and has finally given me the freedom to eat when I'm hungry!"

—Emily, Birmingham, Alabama

So, you've banished all the foods that make you less healthy from your pantry and stocked your kitchen with all the foods that make you healthier. Now what?

The easiest way to transition into your new eating habits is to focus on making meals based on yummy *ingredients* rather than trying to recreate complicated *recipes*. This approach has two advantages. For one thing, you don't have to worry about whether a recipe is compliant because you'll be basing all your meals around what are now familiar, approved ingredients. For another thing, you can create delicious meals that take a minimum amount of time and require only basic cooking skills.

The formula for a meal is simple:

ANIMAL PROTEIN + LOTS OF VEGETABLES + HIGH QUALITY FAT + SEASONINGS

Even if you think you "can't cook," this formula will make it easy for you to adapt your eating habits *without* stress and *with* lots of flavor. Our handy meal charts will help you improvise hundreds of nutritious, satisfying meals during your Whole30 and beyond.

OUR GOOD FOOD MEAL MAP

In this section, we'll give you enough mix-and-match ingredients to create a *year's* worth of meals, all 100 percent approved for your Whole30 program (and beyond). But take note—this is not a set-in-stone, thirty-day meal plan.

We will not decree that you must eat shrimp.

We aren't going to spell out which veggies to eat with each meal.

And we are not going to tell you what to eat a week from Tuesday.

We are all grown-ups, and at this point in our lives, no one should be telling us what to eat and when. As we've mentioned before, we are big fans of the "teach you how to fish" approach, which means that we'll give you all the *tools* you need to comfortably and competently start cooking (and eating) according to your new healthy-eating plan—but but you'll still have to plan and prepare meals yourself. The good news is, you get to eat them all yourself too.

Our basic Meal Map is structured like this:

MASTER RECIPES—PROTEIN AND VEGETABLES is where you'll find scores of easy-to-follow recipes for a variety of protein and vegetable options. We've organized some of our best ideas in our tasty charts, so you'll know exactly how to put together meat, veggies, and seasonings so you can go from cooking to eating in practically no time.

MASTER RECIPES—CURRIES AND SOUPS is your go-to for a complete meal-in-a-bowl. We've given you lots mix-and-match possibilities to suit your tastes and moods—and many can be whipped up in twenty minutes or less.

FINISHING TOUCHES—SAUCES SEASONINGS AND DRESSINGS will satisfy your need for a little drizzle of something flavorful to transform meat-and-vegetables into a feast worthy of a gourmet magazine. Experiment with the master recipes, and get in touch with your inner chef!

We've also given you recipes for three of our favorite when-you're-in-the-mood-to-really-cook-or-entertain meals.

QUICK AND EASY MEAL—A REALLY GREAT STEAK is a classic, and one of the great rewards of eating real food.

QUICK AND EASY MEAL—NO FUSS SALMON CAKES ties all your nutrients up in an eye-catching package. Keep your pantry stocked with the ingredients, and you'll always be just half an hour away from voilà!

FANCYPANTS MEAL—DELICIOUS DINNER PARTY is a mouth-watering menu of entrée, sides, and dessert which never fails to elicit oohs and ahhs, and is perfect for a special occasion or a random Wednesday.

Finally, when you're ready to dig into more detailed recipe creations, we've given you a list of cookbooks and Web sites with *thousands* of Good Food recipes in Appendix B—most of which are also Whole30 approved.

We promise, between our Meal Map and resources, you'll never, ever be bored with healthy eating.

MASTER RECIPES: PROTEIN

GROUND MEAT

Ground meat is very versatile and cooks quickly, so a variety of meals are only a few minutes away at any time. Experiment with beef, lamb, pork, turkey, and bison—we've given you ideas below to get you started. You might just discover a new favorite!

MASTER RECIPE—GROUND MEAT

1-2 Tbsp cooking fat · 1 medium onion, diced · 2 lbs ground meat (beef, bison, lamb, pork, turkey, or chicken) · salt and black pepper · garlic powder

Heat a large skillet over medium-high heat for about 3 minutes. Add cooking fat and allow it to melt. Add the onion, and sauté, stirring with a wooden spoon, until crisp-tender and translucent, about 5 minutes. Crumble the ground meat into the pan with your hands, then break up large chunks using the wooden spoon. Season generously with salt, pepper, and garlic powder. Continue to cook and stir until the meat has no pink spots, about 7-10 minutes. If you're not using grass-fed or pastured meat, drain the excess fat before you dig in.

To make a one-skillet meal, cook 1 to 2 cups of vegetables (see chart) per person. Then, place another 1 to 2 Tbsp cooking fat in a large skillet over medium-high heat. Add cooked ground meat and vegetables, and season according to the chart (seasoning amounts are *per person*). Sauté until heated through.

GROUND MEAT SKILLET RECIPES	NOTES
Asian Beef and Broccoli: ground beef · broccoli · carrots · red bell pepper · 1 tsp coconut aminos · ⅛ tsp each cinnamon and ginger	Serve on a bed of raw baby spinach for extra veggies. Sprinkle with toasted sesame seeds and sliced scallions. Add orange slices for dessert, just like you get in a Chinese restaurant.
Cashew or Almond Beef: ground beef · celery · green bell pepper · ¼ cup cashews or almonds · 1 tsp coconut aminos · pinch each cinnamon and ginger	Toast cashews or almonds in a dry pan over medium-high heat for 3-5 minutes, then chop and sprinkle on top. Add a cup of Bone Broth (see recipe) as a tasty variation.
Morning Mix: ground pork or turkey · diced apple · ⅛ tsp each cinnamon and nutmeg	A great morning meal, or "breakfast for dinner." A real kid pleaser!
Sweet Potato Hash: ground beef or turkey · roasted sweet potatoes · green bell peppers · ⅛ tsp each paprika and cinnamon	Butternut squash is a good stand-in for sweet potatoes. Consider fried or poached eggs on top, along with a sprinkle of dried chives. Great for kids!

GROUND MEAT SKILLET RECIPES	NOTES
Taste of Greece: ground pork or lamb · tomatoes · green beans · ⅛ tsp each oregano and marjoram	Feel free to replace green beans with zucchini, spinach, or eggplant. Drizzle with Classic Pantry Vinaigrette (see recipe) and chopped fresh parsley.
Indian Curry: ground beef or lamb · cauliflower · carrots · ¼ cup coconut milk · 1 tsp curry powder	Trade cauliflower for broccoli and/or raw diced tomatoes for a different flavor sensation.
Thai Basil Beef: ground beef · green beans · red bell pepper · 1 Tbsp each lime juice and coconut aminos · a few fresh basil leaves	Top with a squeeze of lime juice for added zing. Great for breakfast with an egg added to the mix—or in a bowl with lots of broth for instant soup.
Deconstructed Pizza: ground beef · tomato · baby spinach · sliced black olives · ½ tsp each rosemary and oregano	Also tasty: mushrooms, zucchini, and/or kale; drizzle with a little Classic Pesto (see recipe) just before eating.
10-Minute Chili: ground beef · ½ cup canned diced tomatoes · red and green bell peppers · ½ tsp cumin · 1 tsp chili powder	Serve on a bed of baby spinach and top with diced avocado and/or black olives, chopped fresh cilantro, and a light drizzle of Ranch Dressing (see recipe).
Deconstructed Burger: ground beef · green bell pepper · ⅛ tsp paprika	Mound ground beef on a pile of lettuce, then top with: tomatoes, onion, mushrooms, pickles, Olive Oil Mayo (see recipe), mustard, jalapeños, or BBQ Sauce (see recipe).
Mexicali Meat: ground beef · jalapeños · tomatoes · green and red bell pepper · ½ tsp chili powder · ¼ tsp cumin	Drizzle with Dreamy Avocado Dressing (see recipe) and top with sliced scallions and/or chopped fresh cilantro.

CHICKEN, PORK, OR FISH

Tender and oh-so-versatile, chicken breasts — or pork chops, or seafood — can be quickly transformed into one-skillet meals that will satisfy your taste buds without requiring special skills or tons of time. Serve this tender, flavorful protein alongside two bright vegetables for a pretty plate that packs a nutritional punch.

MASTER RECIPE—CHICKEN, PORK, OR FISH

This technique works for chicken breast; pork chops; firm, white fish filets at least 1-inch thick; salmon; and shellfish (like shrimp or scallops).

2 lbs boneless, skinless chicken breasts, cut lengthwise into 1-inch strips · salt and black pepper · 2-4 Tbsp cooking fat · 2 cloves garlic, minced or crushed · ⅓ cup chicken broth

Sprinkle the chicken pieces with salt and pepper. Cook the fat in a large nonstick skillet over high heat for about 3 minutes. Add the chicken and reduce heat to medium-high. Allow the chicken to cook on one side, undisturbed, for 2-3 minutes. Use tongs to flip the chicken over and brown other side, 2-3 minutes. (For pork, cook 3-4 minutes per side.) Remove chicken from pan, reduce heat to medium, add the crushed garlic, and cook until fragrant, about 15 seconds. Then, *deglaze* the pan and finish the dish using the ingredients below. (To deglaze: Add broth to pan, along with additional seasonings. Scrape up any tasty brown bits with a wooden spoon, then bring to a boil.)

CHICKEN/PORK/WHITE FISH RECIPES	NOTES
California Style: ¼ cup organic balsamic · 8 sundried tomatoes (in oil), minced · ½ cup fresh basil leaves, minced	Deglaze the pan with balsamic vinegar, broth, and sundried tomatoes. Return chicken to pan. Simmer until sauce is slightly thickened, 2-3 minutes. Remove pan from heat and stir in basil.

CHICKEN/PORK/WHITE FISH RECIPES	NOTES
Tarragon Cream: 4 thinly sliced scallions · ½ lb sliced mushrooms ·1 tsp tarragon · ⅓ cup coconut milk	After chicken is browned, add scallions and mushrooms; sauté until just softened, about 1-2 minutes. Deglaze with broth, tarragon, and coconut milk. Return chicken to pan. Bring to a boil, then simmer over low heat until sauce is thickened, about 2-3 minutes.
Italian: 1 tsp oregano ·1 tsp rosemary ·1 can (14.5 oz) diced, fire-roasted tomatoes ·½ cup fresh parsley leaves, minced	Deglaze with broth, oregano, and rosemary. Add diced tomatoes, bring to a boil. Return chicken to pan, simmer uncovered until sauce is thickened, 3-5 minutes. Remove from heat, stir in parsley.
Citrus: ⅓ cup lime, lemon, or orange juice · 1 tsp lime, lemon, or orange zest · ½ cup fresh parsley leaves, minced· 1 Tbsp clarified butter	Deglaze the pan with the broth, citrus juice, and zest. Return chicken to pan and simmer until sauce is slightly thickened, 1-2 minutes. Remove pan from heat and stir in parsley, along with clarified butter.
Moroccan: 1 onion, finely diced · an additional ⅔ cup chicken broth · 1 tsp ground cumin · ½ tsp cinnamon · ¼ cup raisins · ½ cup coconut milk	Deglaze the pan with the broth, cumin, and cinnamon. Add the onion and sauté until soft, about 3-4 minutes. Add the raisins and coconut milk to the pan; bring to a boil, then simmer over low until slightly thickened, 2-3 minutes.
Mexican: ¼ cup lime juice ·2 tsp chili powder · 1 tsp ground cumin · an additional ⅔ cup chicken broth ·1 can (4 oz) diced green chilies (mild or hot) ·½ cup fresh cilantro leaves, minced· 1 Tbsp clarified butter	Deglaze the pan with the lime juice, chili powder, and cumin. Add the broth and chilies, then return chicken to pan. Boil until liquid is reduced by about half, 7-10 minutes. Remove pan from heat and stir in the cilantro and clarified butter.

EGGS

Eggs aren't just for Meal 1! In a savory frittata or omelet, hot or at room temperature, they're a perfect comfort food, and a slice of frittata is great for brown-bagging. In a hurry? Make a big scramble instead! Skip the broiling step and cook eggs through during the skillet stage.

MASTER RECIPE—FRITTATA

9 large eggs · ½ tsp salt · ¼ tsp black pepper · seasonings (see chart) · 1-2 Tbsp cooking fat · 1-2 palm-size servings added protein (see chart) · 2-3 cups cooked vegetables (see chart)

Preheat oven to 400° F. Beat eggs, salt, pepper, and seasonings until blended. In a large oven-safe skillet, cook fat over medium heat until shimmering. Place protein and vegetables in the pan, stir to coat with fat, then pour in the beaten eggs. Use a spatula to stir, gently scraping the bottom of the skillet to make large curds, about 2 minutes. Shake the pan to evenly distribute the ingredients and allow to cook undisturbed so the bottom sets, about 30 seconds. Place the pan in the oven and bake until the top is puffed and beginning to brown, 13-15 minutes. Remove skillet from the oven, allow the frittata to set for 5 minutes, then cut into wedges to serve.

Use these protein-vegetable-seasoning ideas to take your frittatas to the next level.

ADDED PROTEIN	VEGETABLES	SEASONINGS	SERVING SUGGESTIONS
Ground beef	Onion Spinach	1 tsp sweet paprika	Sprinkle with finely diced fresh tomato and drizzle with Classic Pantry Vinaigrette.

ADDED PROTEIN	VEGETABLES	SEASONINGS	SERVING SUGGESTIONS
Shrimp or salmon	Mushrooms Asparagus	1 Tbsp chives ½ tsp lemon zest	Sprinkle with fresh lemon juice and chopped fresh parsley or drizzle with Dreamy Avocado Dressing.
Shrimp or salmon	Scallions Fresh basil leaves	½ tsp lemon zest	Drizzle with a little Classic Pesto or Tartar Sauce.
Diced chicken	Broccoli Cabbage	1-2 Tbsp coconut aminos ½ tsp ginger	Sprinkle with chopped scallions and a tiny drizzle of sesame oil.
Ground pork or beef	Red bell peppers Asparagus	1 tsp tarragon	Sprinkle with minced fresh parsley leaves and Classic Pantry Vinaigrette.
Italian or chicken sausage	Bell peppers Onion Zucchini	1 tsp oregano	Drizzle with Classic Pantry Vinaigrette.
Ground pork or beef	Mushrooms Broccoli	½ tsp nutmeg	Drizzle with Classic Pantry Vinaigrette.
Ground lamb	Butternut squash Spinach	1 tsp cinnamon ½ tsp cumin	Drizzle with extra-virgin olive oil, sprinkle with minced fresh parsley.

MASTER RECIPES: VEGETABLES

With these instructions you'll have all the know-how to cook just about any vegetables you find at the grocery store or farmers' market. We've included seasoning ideas for serving the vegetables as a side dish. If you plan to use the vegetables for a frittata, curry, or soup just follow the master recipe and skip the seasonings listed in the chart.

MASTER RECIPE—ROASTED VEGETABLES

Preheat the oven to 425° F. Wash veggies and cut into even-size pieces. In a large bowl, toss with 2 Tbsp clarified butter or coconut oil, 1-2 crushed garlic cloves, and salt and pepper. Spread the vegetables in a single layer on a baking sheet. Bake on the middle racks of the oven, stirring about every 15 minutes to ensure even browning. If veggies are browned to your liking before they've reached your desired tenderness, turn the heat down to 350° F and roast longer, checking for doneness every 5-7 minutes.

MASTER RECIPE—WET SAUTE VEGETABLES

Wash your veggies under running water, then cut according to chart below. Place ½ cup water in a large nonstick skillet. Turn the heat to high, and when the water is boiling, add vegetables to pan, cover with a lid, and allow the vegetables to soften, according to the times below. When most of the water has evaporated, remove the lid and stir with a wooden spoon. Check for doneness and, if necessary, add more water, stirring vigorously, until the vegetables are tender.

MASTER RECIPE—GRILLED VEGETABLES

In a large bowl, toss 1-2 lbs washed and cut vegetables with 2 Tbsp melted clarified butter or coconut oil, 1-2 crushed garlic cloves, and salt and pepper. Let marinate for 20-30 minutes. Heat grill on high with lid closed. Remove vegetables from marinade, wrap in foil (if necessary to avoid falling through the slats), and place on grill. Turn heat down to medium and close lid. Grill for time listed, checking every 5 minutes for browning and tenderness.

Make any veggie in this chart instantly "kid friendly" by serving a little Ranch Dressing, Classic Pantry Vinaigrette, or Dreamy Avocado Dressing alongside for dipping. Healthy fats plus vegetables is a big win!

VEGETABLE	ROAST	WET SAUTÉ	GRILL	SEASON·
Asparagus	Whole, 25 min	Whole, 5-10 min	Whole, 2-3 min	Squeeze of lemon juice and zest after cooking
Beets	1" pieces, 35-45 min	1" pieces, 15-20 min	Halve; wrap in foil, 25-30 min	Squeeze of orange juice and zest after cooking
Bell pepper	1" pieces, 25-35 min	1" pieces, 5-6 min	Halve, 5-6 min per side	Splash of balsamic vinegar after cooking
Broccoli	1" florets, 20-25 min	1" florets, 5-7 min	Large spears, 8-10 min per side	Squeeze of lemon juice and zest after cooking
Brussels sprouts	Halve, 35-40 min	Halve, 6-8 min	Whole, skewered, 7-8 min per side	Dried thyme and lemon zest before cooking
Butternut squash	1" pieces, 45-50 min	1" pieces, 7-9 min	½" slices, 7-8 min per side	Dried thyme before cooking
Cabbage	8 wedges, 25-30 min	8 wedges, 8-10 min	8 wedges; wrap in foil, 30 min	Squeeze of lemon juice and dried chives after cooking

VEGETABLE	ROAST	WET SAUTÉ	GRILL	SEASON
Carrots	1" pieces, 20-25 min	1½" pieces, 6-8 min	Whole, 20-25 min	Squeeze of lemon juice and fresh chopped parsley and mint after cooking
Cauliflower	1" florets, 25-30 min	1" florets, 5-7 min	1" florets; wrap in foil, 20-25 min	Squeeze of lemon juice and dried chives after cooking
Eggplant	½" slices, 20-25 min	1" pieces, 6-8 min	½" slices, 6-7 min per side	Chopped fresh tomatoes and dried oregano after cooking
Fennel	1" pieces, 30-40 min	1" pieces, 8-10 min	Quarter, 5-8 min per side	Squeeze of orange or lemon juice and zest after cooking
Green beans	Whole, 12-15 min	Whole, 5-6 min	Whole; wrap in foil, 30 min	Dried thyme before cooking; squeeze of lemon juice and zest after
Kale	2" pieces, 10-12 min (kale chips!)	2" pieces, 6-8 min	N/A	Squeeze of lemon juice and zest after cooking

VEGETABLE	ROAST	WET SAUTÉ	GRILL	SEASON
Mushrooms	Halve, 30-35 min	Halve, 4-5 min	Halve; skewer, 5-6 min per side	Splash of balsamic vinegar and dried chives after cooking
Onion	8 wedges, 20-25 min	½" slices, 5-7 min	Quarter; skewer, 8-10 min per side	Dried thyme before cooking; squeeze of lemon juice and zest after cooking
Parsnips	1" pieces, 20-25 min	1½" pieces, 6-8 min	Whole, 20-25 min	Dried thyme before cooking
Radishes	Halve, 15-20 min	Sliced thin, 5-7 min	Halve; wrap in foil, 20-25 min	Squeeze of orange juice and fresh parsley after cooking
Snap peas/ snow peas	Whole, 12-14 min	Whole, 4-5 min	Whole; wrap in foil, 12-14 min	Splash of coconut aminos and chopped scallions after cooking
Sweet potatoes	1" pieces, 45-50 min	1" pieces, 7-9 min	N/A	Squeeze of orange juice and a pinch of cinnamon after cooking

VEGETABLE	ROAST	WET SAUTÉ	GRILL	SEASON
Tomatoes	Quarter, 30-40 min	1" pieces, 3-4 min	Halve, 3-5 min per side	Drizzle of extra-virgin olive oil and coarse salt after cooking
Turnips	1" pieces, 45-50 min	1" pieces, 7-9 min	¼" slices, 3-4 min per side	Dried chives after cooking
Zucchini/ summer squash	Quarter, 6-10 min	½" rounds, 5-6 min	½" length-wise slices, 4-5 min per side	Lemon zest and dried chives after cooking

All vegetables benefit from a drizzle of olive oil after cooking.

MASTER RECIPES: CURRIES

A Thai curry made with coconut milk is nutritious, silky, and comforting. When you have prepped ingredients on hand, it's also superfast. You can buy curry paste in most grocery stores, and the different colors lend themselves to different vegetable combinations, so you never have to eat the same dish twice.

MASTER RECIPE FOR THAI CURRY

¼-½ can coconut milk, *per person* · 1-2 Tbsp yellow, green, or red curry paste · protein portion, *per person* (see chart) · 2 cups cooked vegetables, *per person* (see chart)

Place coconut milk and curry paste in a large skillet over medium heat. Stir until combined, then simmer 5 minutes. Add protein (cooked) and vegetables to the skillet. Simmer until heated through, about 5-10 minutes. Mix and match your choice of protein with our vegetable recommendations, garnish, and serve.

PROTEIN	YELLOW CURRY (MILD)	GREEN CURRY (MEDIUM)	RED CURRY (HOT)	GARNISH (MINCED)
Beef Chicken Hard-boiled eggs Lamb Pork Salmon Scallops Shrimp	Butternut squash Cabbage Carrots Cauliflower Mushrooms Onion Pineapple Red peppers Sweet potato	Broccoli Cauliflower Chard Eggplant Green beans Onion Red/green peppers Snow peas Spinach Sugar-snap peas	Eggplant Green beans Mushrooms Onion Pineapple Red peppers Sweet potato Zucchini	Almonds Basil leaves, fresh Cashews Cilantro Raisins Scallions Plus a squeeze of fresh lime juice

MASTER RECIPES: SOUPS

What's better than love eaten with a spoon? Warm, comforting, and easy to throw together, soup is also surprisingly great for breakfast—and packs protein, vegetables, and fat into one steaming bowl. Top with a fried or hard-boiled egg for extra protein.

MASTER RECIPE—BONE BROTH

4 qts water · 1 tsp salt · 2 Tbsp cider vinegar · 2 large onions, unpeeled and coarsely chopped · 2 carrots, scrubbed and coarsely chopped · 3 celery stalks, coarsely chopped · 1 bunch fresh parsley · 2-3 garlic cloves, lightly smashed · 2-4 lbs meat or poultry bones

Place all ingredients in a large slow cooker set on high. Bring to a boil, then reduce setting to low for 12- 24 hours. The longer it cooks, the better it tastes! Strain stock through a fine-mesh strainer or coffee filter and discard the waste. Homemade stock is best stored in the freezer if you're not going to use it within a few days.

MASTER RECIPE—QUICK SOUPS

1-2 Tbsp cooking fat, *per person* · ½ medium onion, finely diced · ¼ tsp seasoning, *per person* (see chart) · protein portion (cooked), *per person* · 2-3 cups cooked vegetables, *per person* · 2 cups Bone Broth, *per person*

Heat fat in a large soup pot until shimmering. Add onion and sauté until tender and translucent, about 5-7 minutes. Add seasoning and stir to coat with fat. Add protein and vegetables, tossing to coat with onions and fat. Add stock, bring to a boil, and partly cover for 5-7 minutes, until flavors meld and soup is piping hot.

Use these themes to add flavor and personality to the basic soup recipe—or just sip on the broth throughout your day to add extra vitamins, minerals, and gut-healing micronutrients to your diet.

SOUP RECIPES	NOTES
Classic Chicken: paprika · chicken · diced sweet potato or butternut squash · carrots · celery · chicken broth	Top with a drizzle of extra-virgin olive oil and a sprinkle of minced fresh parsley.
Classic Beef: paprika · ground or cubed beef · diced sweet potato or butternut squash · carrots · beef broth	Top with a drizzle of extra-virgin olive oil and a sprinkle of minced fresh parsley.
Beef Taco: chili powder · ground beef · bell peppers · zucchini · beef broth	Top with diced avocado, minced cilantro, diced red onion, and a squeeze of lime juice.
Faux Pho: coconut aminos · dried ginger · cinnamon · pork/chicken/beef/lamb/shrimp · green beans · red bell pepper · beef broth	Top with sliced scallions, fresh basil leaves, and a squeeze of lime juice.

SOUP RECIPES	NOTES
Creamy Thai: curry powder · chicken/shrimp · green beans · red bell peppers · mango · chicken broth plus ½ cup coconut milk per person	Top with minced fresh cilantro or basil leaves and a squeeze of lime juice.
Ginger Spinach: dried ginger · chicken · spinach · scallions · chicken broth	Top with a squeeze of fresh lemon juice, black pepper, and a few toasted sesame seeds.

FINISHING TOUCHES: SAUCES, SEASONINGS, AND DRESSINGS

A luscious drizzle of something creamy, fatty, spicy—or all three!—can add extra flavor and satisfaction to simple ingredients and still be healthy. Many of these recipes are equally at home on a meat-and-vegetables sauté or a crisp, fresh salad.

OLIVE OIL MAYO

Perfect for tuna, seafood, and egg salad—and the basis for creamy dressing for tossed salads; makes about 1½ cups. From Well Fed: Paleo Recipes for People Who Love to Eat.

1 large egg · 2 Tbsp lemon juice · ¼ cup plus 1 cup light-tasting olive oil (not extra-virgin!) · ½ tsp dry mustard · ½ tsp salt

Place the egg and the lemon juice in a blender or food processor, cover, and allow to come to room temperature, 30 minutes. Add ¼ cup oil, mustard, and salt, blend on medium speed until the ingredients are combined. With the motor running, drizzle in the remaining 1 cup oil in a very thin stream; this should take about 2-3 minutes. Store covered in the fridge.

RANCH DRESSING

You'll never miss the buttermilk; makes about ½ cup. From Well Fed: Paleo Recipes for People Who Love to Eat.

1 clove garlic, minced · ¼ tsp paprika · ¼ cup fresh parsley leaves, minced · 1 Tbsp dried chives · ½ cup Olive Oil Mayo · 1 tsp lemon juice · salt and black pepper

In a small bowl, mix the garlic, paprika, parsley, chives, and mayo with a fork. Drizzle in the lemon juice while continuing to mix, then taste and season with salt and pepper. If your dressing is too thick, add either lemon juice or water — ¼ tsp at a time — until it's the right consistency.

TARTAR SAUCE
Makes everyday fish taste special; makes about ½ cup.

½ cup Olive Oil Mayo · 1 Tbsp minced cornichons or dill pickle · 2 Tbsp fresh parsley leaves, minced · 2 tsp minced capers · 2 tsp minced chives (fresh) · ½ Tbsp lemon juice · 1 tsp pickle juice · salt and ground black pepper

Place all ingredients in a bowl and mix with a spatula until blended. Allow the flavors to meld for 30 minutes before serving. Store covered in the refrigerator.

DREAMY AVOCADO DRESSING
Luscious on grilled meat or fresh raw veggies; makes about ½ cup.

½ large avocado · 1 Tbsp lime juice · ¼ cup Olive Oil Mayo · 1 small garlic clove · ½ Tbsp pickled jalapeño rings (optional) · 1 Tbsp fresh cilantro leaves (optional) · 2 Tbsp water · salt and black pepper

Place all ingredients in a blender or food processor and purée to desired consistency, adding additional water 1 Tbsp at a time, if necessary. Allow the flavors to meld for 30 minutes before serving. Store covered in the refrigerator.

CLASSIC PANTRY VINAIGRETTE
Makes simple green salads feel dressed up for a special occasion; makes about ½ cup.

2 Tbsp Red- or white-wine vinegar · 1 clove garlic, crushed · 1 tsp Olive Oil Mayo · ½ tsp dried mustard · ¼ tsp salt · ⅛ tsp black pepper · 6 Tbsp extra-virgin olive oil · 2 Tbsp minced fresh parsley · ¼ tsp thyme · ¼ tsp oregano

Place vinegar, garlic, mayo, mustard, salt, and pepper in small bowl. Whisk until milky and smooth. Whisking constantly, slowly drizzle the oil into the vinegar mixture. When the oil is combined, crush the dried herbs into the bowl with your fingers, add parsley, and whisk gently to combine.

CLASSIC PESTO
Tastes indulgent when stirred into soup or freshly cooked vegetables; makes about 1 cup. From Well Fed: Paleo Recipes for People Who Love to Eat.

⅓ cup walnuts or pine nuts · 3 medium cloves garlic, unpeeled · 2 cups packed fresh basil leaves · ½ cup fresh parsley leaves · ⅓ cup extra-virgin olive oil · ½ tsp salt · ⅛ tsp black pepper

Toast the nuts in a heavy skillet over medium heat, stirring until just golden and fragrant, about 5 minutes. Set aside, then add garlic to the skillet and lightly toast over medium heat, about 7 minutes. Set aside to cool. Place all ingredients in a blender or food processor and purée to desired consistency. Allow the flavors to meld for 30 minutes before serving. Store covered in the refrigerator or freeze in ice cube trays for pesto on demand.

BBQ SAUCE
Adapted from Cook's Illustrated's *"Quick BBQ Sauce" (2007); makes about 1 cup.*

1 cup tomato sauce · ⅓ cup unsweetened apple sauce · 2 Tbsp cider vinegar · 2 Tbsp coconut aminos · 1 Tbsp Dijon mustard · 1 tsp hot-pepper sauce · ¼ tsp black pepper · ½ Tbsp clarified butter or coconut oil · 1 clove garlic, minced · 1 tsp chili powder · ½ tsp paprika · ¼ tsp cayenne pepper (optional) · pinch cloves

In a medium bowl, whisk the tomato sauce, apple sauce, vinegar, coconut aminos, mustard, hot-pepper sauce, and black pepper until combined. Heat the clarified butter or coconut oil in a large saucepan over medium-high heat, then add the garlic, chili powder, paprika, and cayenne, stirring until fragrant, about 30 seconds. Whisk in the sauce and bring to a boil. Simmer gently, uncovered, 25 30 minutes, until the sauce is thickened and flavorful. Cool to room temperature before using, and store covered in the fridge for up to a week.

QUICK-AND-EASY MEAL: THE PERFECT STEAK

An organic, grass-fed, beautifully marbled steak—served alongside a crisp salad and a few supporting vegetables—is the ideal "real food" dinner. Follow these instructions for a perfect steak, hot off the stove or gas grill.

DALLAS AND MELISSA'S MOCHA STEAK RUB
The only steak rub you'll ever need; makes enough for about 4 steaks.

1 Tbsp black pepper · 1 Tbsp ground coriander · 2 tsp salt · ½ tsp ground cloves · 1 tsp cinnamon · 1 tsp unsweetened cocoa · 2 tsp ground coffee

Crush all ingredients in a spice grinder or with a mortar and pestle. Massage rub generously into steaks, wrap tightly in plastic wrap, and allow to rest for at least 30 minutes before cooking.

MASTER RECIPE—PAN FRIED STEAK
For pan-frying, choose rib-eye steaks that are 1-1¼" thick. Massage Mocha Steak Rub generously into steaks about 30-60 minutes before you want to start cooking. Heat a large cast-iron skillet over medium heat for about 10 minutes. Add 1-2 Tbsp clarified butter to the pan and swirl to coat the bottom. Add the steak(s) and cook until well browned on one side, about 5 minutes. Turn steak(s) with tongs and cook to desired doneness:

Rare: 3 minutes more.
Medium-rare: 4 minutes more.
Medium: 5 minutes more.

Remove steaks from pan, let rest 5 minutes, then serve.

MASTER RECIPE—GAS GRILLED STEAK

For gas grilling choose strip, T-bone, or rib-eye steaks that are 1-1¼" thick. Massage Mocha Steak Rub generously into them about 30-60 minutes before you want to start grilling. Turn on all burners to high, close the lid, and heat the grill until very hot, about 15 minutes. Scrape the grill grate clean with a grill brush. Leave one burner on high and turn the other burner(s) to medium. Grill the steaks, uncovered, on the hotter part of the grill until well browned on one side, 2-3 minutes. Flip the steaks with tongs and grill until well browned on the other side, 2-3 minutes. Now that the steaks are browned, slide them to the cooler side of the grill. Continue to cook until desired doneness:

Rare (120 degrees): 5-6 minutes.
Medium-rare (125-130 degrees): 6-8 minutes.
Medium (135-140 degrees): 8-9 minutes.

Remove steaks from the grill, let rest for 5 minutes. and serve.

QUICK-AND-EASY MEAL: NO-FUSS SALMON CAKES

Keep recipes for three quick-and-easy meals on your fridge, for those nights when you're too tired to cook. These meals should include ingredients you always have on hand, and will ensure that you still get a delicious, healthy meal when the temptation to order in pizza is strong.

These salmon cakes—inspired by Dallas' mum—should be called protein-fat-veggie cakes cause they've got it all going on. They can be thrown together in just five minutes, and after a brief half-hour in the oven, they're ready to eat. (This recipe can easily be doubled, and they reheat beautifully.)

NO-FUSS SALMON CAKES

Serves 2-3

1 can (14.75 oz) wild-caught pink or red salmon · 1 cup canned sweet potatoes · 1 large egg · ½ cup almond flour · 2 Tbsp minced fresh parsley (or 2 tsp dried) · 2 scallions, white and green, very thinly sliced · 2 Tbsp minced fresh dill (or 2 tsp dried) · 1 tsp hot-pepper sauce · ½ tsp paprika · 1 tsp salt · ¼ tsp black pepper · 2 Tbsp clarified butter or coconut oil, melted

Preheat oven to 425° F and cover a large baking sheet with parchment paper. Drain the liquid from the salmon, and using your fingers, crumble the fish into a large mixing bowl, removing bones. Add all the remaining ingredients—except the butter—and mix with a wooden spoon until well combined. Pop into the fridge to chill for 5-10 minutes. Brush the parchment paper with some of the melted butter, then use a ⅓ cup measuring cup to scoop out salmon mixture and drop onto the parchment. The cakes should be about 2½" wide and about 1" thick. Bake for 20 minutes, then flip each patty with a spatula and return to the oven. Bake 10 minutes more, until golden brown and crisp. Serve with a squeeze of lemon juice and Tartar Sauce.

FANCYPANTS MEAL: DELICIOUS DINNER PARTY

Seems like there's always a special occasion to celebrate, and there's no reason to ditch your healthy new habits in the name of having a good time. This dinner party menu is elegant, easy to prepare, and completely deprivation-free.

HAZELNUT ROASTED SALMON

Adapted from Sur la Table. Serves 4.
2 Tbsp hazelnuts, finely chopped · ½ cup clarified butter, at room temperature, plus 1 Tbsp melted · 1 small shallot or garlic clove, finely minced · 2 tsp fresh thyme leaves, finely minced · ½ tsp salt · ¼ tsp black pepper · 4 (4-5 oz each) wild-salmon filets, 1½" thick

Place a skillet over medium-high heat and add the hazelnuts. Toast until golden, about 3-5 minutes, then set aside to cool. Put ½ cup clarified butter, the garlic, thyme, salt, pepper, and cooled nuts into a small bowl and stir to combine with a spatula. Place a large piece of plastic wrap on a flat surface, transfer the butter mixture to the center of the plastic, and form a rough log shape about 1½" in diameter. Wrap tightly in the plastic and refrigerate until firm, about 2 hours. (You can also do this several days ahead, to save time on the big day.)

Place rack in center of oven and preheat to 400° F. Cover a large baking sheet with parchment paper and brush the parchment with some of the melted clarified butter, then sprinkle generously with salt and pepper. Place the salmon filets in the middle of the parchment, skin side down, leaving at least 1" of space around all sides of each filet. Brush the tops of the fish with the rest of the melted butter and sprinkle with salt and pepper.

Place salmon in oven and roast just until it begins to barely flake when poked with a fork, about 8-10 minutes total. To serve, place each salmon filet on a plate and top with 1-2 thin slices of the hazelnut butter.

BUTTERNUT SQUASH PUREE WITH ROASTED GARLIC

Adapted from Well Fed: Paleo Recipes for People Who Love to Eat.
Serves 4.
2½ lbs butternut squash · 1 head garlic · 1 Tbsp clarified butter · 2 Tbsp coconut milk · ¼ tsp salt · ¼ tsp cinnamon · ⅛ tsp cayenne pepper · ⅛ tsp nutmeg · ⅛ tsp allspice

Preheat oven to 350° F. Cover a baking sheet with parchment paper. Cut the squash into quarters and scoop out seeds and pulp. Place cut side down on baking sheet and sprinkle 2 Tbsp water onto the paper around the squash.

Peel the loose, papery skin off the garlic, and wrap it in a piece of aluminum foil. Put the squash and the garlic in the oven. Bake 40-50 minutes, until the squash is tender. Set both aside until they're cool enough to handle, about 20 minutes.

When the squash is cool, use a spoon to scoop the flesh into the bowl of a food processor. Separate the garlic cloves and squeeze the roasted pulp into the bowl with the squash. Process the mixture to a smooth purée, then add the rest of the ingredients. Taste and adjust seasonings; serve immediately.

GREEN BEANS WITH FIG VINAIGRETTE

Adapted from Sur la Table. Serves 4.

1 lb green beans, trimmed · ¼ cup white-wine or champagne vinegar · 1 small shallot or garlic clove, minced · ½ tsp Dijon mustard · ¼ cup balsamic vinegar · ½ cup extra-virgin olive oil · ¼ cup dried black mission figs, finely chopped · 2 tsp fresh thyme leaves, minced · salt and black pepper

Bring a large pot of salted water to a rolling boil over high heat. Add the green beans and cook until crisp-tender, about 3 minutes. Drain the beans in a colander, then rinse under cold running water until cool to the touch to stop the cooking process and set the color. Set aside.

In a medium bowl, whisk the white-wine vinegar, shallot, mustard, and balsamic vinegar. Continue to whisk and slowly drizzle in the olive oil. Stir in the figs and thyme, and season with salt and pepper.

Return the bean pot to the stove and heat over medium-low heat. Shake excess water off beans and add to pot. Drizzle enough vinaigrette over the beans to coat; toss until evenly dressed. Taste and adjust salt and pepper. Serve immediately.

ALMOND POACHED PEARS WITH RASPBERRY CREAM
Serves 4

½ tsp plus ¼ tsp pure almond or vanilla extract · 10 black peppercorns · 2" piece lemon rind · ¼ tsp salt · 4 ripe Bosc pears, peeled, halved, and cored · 2 Tbsp sliced almonds · 6 oz fresh raspberries · 1 Tbsp balsamic vinegar · 1 cup coconut milk

Place 3 cups water, ½ tsp almond extract, peppercorns, lemon rind, and salt in a medium saucepan, and bring to a boil. Add the pears and bring back to a boil for 5 minutes, then turn off the heat, cover, and set aside until the water returns to room temperature, about 30 minutes. Remove pears from the pot with a slotted spoon and set aside.

While the pears poach, heat a skillet over medium-high heat and add the sliced almonds. Toast until golden, about 3-5 minutes. Set aside to cool.

Place ¾ cup raspberries and the balsamic vinegar in a small saucepan over medium-high heat. Save remaining raspberries for garnish. Bring to a simmer and cook, covered, for 5 minutes, then uncover and simmer an additional minute, crushing the berries with the back of a wooden spoon. Add the coconut milk and ¼ tsp almond extract. Bring to a boil and then simmer until slightly thickened, stirring often, about 5 minutes. The sauce is the right consistency when it coats the spoon.

To serve, place 1-2 Tbsp warm coconut sauce in the bottom of individual dessert dishes and top with a pear. Garnish with a few fresh raspberries and the toasted almonds.

Note: You can poach the pears and store in an airtight container for up to 3 days before serving.

HUNGRY FOR MORE?

Ready to move past our Meal Map and start exploring some fun and creative healthy-eating recipes? In Appendix B you'll find a list of our favorite cookbooks and online resources.

APPENDIX B:
IT STARTS WITH FOOD RESOURCES

Visit our Web site at **http://whole9life.com/itstartswithfood** to download a variety of free PDF reference sheets, including our detailed shopping list, good food buzzwords, and guides to stocking your pantry, managing your food budget, reading labels, dining out, traveling, and more.

COOKING CONVERSIONS

Metric equivalents have been rounded slightly here to make measuring easier.

WEIGHT

US	Metric
¼ oz	7 grams
½ oz	15 g
¾ oz	20 g
1 oz	30 g
8 oz (½ lb)	225 g
12 oz (¾ lb)	340 g
16 oz (1 lb)	455 g
2 lb	900 g
2 ¼ lb	1 kg

VOLUME

US	Metric	Imperial
¼ tsp	1.2 ml	
½ tsp	2.5 ml	
1 tsp	5 ml	
½ Tbsp (1.5 tsp)	7.5 ml	
1 Tbsp (3 tsp)	15 ml	
¼ cup (4 Tbsp)	60 ml	2 fl oz
⅓ cup (5 Tbsp)	75 ml	2½ fl oz
½ cup (8 Tbsp)	125 ml	4 fl oz
⅔ cup (10 Tbsp)	150 ml	5 fl oz
¾ cup (12 Tbsp)	175 ml	6 fl oz
1 cup (16 Tbsp)	250 ml	8 fl oz
1 ¼ cup	300 ml	10 fl oz (½ pint)
1 ½ cup	350 ml	12 fl oz
2 cups (1 pint)	500 ml	16 fl oz
2 ½ cups	625 ml	20 fl oz (1 pint)
1 quart	1 liter	32 fl oz

OVEN CONVERSIONS

Fahrenheit (degrees F)	Celsius (degrees C)	Gas Number	Oven Terms
225	110	¼	Very Cool
250	130	½	Very Slow
275	140	1	Very Slow
300	150	2	Slow
325	165	3	Slow
350	177	4	Moderate
375	190	5	Moderate
400	200	6	Moderately Hot
425	220	7	Hot
450	230	8	Hot
475	245	9	Hot
500	260	10	Extremely Hot
550	290	10	Broiling

HEALTHY-EATING RECIPES

This is a list of Good Food and Whole30-friendly cookbooks and recipe sites perfect for the budding chef, the gourmet cook, and everyone in between.

COOKBOOKS

Well Fed: Paleo Food for People Who Love to Eat, **by Melissa Joulwan** (http://theclothesmakethegirl.com): Melissa Joulwan is not only the culinary genius behind our Meal Map, but she is the author of her own bestselling healthy-eating cookbook. *Well Fed* includes more than 115 mouth-watering recipes from every corner of the world, and is the definitive resource for every Good Food chef (and aspiring chef). In addition, all recipes in *Well Fed* (save one dessert treat) are Whole30-approved.

Paleo Comfort Foods, **by Julie and Charles Mayfield** (http://paleocomfortfoods.com): The Mayfields are two talented chefs with an immense joy of growing, cooking, and eating fantastic food. This husband-and-wife team shows you unique and fun ways to prepare familiar foods to maximize their healthiness. Most recipes in *Paleo Comfort Foods* are Whole30-approved (or can be easily tailored to your Whole30 program).

Everyday Paleo, **by Sarah Fragoso** (http://everydaypaleo.com): Sarah Fragoso is a busy mom of three, a fitness trainer, and an accomplished Paleo chef. During her own healthy-eating journey, she has learned a lot about how to successfully feed a family and specializes in kid-friendly recipes sure to please everyone at the dinner table.

RECIPE SITES

The Whole9 Recipe Collection (http://whole9life.com/recipes): Our own "Steal This Meal" series features Whole30-approved recipes contributed by our readers and Whole30 participants (with a few of our own original creations throw in).

The Clothes Make the Girl (http://theclothesmakethegirl.com): Not only is Melissa Joulwan the author of *Well Fed* and the genius behind our Meal

Map, she's also a brilliant food, fitness, and health blogger, with hundreds of Whole30-friendly recipes available free on her site.

Whole Life Eating (http://wholelifeeating.com): Whole30 expert (and an editor of this book!) Tom Denham has created more than three hundred delicious, easy, often one-pot recipes, *100 percent* of which are Whole30-approved.

Nom Nom Paleo (http://nomnompaleo.com): Nom Nom is the creation of mom, foodie, and self-described "culinary nerd" Michelle Tam. Since the fall of 2010, she has been religiously taking pictures of her Whole30 and Paleo meals, and sharing her kitchen experiments and recipe creations.

The Food Lovers Primal Palate (http://primal-palate.com): Bill Staley and Hayley Mason are a couple with a passion for health and wellness—and their cooking and recipes shout that out loud and clear.

Chowstalker (http://chowstalker.com/whole30): A compilation of some of the best healthy-eating recipes on the Web—with an entire section dedicated to Whole30-approved meals. It's a great place to discover new recipe bloggers and Paleo chefs!

The Foodee Blog (http://thefoodee.com/tag/whole30/): Another fabulous recipe-compilation site, featuring Whole30-approved dishes in their own easy-to-find category.

FINDING GOOD FOOD

Visit these sites to learn more about sourcing your food locally, responsibly, and healthfully.

NATIONWIDE RESOURCES
Center for Food Safety (http://truefoodnow.org): Protecting human health and the environment by curbing the proliferation of harmful food-production technologies and by promoting organic and other forms of sustainable agriculture.

Eat Well Guide (http://eatwellguide.org): Find sustainable food—CSAs, farmers' markets, farmers, meat processors, restaurants, co-ops, and more.

Environmental Working Group (http://ewg.org/foodnews): Visit this site for an annually updated list of "clean" and "dirty" produce items.

Local Harvest (http://localharvest.org): Find sustainable food—CSAs, farmers' markets, farmers, community gardens, restaurants, health-food stores, and more.

Sustainable Table (http://sustainabletable.org): Celebrating local sustainable food, educating consumers about the issues, and building community through food. A fabulous resource for those interested in learning more about the health and environmental consequences of factory farming.

RESPONSIBLY SOURCED PROTEIN

Eatwild (http://eatwild.com and http://eatwild.com/products/canada. html): A comprehensive listing of local, pastured meat and dairy products in all fifty states and Canada. Includes food markets, farms and ranches, restaurants and retail shipping outlets for meat, fish, eggs, and other products.

Gourmet Grassfed (http://gourmetgrassfedmeat.com): Whole30-approved, 100 percent grass-fed, organic jerky, sourced responsibly and produced with integrity, in a variety of delicious flavors.

Heritage Foods (http://heritagefoodsusa.com): Retail food products from heritage and traditionally-raised animals, including grass-fed beef, pastured pork, and other foods.

Primal Pacs (http://primalpacs.com): Whole30-approved, 100 percent grass-fed, organic jerky, sourced responsibly and produced with integrity. Perfect for on-the-go meals; order the complete snack kit (with nuts and dried fruit) or just the jerky.

Pure Indian Foods (http://pureindianfoods.com): Organic ghee from grass-fed, pastured cows, produced according to traditional Ayurvedic principles. All flavors are Whole30-approved.

SFH Whey Protein (http://strongerfasterhealthier.com): Stronger Faster Healthier's whey protein powders are derived from grass-fed, antibiotic- and hormone-free cows—it's the highest-quality whey protein source for vegetarians. **Use the special code "itstartswithfood" to get 10 percent off your total order.**

US Wellness Meats (http://bit.ly/grasslandbeef): Buy the highest-quality grass-fed, pastured, wild-caught, and organic meat, fish, and eggs (including Whole30-approved bacon!) and have it shipped anywhere in the US.

WHOLE30-APPROVED PRODUCTS

Pure Wraps (http://improveat.com): Delicious sandwich-wrap substitute made from coconut meat, original and curry flavor.

SeaSnax (http://seasnax.com): Toasted nori sheets in a variety of flavors. An excellent source of micronutrients (including iodine) unique to sea vegetables. Lightly salted and crunchy—kids love them!

SFH Super Omega-3 Oil (http://strongerfasterhealthier.com): Stronger Faster Healthier's fish oil is of the highest quality, highly concentrated (2.7 grams of EPA and DHA per teaspoon) and comes in five delicious (not-at-all-fishy) flavors. **Use the special code "itstartswithfood" to get 10 percent off your total order.**

Spicehound (http://spicehound.com): Locally and globally sourced, fresh fragrant flavors inspire its line of spices, herbs, blends, salts, and spice accessories. Most spice mixtures are Whole30-approved (although a few have small amounts of added sugar).

Whole30 Approved (http://whole9life.com/whole30-approved): A list of products and producers that meet our Whole30 criteria. These products are healthy and responsibly sourced, and are perfect for your Whole30 and beyond.

GENERAL RESOURCES: WEB SITES, BOOKS, AND MOVIES

For more information about the Paleo diet and our healthy style of eating, visit these Web sites, read these books, and watch these documentaries.

WEB SITES

Whole9 (http://whole9life.com): An integrated system for health and fitness, designed by Dallas and Melissa Hartwig. Check the "9 Blog" for original articles on nutrition, exercise, sleep, stress management, and more. You can also fan us on Facebook (http://facebook.com/whole9) and follow us on Twitter (http://twitter.com/whole9life).

The Whole30 Program (http://whole9life.com/whole30/): The original Whole9 nutrition program that will "change your life in thirty days." Join our community by participating in our free Whole30 forum (http://forum.whole9life.com), or visit our Whole30 Facebook page (http://facebook.com/whole30).

Robb Wolf (http://robbwolf.com): One of the most content-rich and accessible resources for Paleo nutrition and lifestyle (and one of our favorite Web sites on the subject).

Mark's Daily Apple (http://marksdailyapple.com): The home of all things "primal," including diet, exercise, and lifestyle tips, created by Mark Sisson.

Gnolls.org (http://gnolls.org): Nutrition, exercise, and much more from an evolutionary perspective, created by J. Stanton. His "Why Are We Hungry?" series is an especially worthwhile read.

Perfect Health Diet (http://perfecthealthdiet.com): Healing age-related and chronic health problems through diet, from Paul and Shou-Ching Jaminet.

Chris Kresser (http://chriskresser.com): A licensed acupuncturist and practitioner of integrative medicine, Chris Kresser offers a wide range of nutrition-focused articles and customized health and wellness programs.

BOOKS AND MOVIES

- *A Mindful Carnivore,* Tovar Cerulli
- *Big River,* documentary film
- *Eating Animals,* Jonathan Safran Foer
- *Fat Head,* documentary film
- *Food, Inc.,* by Karl Weber
- *Food, Inc.,* documentary film
- *Food Rules,* Michael Pollan
- *In Defense of Food,* Michael Pollan
- *Inflammation Syndrome,* by Jack Challem
- *King Corn,* documentary film
- *Perfect Health Diet,* Paul and Shou-Ching Jaminet
- *Righteous Pork Chop,* Nicolette Hahn Nieman
- *Super Size Me,* documentary film
- *The End of Overeating,* by David Kessler
- *The Ethics of What We Eat, Peter* Singer and Jim Mason
- *The Future of Food,* documentary film
- *The Omnivore's Dilemma,* Michael Pollan
- *The Paleo Diet,* Loren Cordain
- *The Paleo Diet for Athletes,* Loren Cordain and Joe Friel
- *The Paleo Solution,* Robb Wolf

THANKS

We have so many reasons to be grateful, and so many people who deserve our thanks.

To Robb Wolf, our friend and mentor. Without you, there would be no book, and no Whole30 program. We can only hope to change half as many lives as you have. We are eternally grateful.

To Melissa Joulwan, the rock-star genius behind all our recipes and Meal Map creations. We are your biggest fans, and we love you dearly. Thank you for your sass, your motivational speeches, and most importantly, your food.

To Mathieu Lalonde, you radically improved our Science, taught us a lot in the process, and made this book more accurate and more credible. Thank you.

To J. Stanton, for helping us effectively communicate the psychological impact of our food choices, and for so graciously lending us your time, your expertise, and the genius phrase "food with no brakes."

To Jamie Scott, our brilliant friend from the future. Your cheerful assistance, feedback, and encouragement meant more to us than you could ever know.

To Tom Denham and Vanessa Chang, our friends and editors. You made every chapter better, and we are so grateful for your time and your talents.

To Pedro Bastos, for your time, your generosity, and all the work you've done to lay the foundation for books like ours.

To Amy Kubal, Erin Handley, and Emily Deans, for always having just the right research available.

To Robin Strathdee, for all of your help organizing our lives, and the projects you completed for this book. You are appreciated.

To Dr. Luc Readinger, Dr. Chad Potteiger, Dr. Michele Blackwell, Dr. Matt Mechtenberg, Dr. Tim Gerstmar, Dr. Michael Hasz, and Dr. Rick Henriksen for your help, and your personal and professional support.

To Erich Krauss and the Victory Belt team. Thank you for believing in us and bringing this project to life!

To Kathleen Shannon, our amazing graphic designer. We were the worst clients ever, and you still managed to create the most beautiful package we could ever imagine. Thank you.

To Greg White, our illustrator. You made something as boring as the digestive system look sexy. Well done.

To Dave Humphreys, for the gorgeous food photography. Your talent and creativity have no bounds.

To Andy Deas, Badier Velji, Clif Harski, Dan Pardi, and Julie and Charles Mayfield, for your unending support, unwavering faith, motivational speeches, and most important, your snark. #gorgeous #literally

To Jenn Maloney, Melissa's BFF and occasional butt-kicker. You never let me down.

To our parents, sisters, and brother. Thank you for believing in us, even after we quit the highest paying jobs we'll ever have to start this business. We love you. (And we finally have health insurance.)

And finally, to the Whole9 community. *We do this for you.* Thank you, thank you, thank you for providing the inspiration and motivation for this book and for sharing so many of your stories with us.

We are blessed.

MASTER REFERENCES

CHAPTER 1: FOOD SHOULD MAKE YOU HEALTHY

Scientific study that contains you: Used with permission of Brent Pottenger, with thanks to Dave Lull. Pottenger, Brent. "Black Swan Logic for N=1 Health." *epistemocrat.blogspot.com*, The Epistemocrat. February 2010. Web.

CHAPTER 2: OUR NUTRITIONAL FRAMEWORK

The Paleo Diet, defined: Lindeberg Staffan. Palaeolithic diet ("stone age" diet). *Scandinavian Journal of Food & Nutrition* Jun 2005;49(2):75–7

Paleo Diet studies: You can find 35 studies related to the Paleo diet aggregated here: Cordain Loren, Fontes Maelán, Bastos Pedro Carrera. "Rebuttal to U.S. News and World Top 20 Diets." *robbwolf.com*, Robb Wolf. Jun 11, 2011. Web.

CHAPTER 4: YOUR BRAIN ON FOOD

Dieting doesn't work: Jeffery R W, Drenowski A, Epstein L H, Stunkard A J, Wilson G T, Wing R R, et al. Long-term maintenance of weight loss; current status. *Health Psychol* 2000;19:5-16

Calorie-restrictive: Joseph R J, Alonso-Alonso M, Bond D S, Pascual-Leone A, Blackburn G L. The neurocognitive connection between physical activity and eating behavior. *Obes Rev* 2011;12:800-812

The vast majority : Mann T, Tomiyama J A, Westling E, Lew A M, Samuels B, Chatman J. Medicare's search for effective obesity treatments: Diets are not the answer. *American Psychologist* Apr 2007;62(3):220-233

Simply reducing your calories: Martin C K, Rosenbaum D, Han H, Geiselman P, Wyatt H, Hill J, Brill C, et al. Change in food cravings, food preferences and appetite during a low-carbohydrate and low-fat diet. *Obesity* 2011;19(10):1963-1970

Food craving: White M A, Whisenhunt B L, Williamson D A, Greenway F L, Netemeyer R G. Development and validation of the food-craving inventory. *Obes Res* 2001;10:107-114

More closely related to mood | Capacity to visualize: Hill, Andrew J. The psychology of food cravings. *Proceedings of the Nutrition Society.* 2007;66:277–285

In just a few days: Kessler, David M. *The End of Overeating.* New York: Rodale, 2009.

A safer choice: Eaton S B, Shostak M, Konner M. *The Paleolithic Prescription: A program of diet & exercise and a design for living.* New York, NY: Harper & Row, 1988.

Supernormal: Sørensen LB, Møller P, Flint A, Martens M, Raben A. Effect of sensory perception of foods on appetite and food intake: a review of studies on humans. *Obesity* 2003;27:1152–1166

Yeomans MR. Taste, palatability and the control of appetite. *Proceedings of the Nutrition Society* 1998;57:609-615

Flavor restriction: van Koningsbruggen G M, Stroebe W, Aarts H. Mere exposure to palatable food cues reduces restrained eaters' physical effort to obtain healthy food. *Appetite* Apr 2012;58(2):593-596

Satiety and satiation: Benelam, B. Satiation, satiety and their effects on eating behaviour. *Nutrition Bulletin* 2009;34:126–173

Makes protein even more satiating: Thouvenot Pierre, Latge C, Laurens M H, Antoine J M. Fat and starch gastric emptying rate in humans: a reproducibility study of a double-isotopic technique. *Am J Clin Nutr* 1994;59(suppl):781S

Oreo is a registered trademark of Kraft Foods.

Pleasure, emotion and reward: Stefano, G B. The neurobiology of pleasure, reward processes, addiction and their health implications. *Neuroendocrinol Lett* 2004;25(4):235-251

Kessler, David M. *The End of Overeating.* New York, NY: Rodale, 2009.

The foods in question: Kessler, David M. *The End of Overeating.* New York: Rodale, 2009.

Chronic stress: George Sophie A, Khan Samir, Briggs Hedieh, Abelson James L. CRH-stimulated cortisol release and food intake in healthy, non-obese adults. *Psychoneuroendocrinology* May 2010;35(4):607–612

Stress affects the activation | Absence of active stress: Epel E, Tomiyama J, Dallman M. "Stress and Reward Neural Networks, Eating, and Obesity." Handbook of Food and Addiction. Oxford: Oxford University Press. Print.

CHAPTER 5: HEALTHY HORMONES, HEALTHY YOU

Highly damaging: Gastaldelli A, Ferrannini E, Miyazaki Y, Matsuda M, De Fronzo R A. Beta-cell dysfunction and glucose intolerance: results from the San Antonio metabolism (SAM) study. *Diabetologia* Jan 2004;47(1):31-9

Singleton, J R Smith A G, Bromberg, M B. Increased prevalence of impaired glucose tolerance in patients with painful sensory neuropathy. *Diabetes Care* 2001;24(8)1448-1453

Gianluca Bardini, et al. Inflammation markers and metabolic characteristics of subjects with one-hour plasma glucose levels. *Diabetes Care* Feb 2010;33(2):411-413

Held C, Gerstein H C, Zhao F, et al. Fasting plasma glucose is an independent predictor of hospitalization for congestive heart failure in high-risk patients. *American Heart Association 2006 Scientific Sessions* 13 Nov 2006. Abstract 2562.

Pär Stattin, Ove Björ, Pietro Ferrari, Annekatrin Lukanova, Per Lenner, Bernt Lindahl, Göran Hallmans, Rudolf Kaaks. Prospective Study of Hyperglycemia and Cancer Risk. *Diabetes Care* 2007;30:561-567

D. Batty, et al. Post-challenge blood glucose concentration and stroke mortality rates in non-diabetic men in London: 38-year follow-up of the original Whitehall prospective cohort study. *Diabetologia* Jul 2008;51(7):1123–1126

90 minutes: "NISMAT Exercise Physiology Corner: Energy Supply for Muscle." *nismat.org,* Nicholas Institute of Sports Medicine and Athletic Trauma. March 2007. Web.

Stomach cells secrete: Beckerman Martin. *Cellular Signaling in Health and Disease.* New York: Springer, 2009. Print.

Normal daily cycle: Schoeller D A, Cella L K, Sinha M K, Caro J F. Entrainment of the diurnal rhythm of plasma leptin to meal timing. *J Clin Invest* 1 Oct 1997;100(7):1882-1887

Wake up hungry | Higher at night: Richards, Byron J. *Mastering Leptin.* Minneapolis: Wellness Resources Books, 2009. Print.

Survive the coming famine: MacLean Paul S, Bergouignan Audrey, Cornier Marc-Andre, Jackman Matthew R. Biology's response to dieting: the impetus for weight regain. *Am J Physiol Regul Integr Comp Physiol* Sep 2011;301(3):R581-600

Secreted by fat cells: Beckerman, Martin. *Cellular Signaling in Health and Disease.* New York: Springer, 2009. Print.

Leptin resistance: Sahu A. Leptin signaling in the hypothalamus: emphasis on energy homeostasis and leptin resistance. *Front Neuroendocrin* Dec 2003;24(4):225-253

Knight Z A, Hannan K S, Greenberg M L, Friedman J M. Hyperleptinemia Is Required for the Development of Leptin Resistance. *PLoS One* Jun 29 2010;5(6):e11376

Gray Sarah L, Donald Christine, Jetha Arif, Covey Scott D, Kieffer Timothy J. Hyperinsulinemia Precedes Insulin Resistance in Mice Lacking Pancreatic B-Cell Leptin Signaling. *Endocrinology* Sep 2010;151(9):4178-86

Morioka Tomoaki, Asilmaz Esra, Hu Jiang, Dishinger John F, Kurpad Amarnath J, Elias Carol F, Li Hui, Elmquist Joel K, Kennedy Robert T, Kulkarni Rohit N. Disruption of leptin receptor expression in the pancreas directly affects B cell growth and function in mice. *J Clin Invest* Oct 2007;117(10):2860-68

Seufert Jochen. Leptin Effects on Pancreatic B-Cell Gene Expression and Function. *Diabetes* Feb 2004;53(1):S153-58

Tuduri Eva, Marroqui Laura, Soriano Sergi, Ropero Ana B, Batista Thiago M, Piquer Sandra, Lopez-Boado Miguel A, Carneiro Everardo M, Gomis Ramon, Nadal Angel, Quesada Ivan. Inhibitory Effects of Leptin on Pancreatic a-Cell Function. *Diabetes* Jul 2009;58 :1616-24

Kieffer Timothy J, Heller R Scott, Leech Colin A, Holz George G, Habener Joel F. Leptin Suppression of Insulin Secretion by the Activation of ATP-Sensitive K+ Channels in Pancreatic B-Cells. *Diabetes* Jun 1997;46(6):1087-93

Leptin resistance leads to insulin resistance: Savage D B, Petersen K F, Shulman G I. Disordered lipid metabolism and the pathogenesis of insulin resistance. *Physiol Rev* 2007;87(2):507–520

Kieffer T J, Heller R S, Leech C A, Holz G G, Habener J F. Leptin suppression of insulin secretion by the activation of ATP-sensitive K+ channels in pancreatic beta-cells. *Diabetes* Jun 1997;46(6):1087–1093

Tuduri E, et al. Inhibitory effects of leptin on pancreatic alpha-cell function. *Diabetes* Jul 2009;58(7):1616–1624

Insulin resistance: Corcoran M P, Lamon-Fava S, Fielding R A. Skeletal muscle lipid deposition and insulin resistance: effect of dietary fatty acids and exercise. *Am J Clin Nutr* 2007;85(3):662- 677

Reaven G M. Role of insulin resistance in human disease. *Diabetes* Dec 1988;37(12): 1595-1607

Elevated fat levels in the blood: Boden, Guenther. Obesity, insulin resistance and free fatty acids. *Curr Opin Endocrinol Diabetes* Apr 2011;18(2):139–143.

Delarue Jacques, Magnan Christophe. Free fatty acids and insulin resistance. *Curr Opin Clinic Nutr Metab Care* Mar 2007;10(2):142-148

Pancreatic beta cells: Robertson R Paul. Chronic Oxidative Stress as a Central Mechanism for Glucose Toxicity in Pancreatic Islet Beta Cells in Diabetes. *J Biol Chem* 8 Oct 2004;279(41): 42351-42354

Prentki M, Joly E, El-Assaad W, Roduit R. Malonyl-CoA signaling, lipid partitioning, and glucolipo-toxicity: role in β-cell adaptation and failure in the etiology of diabetes. *Diabetes* Dec 2002;51(Suppl. 3):S405-S413

Robertson R Paul, Harmon Jamie S. Diabetes, glucose toxicity, and oxidative stress: A case of double jeopardy for the pancreatic islet β cell. *Free Radical Bio Med* 15 Jul 2006;41(2):177-184

Unger R H, Grundy, S. Hyperglycaemia as an inducer as well as a consequence of impaired Islet cell function and insulin resistance: implications for the management of diabetes. *Diabetologia* 1985;28:119-121

Leahy, J L, Cooper, H E, Deal, D A, Weir, G C. Chronic hyperglycemia is associated with impaired glucose influence on insulin secretion. A study in normal rats using chronic in vivo glucose infusions. *J Clin Invest* 1986;77:908-915

Rossetti L, Giaccari A, DeFronzo RA. Glucose toxicity. *Diabetes Care* 1990;13:610-630

Clear risk factor: Fahim Abbasi, Byron William Brown Jr, Cindy Lamendola, Tracey McLaughlin, Gerald M Reaven. Relationship between obesity, insulin resistance, and coronary heart disease risk. *J Am Coll Cardiol* 4 Sep 2002;40(5):937-943

Zunker Peter, Schick Achim, Buschmann Hans-Christian, Georgiadis Dimitrios, Nabavi Darius G., Edelmann Michael, Ringelstein E. Bernd. Hyperinsulinism and Cerebral Microangiopathy. *Stroke*1996;27:219-223

Luchsinger J A. Adiposity, hyperinsulinemia, diabetes and Alzheimer's disease: an epidemiological perspective. *Eur J Pharmacol* 6 May 2008;585(1):119-29

Too far in the other direction: Hofeldt Fred, Dippe Stephen, Forsham Peter. Diagnosis and classification of reactive hypoglycemia based on hormonal changes in response to oral and intravenous glucose administration. *Am J Clin Nutr* Nov 1972;25(11):1193-1201

Must. Eat. Sugar: Page Kathleen, et al. Circulating glucose levels modulate neural control of desire for high-calorie foods in humans. *J Clin Invest* 2011;121(10):4161-4169

When insulin levels are elevated: Paulev Poul-Erik , Zubieta-Calleja Gustavo. New Human Physiology, 2nd Edition. *zuniv.net, Zubieta University Library*. Web.

Bansal Pritpal, Wang Qinghua. Insulin as a physiological modulator of glucagon secretion. *Am J Physiol Endocrinol Metab* 2008;295:E751-E761

Impairs glucose uptake | Inhibits insulin secretion: Andrews Robert C, Walker Brian R. Glucocorticoids and insulin resistance: old hormones, new targets. *Clinical Science* 1999;96:513-523

Stress-related overeating: Dallman Mary F, Pecoraro Norman C, la Fleur Susanne E. Chronic stress and comfort foods: self-medication and abdominal obesity *Brain Behav Immun* Jul 2005;19(4):275-280

Preferentially directs body fat: Talbott Shawn. *The Cortisol Connection*. Alameda: Hunter House, 2007. Print.

Epel E S, McEwen B, Seeman T, Matthews K, Castellazzo G, Brownell K D, Bell J, Ickovics J R. Stress and body shape: stress-induced cortisol secretion is consistently greater among women with central fat. *Psychosom Med* Sep-Oct 2000;62(5):623-32

Fraser Robert, Ingram Mary C, Anderson Niall H, Morrison Caroline, Davies Eleanor, Connell John M C. Cortisol Effects on Body Mass, Blood Pressure, and Cholesterol in the General Population. *Hypertension* 1999;33:1364-1368

Peeke P M, Chrousos G P. Hypercortisolism and Obesity. *Ann NY Acad Sci* 29 Dec 1995;771:665-76

Increased central obesity: Donahue Richard P, Bloom Ellen, Abbott Robert D, Reed Dwayném, Yano Katsuhiko. Central obesity and coronary heart disease in men. *Lancet* 11 Apr 1987;329(8537):821-824

Brunzell John D, Hokanson John E. Dyslipidemia of Central Obesity and Insulin Resistance. *Diabetes Care* 1999;22(Suppl 3):C10-3

Krotkiewski M, Björntorp P, Sjöström L, Smith U. Impact of obesity on metabolism in men and women: importance of regional adipose tissue distribution. *J Clin Invest* 1983;72:1150-1162

Desprès J P, Moorjani S, Ferland M, Tremblay A, Lupien P J, Nadeau A, Pinault S, Theriault G, Bouchard C. Adipose tissue distribution and plasma lipoprotein levels in obese women, importance of intra-abdominal fat. *Arteriosclerosis* 1989;9:203-210

Ashwell M, Cole T J, Dixon A K. Obesity: new insight into the anthropometric classification of fat distribution shown by computed tomography. *BMJ* 1985;290:1692-1694

Terry R B, Wood P D S, Haskell W L, Stefanick M L, Krauss R M. Regional adiposity patterns in relation to lipids, lipoprotein cholesterol, and lipoprotein subfraction mass in men. *J Clin Endocrinol Metab* 1989;68:191-199

Welborn T A. Preferred clinical measures of central obesity for predicting mortality. *Eur J Clin Nutr* 2007;61:1373-1379

Normal thyroid function: Lee, John R. *What Your Doctor May Not Tell You about Menopause: The Breakthrough Book on Natural Progesterone*. New York: Grand Central Publishing. 2004. eBook.

Talbott Shawn. *The Cortisol Connection*. Alameda: Hunter House, 2007. Print.

CHAPTER 6: THE GUTS OF THE MATTER

Sensor for satiety: Koopmans H S. Satiety signals from the gastrointestinal tract. *Am J Clin Nutr* Nov 1985;42(5):1044-1049

Tennis court: Bowen R. Gross and Microscopic Anatomy of the Small Intestine. *vivo.colostate.edu*, Colorado State University Biomedical Hypertexts. April 18, 2000. Web.

70% - 80% of your immune system: Furness John B, Kunzel Wolfgang A A, Clerc Nadine. The intestine as a sensory organ: neural, endocrine, and immune responses. *AJP-GI* Nov 1999;299(5):G922-G928

Leaky gut: Arrieta M C, Bistritz L, Meddings J B. Alterations in intestinal permeability. *Gut* 2006;55(10):1512-20

Liu Z, Li N, Neu J. Tight junctions, leaky intestines, and pediatric diseases. *Acta Paediatr* Apr 2005;94(4):386-93

Laukoetter M G, Nava P, Nusrat A. Role of the intestinal barrier in inflammatory bowel disease. *World J Gastroenterol* Jan 2008;14(3):401-7

Shen L, Turner J R. Role of epithelial cells in initiation and propagation of intestinal inflammation. Eliminating the static: tight junction dynamics exposed. *Am J Physiol Gastrointest Liver Physiol* Apr 2006;290(4):G577-82

Fasano A, Shea-Donohue T. Mechanisms of disease: the role of intestinal barrier function in the pathogenesis of gastrointestinal autoimmune diseases. *Nat Clin Pract Gastroenterol Hepatol* Sep 2005;2(9):416-22

Berkes J, Viswanathan V K, Savkovic S D, Hecht G. Intestinal epithelial responses to enteric pathogens: effects on the tight junction barrier, ion transport, and inflammation. *Gut* Mar 2003;52(3):439-51

Alliance with gut bacteria: Mazmanian Sarkis K, Liu Cui Hua, Tzianabos Arthur O, Kasper Dennis L. An immunomodulatory molecule of symbiotic bacteria directs maturation of the host immune system. *Cell* 15 Jul 2005;122(1):107-118

Kelly Denise, Conway Shaun, Aminov Rustam. Commensal gut bacteria: mechanisms of immune modulation. *Trends in Immunology* Jun 2005;26(6):326-333

Intestinal inflammatory diseases: Oriishi T, Sata M, Toyonaga A, Sasaki E, Tanikawa K. Evaluation of intestinal permeability in patients with inflammatory bowel disease using lactulose and measuring antibodies to lipid A. *Gut* Jun 1995;36(6):891–896

Welcker K, Martin A, Kölle P, Siebeck M, Gross M. Increased intestinal permeability in patients with inflammatory bowel disease. *Eur J Med Res* 2004;9:456-460

Chronic diseases: Anja Sandek, et al. Altered intestinal function in patients with chronic heart failure. *J Am Coll Cardiol* Oct 2007; 50(16);1561-1569

Pradhan Aruna D, Manson JoAnn E, Rifai Nader, et al. C-reactive protein, interleukin 6, and risk of developing type 2 diabetes mellitus. *JAMA* 2001;286(3):327-334

Cani Patrice D, et al. Metabolic endotoxemia initiates obesity and insulin resistance. *Diabetes* Jul 2007;56(7):1761-1772

Arrieta, M C, L Bistritz, J B Meddings. Alterations in intestinal permeability. *Gut* 2006; 55:1512-1520

Hypersensitivities: Forbes Elizabeth E et al. IL-9– and mast cell–mediated intestinal permeability predisposes to oral antigen hypersensitivity. *J Exp Med* 14 Apr 2008;205(4):897–913

Ventura M T, Polimeno L, Amoruso A C, Gatti F, Annoscia E, Marinaro M, Di Leo E, Matino M G, Buquicchio R, Bonini S, Tursi A, Francavilla A. Intestinal permeability in patients with adverse reactions to food. *Digest Liv Dis* Oct 2006;38(10):732-736

Autoimmune conditions: Fasano A, Shea-Donohue T. Mechanisms of disease: the role of intestinal barrier function in the pathogenesis of gastrointestinal autoimmune diseases. *Nat Clin Pract Gastroenterol Hepatol* Sep 2005;2(9):416-22

Fasano Alessio. Leaky Gut and Autoimmune Diseases. Clinical Reviews in Allergy and Immunology. *Nature* Sep 2005;2(9):416-422

Visser J, Rozing J, Sapone A, Lammers K, Fasano A. Tight Junctions, Intestinal Permeability, and Autoimmunity. *Ann NY Acad Sci* 2009;1165:195–205

Bosi E, Molteni L, Radaelli M G, Folini L, Fermo I, Bazzigaluppi E, Piemonti L, Pastore M R, Paroni R. Increased intestinal permeability precedes clinical onset of type 1 diabetes. *Diabetologia* 2006;49(12):2824-2827

Deposition of visceral fat: Lam Yan Y, et al. Role of the Gut in Visceral Fat Inflammation and Metabolic Disorders. *Obesity* 2011;19(11):2113-2120

Gummesson A, et al. Intestinal permeability is associated with visceral adiposity in healthy women. *Obesity* 2011;19(11):2280-2

CHAPTER 7: INFLAMMATION: NO ONE IS IMMUNE

Heart attack, cancer and diabetes: Espinola-Klein C, Gori T, Blankenberg S, Munzel T. Inflammatory markers and cardiovascular risk in the metabolic syndrome. *Front Biosci* 2011;16:1663–1674

Antigens: Holgersson Jan, Gustafsson Anki, Breimer Michael E. Characteristics of protein–carbohydrate interactions as a basis for developing novel carbohydrate-based antirejection therapies. *Immunol Cell Biol* 2005;83:694–708

Metabolic Syndrome: "What is Metabolic Syndrome?" *nhlbi.nih.gov,* U.S. Department of Health and Human Services. November 3, 2011. Web.

Inflammation contributes directly: Espinola-Klein C, Gori T, Blankenberg S, Munzel T. Inflammatory markers and cardiovascular risk in the metabolic syndrome. *Front Biosci* 2011;16:1663–1674

Rocha Viviane Z, Libby Peter. Obesity, inflammation, and atherosclerosis. *NatRev Cardiol* Jun 2009;6:399-409

Haffner Steven M. The Metabolic Syndrome: Inflammation, diabetes mellitus, and cardiovascular disease. *Am Jour Cardiol* Jan 2006;97(2)Supp 1:3-11

Ridker Paul, Wilson Peter W F, Grundy Scott. Should C-reactive protein be added to metabolic syndrome and to assessment of global cardiovascular risk? *Circulation* 2004; 109:2818-2825

Cirillo Pietro, Sautin Yuri Y, Kanellis John, Kang Duk-Hee, Gesualdo Loreto, Nakagawa Takahiko, Johnson Richard J. Systemic inflammation, metabolic syndrome and progressive renal disease. *Nephrol Dial Transplant* 2009;24(5):1384-1387

Adipose tissue: Wisse Brent E. The inflammatory syndrome: the role of adipose tissue cytokines in metabolic disorders linked to obesity. *J Am Soc Nephrol* 2004;15(11):2792-2800

Wajchenberg Bernardo Léo, Nery Marcia, Cunha Maria Rosaria, Silva Maria Elizabeth Rossi da. Adipose tissue at the crossroads in the development of the metabolic syndrome, inflammation and atherosclerosis. *Arq Bras Endocrinol Metab* Mar 2009; 53(2):145-150

Wellen Kathryn E, Hotamisligil Gökhan S. Obesity-induced inflammatory changes in adipose tissue. *J Clin Invest* 2003;112(12):1785–1788

Lam, Yan Y, et al. Role of the gut in visceral fat inflammation and metabolic disorders. *Obesity* 2011;19(11):2113-2120

Belly fat: Berg Anders H, Scherer Philipp E. Adipose Tissue, Inflammation, and Cardiovascular Disease. *Circulation Research* 2005;96:939-949

CHAPTER 8: SUGAR, SWEETENERS, AND ALCOHOL

Health destroyer: Gucciardi, Anthony. "Experts agree - Sugar is a health destroyer." *naturalnews.com,* Natural News. May 09, 2011. Web.

Sugar is addictive: Katz, David. "Sugar *Isn't* Evil: A Rebuttal." *huffingtonpost.com.* The Huffington Post Internet Newspaper. April 18, 2011. Web.

Artificial sweeteners compared to sugar: Artificial Sweeteners: No Calories... Sweet! *FDA Consum* Jul-Aug 2006;40(4):27-8

Leptin and taste buds: Kawai K, Sugimoto K, Nakashima K, Miura H, Ninomiya Y. Leptin as a modulator of sweet taste sensitivities in mice. *Proc Natl Acad Sci U S A* 26 Sep 2000;97(20):11044-9

Splenda and gut bacteria: Abou-Donia M B, El-Masry E M, Abdel-Rahman A A, McLendon R E, Schiffman S S. Splenda alters gut microflora and increases intestinal p-glycoprotein and cytochrome p-450 in male rats. *J Toxicol Environ Health A* 2008;71(21):1415-29

Clinical definition of addiction: Per the American Psychiatric Association's Diagnostic and Statistical Manual of Mental Disorders (DSM-IV)

Temporary hypoglycemia: O'Keefe S J, Marks V. Lunchtime gin and tonic a cause of reactive hypoglycemia. *Lancet* 1977;1(8025):1286-1288

Huang Zhen, Sjöholm Åke. Ethanol acutely stimulates islet blood flow, amplifies insulin secretion, and induces hypoglycemia via NO and vagally mediated mechanisms. *Endocrinology* 2008;149:232-236

Intestinal permeability: Vishnudutt Purohit, et al. Alcohol, intestinal bacterial growth, intestinal permeability to endotoxin, and medical consequences: Summary of a symposium. *Alcohol* Aug 2008;(42)5:349-361

Impairs cellular immunity: Szabo Gyongyi. Consequences of alcohol consumption on host defence. *Alcohol and Alcoholism* 1999;34(6):830-841

Pro-oxidative: Brocardo PS, Gil-Mohapel J, Christie BR. The role of oxidative stress in fetal alcohol spectrum disorders. *Brain Res Rev* 24 Jun 2011;67(1-2):209-25

Resveratrol: Kahn, Amina. "Resveratrol researcher faked data, report says; what drives academic fraud?" *articles.latimes.com*, Los Angeles Times. January 12, 2012. Web.

160 micrograms: Sanders T H, McMichael R W. "Occurrence of resveratrol in edible peanuts." American Oil Chemists Society, Las Vegas, Nevada, 1998. Presentation.

60 liters: "Red wine and resveratrol: Good for your heart?" *mayoclinic.com*, The Mayo Clinic. March 4 2011. Web.

CHAPTER 9: SEED OILS

Specifically from these seed oils: Ikemoto S, Takahashi M, Tsunoda N, Maruyama K, Itakura H, Ezaki O. High-fat diet-induced hyperglycemia and obesity in mice: differential effects of dietary oils. *Metabolism* Dec 1996;45(12):1539-46

Jen KL, Buison A, Pellizzon M, Ordiz Jr. F, Santa Ana L, Brown J. Differential effects of fatty acids and exercise on body weight regulation and metabolism in female Wistar rats. *Exp Biol Med (Maywood)* Jul 2003;228(7):843-9

Simopoulos, Artemis P. Omega-3 Fatty Acids in Inflammation and Autoimmune Diseases. *Am J Clin Nutr* 2002;21(6):495–505

EPA and DHA: Calder Phillip C. n–3 Polyunsaturated fatty acids, inflammation, and inflammatory diseases. *Am J Clin Nutr* Jun 2006;83(6):S1505-1519S

10% of total calories: Gupta Sanjay. "If we are what we eat, Americans are corn and soy." *cnn.com*, CNN Health. September 22, 2007. Web.

PUFA intake from seed oils: Simopoulos A P, The importance of the ratio of omega-6/omega-3 essential fatty acids. *Biomed Pharmacother* Oct 2002;56(8):365-379

Simopoulos Artemis P, Cleland Leslie G. *Omega-6/Omega-3 Essential Fatty Acid Ratio: The Scientific Evidence (World Review of Nutrition and Dietetics)*. Basel: Karger, 2003.

Simopoulos, Artemis. Evolutionary Aspects of Diet: The Omega-6/Omega-3 Ratio and the Brain. *Mol Neurobiol* 1 Oct 2011;44(2)203-215

Most of the diseases of modern civilization: Gupta Sanjay. "If we are what we eat, Americans are corn and soy." *CNN.com*. CNN Health, September 22, 2007. Web.

Blasbalg T L, Hibbeln J R, Ramsden C E, Majchrzak S F, Rawlings R R. Changes in consumption of omega-3 and omega-6 fatty acids in the United States during the 20th century. *Am J Clin Nutr* May 2011;93(5):950-62

Simopoulos A P. The importance of the omega-6/omega-3 fatty acid ratio in cardiovascular disease and other chronic diseases. *Exp Biol Med (Maywood)* Jun 2008;233(6):674-88

Ramsden C E, et al. n–6 fatty acid-specific and mixed polyunsaturate dietary interventions have different effects on CHD risk: a meta-analysis of randomised controlled trials. *Br J Nutr* 2010;104(11):1586–1600

Russo G L. Dietary n-6 and n-3 polyunsaturated fatty acids: from biochemistry to clinical implications in cardiovascular prevention. *Biochem Pharmacol* 15 Mar 2009;77(6):937-46

Free radicals: Aruoma, Okezie I. Free Radicals, Oxidative Stress, and Antioxidants in Human Health and Disease. *JAOCS*. 1998;75(2):199-212

Ames B N, Shigenaga M K, Hagen T M. Oxidants, antioxidants, and the degenerative diseases of aging. *PNAS* Sep 1993;90(17)7915-7922

Tuppo and Forman. Free radical oxidative damage and Alzheimer's disease. *JAOA* Dec 2001;101(12) S11-S15

Touyz Rhian M. Reactive Oxygen Species, Vascular Oxidative Stress, and Redox Signaling in Hypertension. *Hypertension* 2004; 44:248-252

Dreher D, Junod A F. Role of oxygen free radicals in cancer development. *Eur J Canc* Jan 1996;32(1):30-38

Supplemented antioxidants: Melton, Lisa. "The antioxidant myth: a medical fairy tale." *New Scientist* August 5, 2006:40-43. Print

Oxidized PUFA health risk: Esterbauer, H. Cytotoxicity and genotoxicity of lipid-oxidation products. *Am J Clin Nutr* May 1993;57(5):779S-785S

Hayam Israela, Cogan Uri, Mokady Shoshana. Dietary oxidized oil and the activity of antioxidant enzymes and lipoprotein peroxidation in rats. *Nutrition Research* Jul 1995;15(7):1037-1044

Kanazawa K, Ashida H, Minamoto S, Natake M. The effect of orally administered secondary autoxidation products of linoleic acid on the activity of detoxifying enzymes in the rat liver. *Biochim Biophys Acta* 24 Oct 1986;879(1):36-43

Kanazawa Kazuki. Tissue injury induced by dietary products of lipid peroxidation. *Free Radicals Antioxid Nutr* 1993;383-99

Reflected in the makeup of our cell walls: Baylin A, Kabagambe E K, Siles X, Campos H. Adipose tissue biomarkers of fatty acid intake. *Am J Clin Nutr* Oct 2002;76(4):750-7

Dayton S, Hashimoto S, Dixon W, Pearce M L. Composition of lipids in human serum and adipose tissue during prolonged feeding of a diet high in unsaturated fat. *J Lipid Res* Jan 1966;7(1):103-11

High levels of Omega 6: Simopoulos A P, The importance of the ratio of omega-6/omega-3 essential fatty acids. *Biomed Pharmacother* Oct 2002;56(8):365-379

Weaver Kelly L, Ivester Priscilla, Seeds Michael, Arm Jonathan P, Chilton Floyd H. Effect of Dietary Fatty Acids on Inflammatory Gene Expression in Healthy Humans. *J Biol Chem* 5 Jun 2009; 284(23):15400–15407

Staprans I, Rapp J H, Pan X M, Kim K Y, Feingold K R. Oxidized lipids in the diet are a source of oxidized lipid in chylomicrons of human serum. *Arterioscl Throm Vas* 1994;14:1900-1905

Massiera, et al. A Western-like fat diet is sufficient to induce a gradual enhancement in fat mass over generations. *Journal Lipid Res* 2010;51(8):2352

CHAPTER 10: GRAINS AND LEGUMES

Whole grains: "Draft Guidance: Whole Grain Label Statements." *fda.gov*, U.S. Food and Drug Administration. February 17, 2006. Web.

Good Day vs. Bad Day: Nutritional analysis performed in FoodWorks, Version 13.

Dietary fiber in foods: Reprinted with express permission by Jennifer Anderson Ph.D., R.D., Department of Food Science and Human Nutrition, Colorado State University. Anderson J, Perryman S, Young L, Prior S. "Dietary Fiber." *ext.colostate.edu,* Colorado State University. December 2010. Web.

Phytic acid: Cordain Loren. Cereal grains: humanity's double-edged sword. *World Rev Nutr Diet* 1999;84:19-73

Munir Cheryana, Rackisb Joseph J. Phytic acid interactions in food systems. *Crit Rev Food Sci Nutr* 1980;13(4):297-335

Torrea M, Rodrigueza A R, Saura-Calixtob F. Effects of dietary fiber and phytic acid on mineral availability. *Crit Rev Food Sci Nutr* 1991;30(1):1-22

Schlemmer Ulrich, Frølich Wenche, Prieto Rafel M, Grases Felix. Phytate in foods and significance for humans: Food sources, intake, processing, bioavailability, protective role and analysis. *Mol Nut Food Res* 2009;53:S330 –S375

Hallberg L, Rossander L, Skånberg A B. Phytates and the inhibitory effect of bran on iron absorption in man. *Am J Clin Nutr* May 1987;45(5):988-96

Meta-analysis: Kelly S A M, Summerbell C D, Brynes A, Whittaker V, Frost G. Wholegrain cereals for coronary heart disease (Review). *The Cochrane Library* 2009;1:1-61

Whole grain labeling: "Draft Guidance: Whole Grain Label Statements." *fda.gov,* U.S. Food and Drug Administration. February 17, 2006. Web.

Whole Grains Council: "Government Guidance." *wholegrainscouncil.org,* Whole Grains Counsel. n.d. Web.

Gluten: Shewry Peter R, Halford Nigel G, Belton Peter S, Tatham Arthur S. The structure and properties of gluten: an elastic protein from wheat grain. *Philos Trans R Soc Lond B Biol Sci* 28 Feb 2002;357(1418):133–142

Biesiekierski J R, Newnham E D, Irving P M, Barrett J S, Haines M, Doecke J D, Shepherd S J, Muir J G, Gibson P R. Gluten causes gastrointestinal symptoms in subjects without celiac disease: a double-blind randomized placebo-controlled trial. *Am J Gastroenterol* Mar 2011;106(3):508-14

Visser J, Rozing J, Sapone A et al. Tight junctions, Intestinal permeability and Autoimmunity. *Ann NY Acad Sci* 2009;1165:195-205

Shan L, Qiao SW, Arentz-Hansen H, et al. Identification and Analysis of Multivalent Proteolytically Resistant Peptides from Gluten: Implications for Celiac Sprue. *J Proteome Res* 2005;4(5):1732–1741

Drago S, Asmar R, Di Pierro M, et al. Gliadin, zonulin and gut permeability: Effects on celiac and non-celiac intestinal mucosa and intestinal cell lines. *Scandinavian Journal of Gastroenterology* 2006; 41:408/419

Problematic proteins: Gálová Zdenka, Palenčárová Eva, Chňapek Milan, Balážová Želmíra. Gastrointestinal digestion of wheat celiac active proteins. *JMBFS* Feb 2012;1:601-609

Battais F, Richard C, Jacquenet S, Denery-Papini S, Moneret-Vautrin D A. Wheat grain allergies: an update on wheat allergens. *Eur Ann Allergy Clin Immunol* 2008;40(3):67-76

Visser J et al. Tight junctions, intestinal permeability, and autoimmunity: celiac disease and type 1 diabetes paradigms. *Ann N Y Acad Sci* May 2009;1165:195-205

Dieterich W et al. Cross linking to tissue transglutaminase and collagen favours gliadin toxicity in coeliac disease. *Gut* Apr 2006;55(4):478-84

Fasano A, et al. Gliadin, zonulin and gut permeability: Effects on celiac and non-celiac intestinal mucosa and intestinal cell lines. *Scand J Gastroenterol* Apr 2006;41(4):408-19

Alaedini A et al. Immune cross-reactivity in celiac disease: anti-gliadin antibodies bind to neuronal synapsin I. *J Immunol* 15 May 2007 15;178(10):6590-5

Alaedini A, Green PH. Autoantibodies in celiac disease. *Autoimmunity* Feb 2008;41(1):19-26

Shaoul R, Lerner A. Associated autoantibodies in celiac disease. *Autoimmun Rev* Sep 2007;6(8):559-65

Simonato Barbara, Pasini Gabriella, Giannattasio Matteo, Peruffo Angelo D B, De Lazzari Franca, Curioni Andrea. Food Allergy to Wheat Products: The Effect of Bread Baking and in Vitro Digestion on Wheat Allergenic Proteins. A Study with Bread Dough, Crumb, and Crust. *J Agric Food Chem* 2001;49(11):5668–5673

Celiac disease: Used with express permission of The Celiac Disease Foundation. "What Happens With Celiac Disease." *celiac.org*, The Celiac Disease Foundation. n.d. Web.

Gluten sensitivity: Fasano Alessio, et al. Divergence of gut permeability and mucosal immune gene expression in two gluten-associated conditions: celiac disease and gluten sensitivity. *BMC Medicine* 2011;9:23

Soaking, sprouting, fermenting: Haard Normal F, et al. "Fermented cereals. A global perspective." *fao. org*, FAO Agricultural Services Bulletin, No. 138. 1999. Web.

Egli I, Davidsson L, Juillerat M A, Barclay D, Hurrell R F. The Influence of Soaking and Germination on the Phytase Activity and Phytic Acid Content of Grains and Seeds Potentially Useful for Complementary Feedin. *J Food Sci* Nov 2002;67(9):3484–3488

Ruiz R G, Price K, Rose M, Rhodes M, Fenwick R. A preliminary study on the effect of germination on saponin content and composition of lentils and chickpeas. *Z Lebensm Unters Forsch* 1996;203:366-369

Ruiz R G, Price K R, Arthur A E, Rose M E, Rhodes M J, Fenwick R G. Effect of soaking and cooking on the saponin content and composition of chickpeas (Cicer arietinum) and lentils (Lens culinaris). *J Agric Food Chem* 1996;44:1526-1530

FODMAPs: Levitt M D, Hirsh P, Fetzer C A, Sheahan M, Levine A S. H2 excretion after ingestion of complex carbohydrates. *Gastroenterology* Feb 1987;92(2):383-9

Gibson P R, Shepherd S J. Personal view: food for thought—western lifestyle and susceptibility to Crohn's disease. The FODMAP hypothesis. *Aliment Pharmacol Ther* 2005;21:1399–409

Clausen M R, Jorgensen J, Mortensen P B. Comparison of diarrhea induced by ingestion of fructooligosaccharide Idolax and disaccharide lactulose: role of osmolarity versus fermentation of malabsorbed carbohydrate. *Dig Dis Sci* 1998;43:2696–707

Rumessen J J, Gudmand-Hoyer E. Fructans of chicory: intestinal transport and fermentation of different chain lengths and relation to fructose and sorbitol malabsorption. *Am J Clin Nutr* 1998;68:357–64

Davidson M H, Maki K C. Effects of dietary inulin on serum lipids. *J Nutr* 1999;129:1474S–1474TS

Pedersen A, Sandstrom B, van Amelsvoort J M M. The effect of ingestion of inulin on blood lipids and gastrointestinal symptoms in healthy females. *Br J Nutr* 1997;78:215–22

Nilsson U, Dahlqvist A. Cereal fructosans: Part 2—characterisation and structure of wheat fructosans. *Food Chem* 1986;22:95–106

Soy: Humfrey Charles, Holmes Philip. *Phytoestrogens in the Human Diet. le.ac.uk*, Institute for Environment and Health. October 2000. Web.

Sacks Frank M, Lichtenstein Alice, Van Horn Linda, Harris William, Kris-Etherton Penny, Winston Mary. Soy Protein, Isoflavones, and Cardiovascular Health. *Circulation* 2006;113:1034-1044

Ginsburg J, Prelevic G M. Is there a proven place for phytoestrogens in the menopause? *Climacteric* 1999;2:75-78

Newton Katherine M, Grady Deborah. Soy Isoflavones for Prevention of Menopausal Bone Loss and Vasomotor Symptoms. *Archives of Internal Medicine (AMA)* Aug 2011;171(15):1369–1370

Irvine CH and others. Phytoestrogens in soy-based infant foods: concentrations, daily intake and possible biological effects. *Proc Soc Exp Biol Med* Mar 1998;217(3):247-53.

Peanuts: Wang Q, Yu L G, Campbell B J, Milton J D, Rhodes J M. Identification of Intact Peanut Lectin in Peripheral Venous Blood. *Lancet* 1998;352,1831–1832

Beans and cooking: Bender A E. Haemagglutinins (Lectins in Beans). *Food Chemistry* 1983;11:309–320.

Boufassa C, Lafont J, Rouanet, J M, Besançon P. Thermal Inactivation of Lectins (PHA) Isolated from Phaseolus vulgaris. *Food Chemistry* 1986;20:295–304

CHAPTER 11: DAIRY

Children and dairy: Cordain L, Eades M R, Eades M D. Hyperinsulinemic diseases of civilization: more than just syndrome X. *Comp Biochem Physiol Part A* 2003;136:95-112

Adebamowo C A, et al. High school dietary dairy intake and teenage acne. *J Am Acad Dermatol* 2005;52(2):99-106

Kostraba J N, Cruickshanks K J, Lawler-Heavner J, Jobin L F, Rewers M J, Gay E C, Chase H P, Klingensmith G, Hamman R F. Early exposure to cow's milk and solid foods in infancy, genetic predisposition, and risk of IDDM. *Diabetes* Feb 1993;42(2):288-95

Casomorphins and gut motility: Hannelore Daniel, Vohwinkel Margret, Rehner Gertrud. Effect of casein and β-casomorphins on gastrointestinal motility in rats. *J Nutr* Mar 1990;120(3):252-7

Histamine: Kurek M, Przybilla B, Hermann K, Ring J (1992). A naturally occurring opioid peptide from cow's milk, beta-casomorphine-7, is a direct histamine releaser in man. *Int Arch Allergy Immunol* 1997;(2): 115–120

Miller M J, Zhang X J, Gu X, Tenore E, Clark D A. Exaggerated intestinal histamine release by casein and casein hydrolysate but not whey hydrolysate. *Scand J Gastroentero* 1991;26(4):379-384

Maintz Laura, Novak Natalija. Histamine and histamine intolerance. *Am J Clin Nutr* May 2007;85(5):1185-1196

Casein and celiac: Kristjánsson G, Venge P, Hällgren R. Mucosal reactivity to cow's milk protein in coeliac disease. *Clin Exp Immunol* Mar 2007;147(3):449-55

Casein and postpartum/schizophrenia: Millward C, Ferriter M, Calver S, Connell-Jones G. Gluten- and casein-free diets for autistic spectrum disorder. *Cochrane Database of Systematic Reviews* 2004;2:CD003498

Autism and casein: Whiteley Paul, Rodgers Jacqui, Savery Dawn, Shattock Paul. A gluten-free diet as an intervention for autism and associated spectrum disorders: preliminary findings. *Autism* 1999; 3(1):45-65

Swinburn Boyd. "Beta casein A1 and A2 in milk and human health." Report to New Zealand Food Safety Authority. July 13, 2004. Print.

Milk and insulin response: Gannon M C, Nuttall F Q, Krezowski P A, Billington C J, Parker S. The serum insulin and plasma glucose responses to milk and fruit products in Type 2 (non-insulin-dependent) diabetic patients. *Diabetologia* 1986;29(11):784-791

Holt S H, et al. An insulin index of foods: the insulin demand generated by 1000-kj portions of common foods. *Am J Clin Nutr* Nov 1997;66(5):1264-76

Ostman EM, Liljeberg Elmstahl HGM, Bjorck IME. Inconsistency between glycemic and insulinemic responses to regular and fermented milk products. *Am J Clin Nutr* 2001;74:96–100

Milk and insulin resistance: Hoppe C, et al. High intakes of milk, but not meat increase s-insulin and insulin resistance in 8-year old boys. *Eur J Clin Nutr* Mar 2005;59(3):393-8

More insulin sensitive: Borghouts L B, Keizer H A. Exercise and insulin sensitivity: a review. *Int J Sports Med* 2000 Jan;21(1):1-12

IGF-1 and cancer: Renehan A G, Zwahlen M, Minder C, O'Dwyer S T, Shalet S M, Egger M. Insulin-like growth factor (IGF)-I, IGF binding protein-3, and cancer risk: systematic review and meta-regression analysis. *Lancet* 2004;363:1346-1353

Wolk A. The growth hormone and insulin-like growth factor I axis, and cancer. *Lancet* 2004;363:1336-1337

Grimberg A. Mechanisms by which IGF-I may promote cancer. *Cancer Biol Ther* 2003 Nov-Dec;2(6):630-5

Milk and estrogen: Ganmaa D, Sato A. The possible role of female sex hormones in milk from pregnant cows in the development of breast, ovarian and corpus uteri cancers. *Med Hypotheses* 2005;65(6):1028-37

Farlow D W, Xu X, Veenstra T D. Quantitative measurement of endogenous estrogen metabolites, risk factors for development of breast cancer, in commercial milk products. *J Chromatogr B* May 2009;877(13):1327–1334

Lactose intolerance in adults: Swallow D M. Genetics of lactase persistence and lactose intolerance. *Ann Rev Genet* 2003;37:197-219

"Lactose intolerance." *nlm.nih.gov,* U.S. National Library of Medicine, National Institute of Health. July 7, 2010. Web.

Lomer M C E, Parkes G C, Sanderson J D. Lactose intolerance in clinical practice – myths and realities. *Aliment Pharmacol Ther* Jan 2008;27(2)93-103

Milk and disease: Agranoff B W, Goldberg D. Diet and the geographical distribution of multiple sclerosis. *Lancet* 1974;2:1061-66

Butcher P J. Milk consumption and multiple sclerosis – an etiological hypothesis. *Med Hypothesis* 1986;19(2):169-78

Lauren K. Diet and multiple sclerosis. *Neurology* Aug 1997;49(2)S55-61

Cordain L, Toohey L, Smith M J, Hickey M S. Modulation of immune function by dietary lectins in rheumatoid arthritis. *Brit J Nutr* 2000;83:207-217

McLachlan C N. Beta-casein A1, ischaemic heart disease mortality, and other illnesses. *Med Hypotheses* Feb 2001;56(2):262-72

More than just calcium: Other Nutrients and Bone Health at a Glance. *niams.nih.gov.* National Institutes of Health. Dec 2004. Web.

Vitamin K and bone loss: Feskanich D, Weber P, Willett WC, Rockett H, Booth SL, Colditz GA. Vitamin K intake and hip fractures in women: a prospective study. *Am J Clin Nutr* 1999;69(1):74-79

Bügel S. Vitamin K and bone health in adult humans. *Vitam Horm* 2008;78:393-416

Magnesium: Abraham GE, Grewal H. A total dietary program emphasizing magnesium instead of calcium. Effect on the mineral density of calcaneous bone in postmenopausal women on hormonal therapy. *J Reprod Med* 1990;35(5):503-7

Vitamins D and K work together: Adams J, Pepping J. Vitamin K in the treatment and prevention of osteoporosis and arterial calcification. *Am J Health Syst Pharm* Aug 2005; 62 (15): 1574-81

Tanaka, K, Kuwabara, A. Fat soluble vitamins for maintaining bone health. *Clin Calcium* Sep 2009; 19(9):1354-60

Schaafsma A, Muskiet FA, Storm H, Hofstede GJ, Pakan I, Van der Veer E. Vitamin D(3) and vitamin K(1) supplementation of Dutch postmenopausal women with normal and low bone mineral densities: effects on serum 25-hydroxyvitamin D and carboxylated osteocalcin. *Eur J Clin Nutr* Aug 2000;54(8):626-31

Okano T. Vitamin D, K and bone mineral density. *Clin Calcium* Sep 2005;15(9):1489-94

Weber P. Vitamin K and bone health. *Nutrition* Oct 2001;17(10):880-7

Free radicals and bone health: Watkins BA et al, "Importance of Vitamin E in Bone Formation and in Chondrocyte Function" Purdue University, W. Lafayette, IN 47907

Blood sugar and bone health: Burckhardt Peter, Dawson-Hughes Bess, Weaver Connie M. *Nutritional Influences on Bone Health.* New York: Springer, 2010. Print.

Cortisol and bone health: Talbott Shawn. *The Cortisol Connection.* Alameda: Hunter House, 2007. Print.

Homocysteine and bone health: Cordain Loren. *The Paleo Answer.* Hoboken: John Wiley & Sons, 2012. Print.

United States/calcium: Cordain Loren. *The Paleo Answer.* Hoboken: John Wiley & Sons, 2012. Print.

Whole grains and bone health: Cordain Loren. *The Paleo Answer.* Hoboken: John Wiley & Sons, 2012. Print.

Mellanby, Edward. The Rickets-Producing and Anti-Calcifying Action of Phytate. *J. Physiol* 1949;109:488-533

Batchelor A J, Compston J E. Reduced plasma halflife of radio-labelled 25-hydroxyvitamin D3 in subjects receiving a high-fibre diet. *Brit J Nutr* 1983;49:213

Clements Mr, Johnson L, Fraser Dr. A new mechanism for induced vitamin D deficiency in calcium deprivation. *Nature* 1987;324:62-65

Protein and bone health: Kerstetter Jane E, O'Brien Kimberly O, Insogna Karl L. Dietary protein, calcium metabolism, and skeletal homeostasis revisited. *Am J Clin Nutr* Sep 2003;78(3):584S-592S

Cao J J, Nielsen F H. Acid diet (high-meat protein) effects on calcium metabolism and bone health. *Curr Opin Clin Nutr Metab Care* Nov 2010;13(6):698-702

Age and calcium absorption: Heaney Robert P, Recker Robert R, Stegman Mary Ruth, Moy Alan J. Calcium absorption in women: Relationships to Calcium intake, Estrogen status, and age. *J Bone Min Res* Aug 1989;4:(4)469–475

Calcium does not prevent bone fractures: Freskanich D, et al., Milk, dietary calcium, and bone fractures in women: a 12-year prospective study. *Am J Pub Health* 1997 Jun; 87(6): 992-997

Cumming RG, et al., Case-control study of risk factors for hip fractures in the elderly. *Am J Epidem* 1994 Mar 1; 139(5): 493-503

Grant AM, et al. Calcium/vitamin D not effective for secondary prevention of fracture. *Lancet* 2005; 365:1621-1628

Too much calcium: Patel AM, Goldfarb S. Got Calcium? Welcome to the Calcium-Alkali Syndrome. *JASN* 1 Sep 2010;(21):9,1440-1443

Bolland Mark J, Avenell Alison, Baron John A, Grey Andrew, MacLennan Graeme S, Gamble Greg D, Reid Ian R. Effect of calcium supplements on risk of myocardial infarction and cardiovascular events: meta-analysis. *BMJ* 2010;341:c3691

Bolland Mark J, Grey Andrew, Avenell Alison, Gamble Greg D, Reid Ian R. Calcium supplements with or without vitamin D and risk of cardiovascular events: reanalysis of the Women's Health Initiative limited access dataset and meta-analysis. *BMJ* 2011;342:d2040.

Spinach and calcium: Chai W, et al. Effect of Different Cooking Methods on Vegetable Oxalate Content. *J Agric Food Chem* Apr 2005; 53(8):3027–3030

Savage G P, et al. Effect of Cooking on the Soluble and Insoluble Oxalate Content of Some New Zealand Foods. *J Food Comp Anal* Jun 2000;13(3):201-206

Calcium from kale: Heaney RP, Weaver CM. Calcium absorption from kale. *Am J Clin Nutr* 1990; 51:656-657

Plant calcium in particular: Park HM, Heo J, Park Y. Calcium from plant sources is beneficial to lowering the risk of osteoporosis in postmenopausal Korean women. *Nutr Res* Jan 2011;31(1):27-32

"Go Green for Bone Health." *Taste For Life.* May 2011:6. Print.

Tucker Katherine L, Hannan Marian T, Chen Honglei, Cupples L Adrienne, Wilson Peter WF, Kiel Douglas P. Potassium, magnesium, and fruit and vegetable intakes are associated with greater bone mineral density in elderly men and women. *Am J Clin Nutr* Apr 1999;69(4):727-736

New Susan A, Robins Simon P, Campbell Marion K, Martin James C, Garton Mark J, Bolton-Smith Caroline, Grubb David A, Lee Sue J, Reid David M. Dietary influences on bone mass and bone metabolism: further evidence of a positive link between fruit and vegetable consumption and bone health? *Am J Clin Nutr* Jan 2000;71(1):142-151

Magnesium: Marier JR. Magnesium Content of the Food Supply in the Modern-Day World. *Magnesium* 1986;5:1-8

Weight-bearing activity: Kohrt Wendy, Bloomfield Susan, Little Kathleen, Nelson Miriam E, Yingling, Vanessa R. Physical Activity and Bone Health. *Strength training: Medicine & Science in Sports & Exercise* Nov 2004;36(11):1985-1996

Don't need as much calcium: Prentice Ann, Laskey Ann, Shaw Jacquie, Hudson Geoffrey, Day Kenneth, Jarjou Landing, Dibba Bakary, Paul Alison A. The calcium and phosphorus intakes of rural Gambian women during pregnancy and lactation. *Brit J Nutr* 1993;(69)885-896

De Souza Genaro P, Martini LA. Effect of Protein Intake on Bone and Muscle Mass in the Elderly. *Nutr Rev* 2010;68(10):616–623

Sellers EAC, Sharma A, Rodd C. Adaptation of Inuit Children to a Low-Calcium Diet. *Can Pub Health J* 2003;168(9):1141–1143

CHAPTER 12: IT ALL ADDS UP

Autoimmune: "What is autoimmunity?" and "What causes autoimmunity?" *aarda.org*, The American Autoimmune Related Diseases Association. n.d. Web.

Fasano Alessio: Zonulin and Its Regulation of Intestinal Barrier Function: The Biological Door to Inflammation, Autoimmunity, and Cancer. *Physiol Rev* Jan 2011;91(1):151-175

Thought to develop: Cordain Loren. Cereal grains: humanity's double-edged sword. *World Rev Nutr Diet* 1999;84:19-73

Molecular mimicry: "Molecular Mimicry." *direct-ms.org* Direct-MS. n.d. Web.

Oldstone M B. Molecular mimicry and immune-mediated diseases. *FASEB J* Oct 1998;12(13):1255-65

Ostenstad B, Dybwad A, Lea T, Forre O, Vinje O, Sioud M. Evidence for monoclonal expansion of synovial T cells bearing V alpha 2.1/V beta 5.5 gene segments and recognizing a synthetic peptide that shares homology with a number of putative autoantigens. *Immunology* Oct1995;86(2):168-75

Wucherpfennig K W, Strominger J L. Molecular mimicry in T cell-mediated autoimmunity: viral peptides activate human T cell clones specific for myelin basic protein. *Cell* 10 Mar 1995;80(5):695-705

Honeyman M C, Stone N L, Harrison L C. T-cell epitopes in type 1 diabetes autoantigen tyrosine phosphatase IA-2: potential for mimicry with rotavirus and other environmental agents. *Mol Med* Apr 1998;4(4):231-9

Chervonsky Alexander V. Influence of microbial environment on autoimmunity. *Nature Immunology* 2010;11:28-35

Autoimmune/reversible: Fasano Alessio. Leaky Gut and Autoimmune Diseases. *Clin Rev Allerg Immun* 2011;42(1):71-78

CHAPTER 13: MEAT, SEAFOOD, AND EGGS

Most satiating: Astrup A. The satiating power of protein—a key to obesity prevention? *Am J Clin Nutr* Jul 2005;82(1):1-2

Healthy body weight: Astrup A. The satiating power of protein—a key to obesity prevention? *Am J Clin Nutr* Jul 2005;82(1):1-2

Natural: Ikerd, John. "The New American Food Economy." *web.missouri.edu*, University of Missouri. January 2008. Web.

Measurably healthier: Duckett S K, Neel J P S, Fontenot J P, Clapham W M. Effects of winter stocker growth rate and finishing system on: III. Tissue proximate, fatty acid, vitamin and cholesterol content. *J Anim Sci* 5 Jun 2009;jas.2009-1850

Pastured eggs: Alterman Tabitha. "More Great News About Free-Range Eggs." *motherearthnews.com*, Mother Earth News. February/March 2009. Web.

Wild-caught fish: "PCBs in Farmed Salmon: Wild versus farmed." *ewg.org*, Environmental Working Group. n.d. Web

E. Coli bacteria: Diez-Gonzalez Francisco, Callaway Todd R, Kizoulis Menas G, Russell James B. Grain-feeding and the dissemination of acid-resistant Escherichia coli from Cattle. *Science* 11 Sep 1998;281:1666-8

99%: Farm Forward calculation based on U.S. Department of Agriculture, 2002 *Census of Agriculture*, June 2004; and *ibid.*

Factory farming: Reprinted with the express permission of Sustainable Table. "Factory Farming." *sustainabletable.org*, Sustainable Table. n.d. Web

Residues in meat: Pearson A M, Dutson T R. *Quality Attributes and Their Measurement in Meat, Poultry and Fish Products*. New York: Springer, 1995. Print.

Two to ten times the cholesterol: Ravnskov Uffe. "The Cholesterol Myths." *ravnskov.nu*, Uffe Ravnskov, MD, PhD. n.d. Web.

Triglycerides and HDL: El Harchaoui Karim, et al. Value of Low-Density Lipoprotein Particle Number and Size as Predictors of Coronary Artery Disease in Apparently Healthy Men and Women. *J Am Coll Cardiol* 2007;49:547-553

Ratio: Bittner Vera, Johnson B. Delia, Zineh Issam, Rogers William J, Vido Diane, Marroquin Oscar C, Bairey-Merz C Noel, Sopko George. The Triglyceride/High-Density Lipoprotein Cholesterol Ratio Predicts all-Cause Mortality in Women With Suspected Myocardial Ischemia: A Report From the Women's Ischemia Syndrome Evaluation (WISE). *Am Heart J* 2009;157(3):548-555

Gaziano J M, Hennekens C H, O'Donnell C J, Breslow J L, Buring J E. Fasting triglycerides, high-density lipoprotein, and risk of myocardial infarction. *Circulation* 1997;96:2520-2525

One 2008 study: "Two-egg diet cracks cholesterol issue." *physorg.com*, PhysOrg. Aug 28 2008. Web.

Processed meats: Ward M, Cross A. Processed meat intake, CYP2A6 activity, and risk of colorectal adenoma. *Carcinogenesis* 2007;28(6):1210-1216

Santarelli R L, Pierre F, Corpet D E. Processed meat and colorectal cancer: a review of epidemiologic and experimental evidence. *Nutr Cancer* 2008;60(2):131-44

CHAPTER 14: VEGETABLES AND FRUIT

Stroke: Dauchet L, Amouyel P, Dallongeville J. Fruit and vegetable consumption and risk of stroke: A meta-analysis of cohort studies. *Neurology* 25 Oct, 2005;65(8):1193-1197

Coronary heart disease: Hu F B, Willett W C. Optimal diets for prevention of coronary heart disease. *JAMA* 2002;288:2569–2578

Cancer: Shacter E, Weitzman S. Chronic Inflammation and Cancer. *Oncology* 31 Jan 2002; 16(2):217-232

Meat and antioxidants: Rizzo AM, Berselli P, Zava S, Montorfano G, Negroni M, Corsetto P, Berra B. Endogenous antioxidants and radical scavengers. *Adv Exp Med Biol* 2010;698:52-67

Fats and oils: Ramachandra Prabhu H. Lipid peroxidation in culinary oils subjected to thermal stress. *Indian J Clin Biochem* 2000;15(1):1-5

Strenuous exercise: Ji Li. Free radicals and exercise: implications in health and fitness. *JESF* 2003;1(1):15-22

Fight free radicals: Shen J. Impact of genetic and environmental factors on hsCRP concentrations and response to therapeutic agents. *Clin Chem* 2009;55(2):256-264

Diets rich in fruit: Wannamethee S, Lowe G, Rumley A, Burckdorfer K, Whincup P. Associations of vitamin C status, fruit and vegetable intakes, and markers of inflammation and hemostasis. *Am J Clin Nutr.* Mar 2006; 83(3):567-574

Certified organic: Allen, Gary J. and Albala, Ken. *The business of food: encyclopedia of the food and drink industries.* Santa Barbara: ABC-Clio/Greenwood, 2007.

Effects of a diet too high in fructose: Skerrett P J. "Is fructose bad for you?" *health.harvard.edu*, Harvard Health Blog. April 26, 2011. Web.

"A Special Interview with Dr. Richard Johnson By Dr. Mercola." *mercola.com*, Mercola. May 18 2010. Web.

Johnson R, et al. Potential role of sugar (fructose) in the epidemic of hypertension,obesity and the metabolic syndrome, diabetes, kidney disease, and cardiovascular disease. *Am J Clin Nutr* 2007;86:899-906

Nakagawa T, et al. A causal role for uric acid in fructose-induced metabolic syndrome. *AJP - Renal Physiol* Mar 2006;290(3):F625-F631

Most fructose in the American diet: Bray George A. How bad is fructose? *Am J Clin Nutr* Oct 2007;86(4):895-896

A 20 oz. soda: Calculated from *nutritiondata.com.*

Consumption of HFCS: Bocarsly M E, et al. High-fructose corn syrup causes characteristics of obesity in rats: Increased body weight, body fat and triglyceride levels. *Pharmacol Biochem Behav* Nov 2010;97(1):101–106

FDA and HFCS: Heller Lorraine. "HFCS is not 'natural', says FDA." *FoodNavigator-USA.com*, Food Navigator USA. April 2, 2008. Web.

Liquid foods aren't as satiating: Walikea Barbara C, Jordan Henry A, Stellar Eliot. Preloading and the regulation of food intake in man. *J Comp Physiol Psych* Jul 1969;68(3):327-333

CHAPTER 15: THE *RIGHT* FATS

Suppress hunger better long term: Foster-Schubert K E, et al. Acyl and total ghrelin are suppressed strongly by ingested proteins, weakly by lipids, and biphasically by carbohydrates. *J Clin Endocrinol Metab* May 2008;93(5):1971-9

Run 20 marathons: Rapoport B I. Metabolic Factors Limiting Performance in Marathon Runners. *PLoS Comput Biol* 2010;6(10):e1000960

Trans fats: Kyungwon Oh, et al. Dietary Fat Intake and Risk of Coronary Heart Disease in Women: 20 Years of Follow-up of the Nurses' Health Study. *Am J Epidemiol* 2005;161(7):672-679

Rich in MUFAs: Appel L, et al. Effects of Protein, Monounsaturated Fat, and Carbohydrate Intake on Blood Pressure and Serum Lipids. *JAMA* 2005;294(19):2455-2464

MUFA, insulin and blood sugar: Garg A. High-monounsaturated-fat diets for patients with diabetes mellitus: a meta-analysis. *Am J Clin Nutr* Mar 1998;(67):3,577S-582S

MUFA and anti-inflammatory effect: Miles E, Zabout P, Calder P. Differential anti-inflammatory effects of phenolic compounds from extra virgin olive oil identified in human whole blood cultures. *Nutrition* Mar 2005;21(3):389-394

Journal of Clinical Nutrition: Siri-Tarino P, Sun Q, Hu F, Krauss R. Meta-analysis of prospective cohort studies evaluating the association of saturated fat with cardiovascular disease. *Am J Clin Nutr* Mar 2010;91(3):535–546

Low-grade inflammation/CHD: Koenig W, Sund M, Fröhlich M, Fischer H G, Löwel H, Döring A, Hutchinson W L, Pepys M B. C-Reactive protein, a sensitive marker of inflammation, predicts future risk of coronary heart disease in initially healthy middle-aged men: results from the MONICA (Monitoring Trends and Determinants in Cardiovascular Disease) Augsburg Cohort Study, 1984 to 1992. *Circulation* 19 Jan 1999;99(2):237-42

Low-grade inflammation/obesity and diabetes: Wellen K, Hotamisligil G. Inflammation, stress, and diabetes. *J Clin Invest* 2005;115(5):1111–1119

Palmitic acid: Benoit Stephen C. et al. Palmitic acid mediates hypothalamic insulin resistance by altering PKC-θ subcellular localization in rodents. *J Clin Invest* 1 Sep 2009;119(9):2577–2589.

Oleic acid: Kennedy Arion, Martinez Kristina, Chuang Chia-Chi, LaPoint Kathy, McIntosh Michael. Saturated Fatty Acid-Mediated Inflammation and Insulin Resistance in Adipose Tissue: Mechanisms of Action and Implications. *J Nutr* Jan 2009;139(1):1-4.

High-carbohydrate diets: German J, and Dillard C. Saturated fats: what dietary intake? *Am J Clin Nutr* Sep 2004;(80):3,550-559

Wood A, et al. Dietary carbohydrate modifies the inverse association between saturated fat intake and cholesterol on very low-density lipoproteins. *Lipid Insights* 2011;(4):7-15

More rapidly absorbed: Dean Ward, English Jim. Medium Chain Triglycerides (MCTs) "Beneficial Effects on Energy, Atherosclerosis and Aging." *nutritionreview.org*, Nutrition Review. n.d. Web.

Digestive malabsorption conditions: Bach A C, Babayan V K. Medium-chain triglycerides: An update. *Am J Clin Nutr* 1982;36:950-962.

Prevent oxidation: Kay Colin D, Gebauer Sarah K, West Sheila G, Kris-Etherton Penny M. Pistachios Increase Serum Antioxidants and Lower Serum Oxidized-LDL in Hypercholesterolemic Adults. *J. Nutr* Jun 2010;140(6):1093-1098

Improve cholesterol numbers: Hu F B; Stampfer M J. Nut consumption and risk of coronary heart disease: a review of epidemiologic evidence. *Curr Atheroscler Rep* Nov 1999;1(3): 204-9

Reduce inflammation: Jiang Rui, Jacobs David R, Mayer-Davis Elizabeth, Szklo Moyses, Herrington David, Jenny Nancy S, Kronmal Richard, Barr R Graham. Nut and Seed Consumption and Inflammatory Markers in the Multi-Ethnic Study of Atherosclerosis. *Am J Epidemiol* 1 Feb 2006;163(3):222-231

Mukuddem-Petersen J, Oosthuizen W, Jerling J C. A systematic review of the effects of nuts on blood lipid profiles in humans. *J Nutr* 2005;135(9):2082-9

Lamarche B, Desroche S, Jenkins D J, et al. Combined effects of a dietary portfolio of plant sterols, vegetable protein, viscous fiber and almonds on LDL particle size. *Br J Nutr* 2004:92(4):654-63

Nut and seed nutritional information: Adapted from USDA National Nutrient Database Reference, Release 18.

Can be blocked: Fallon Sally, Enig Mary G. "Tripping Lightly Down the Prostaglandin Pathways." *westonaprice.org*, The Weston A Price Foundation. 2000. Web.

Amount of EPA and DHA: Sanders T A B, Younger Katherine M. The effect of dietary supplements of omega-3 polyunsaturated fatty acids on the fatty acid composition of platelets and plasma choline phosphoglycerides. *Br J Nutr* 1981;45:613-616

Salem Jr N, Wegher B, Mena P, Uauy R. Arachidonic and docosahexaenoic acids are biosynthesized from their 18-carbon precursors in human infants. *Proc Natl Acad Sci U S A* 9 Jan 1996;93(1):49–54

Vegetable sources like flax: Duda Monika K, et al. Fish oil, but not flaxseed oil, decreases inflammation and prevents pressure overload-induced cardiac dysfunction. *Cardiovasc Res* 2009;81(2):319-327

CHAPTER 16: MEAL PLANNING MADE EASY

Receptors in the stomach: MacDonald Ann. Why eating slowly may help you feel full faster. *health. harvard.edu*, Harvard Health Publications. October 19, 2010, Web.

High level of dietary protein: Skov A R, Toubro S, Bulow J, Krabbe K, Parving H H, Astrup A. Changes in renal function during weight loss induced by high vs. low-protein low-fat diets in overweight subjects. *Int J Obes Relat Metab Disord* Nov 1999;23(11):1170-7

Liquid food: Walikea, Barbara C, Henry A. Jordana, Eliot Stellara. Preloading and the regulation of food intake in man. *J Comp Physiol Psychol* Jul 1969;(68)3:327-333

More sensitive to fructose: David E S, Cingari D S, Ferraris R P. Dietary induction of intestinal fructose absorption in weaning rats. *Pediatr Res* Jun 1995;37(6):777-82

Shu Rong, David Elmer S, Ferraris Ronaldo P. Luminal fructose modulates fructose transport and GLUT-5 expression in small intestine of weaning rats. *AJP - GI* Feb 1998;274(2):G232-G239

Sakar Y, Nazaret C, Lettéron P, Ait Omar A, Avenati M, Viollet B, Ducroc R, Bado A. Positive regulatory control loop between gut leptin and intestinal GLUT2/GLUT5 transporters links to hepatic metabolic functions in rodents. *PLoS One* 30 Nov 2009;4(11):e7935

CHAPTER 17: THE WHOLE30: PREFACE TO THE PROGRAM

10mg: Akobeng A K, Thomas A G. Systematic Review: Tolerable Amount of Gluten for People With Coeliac Disease. *Aliment Pharmacol Ther* 2008;27:1044-1052

Habit research: Barrett, Deirdre. *Waistland: A (R)evolutionary View of Our Weight and Fitness Crisis.* New York: W.W. Norton & Co., Inc. 2007.

Ouellette Judith A, Wood Wendy. Habit and intention in everyday life: The multiple processes by which past behavior predicts future behavior. *Psychol Bull* Jul 1998;24(1):54-74

Lally P, van Jaarsveld C, Potts H, Wardle, J. How are habits formed: Modelling habit formation in the real world. *Eur J Soc Psych* Oct 2010;40(6):998–1009

CHAPTER 18: THE WHOLE30: PROCESS OF ELIMINATION

MSG: Sant' Diniz Yeda, Faine Luciane A, Galhardi Cristiano M, Rodrigues Hosana G, Ebaid Geovana X, Burneiko Regina C, Cicogna Antonio C, Novelli Ethel LB. Monosodium glutamate in standard and high-fiber diets: metabolic syndrome and oxidative stress in rats. *Nutrition* Jun 2005;21(6):749-755

Sulfites: Knodel LC. Current Issues in Drug Toxicity; Potential health hazards of sulfites. *Toxic Subst. Mech* 1997;16(3): 309-311

Lester M R. Sulfite sensitivity: Significance in human health. *J Am Coll Nutr* 1995;14(3):229-232

Carrageenan: Bhattacharyya Sumit, Gill Ravinder, Chen Mei Ling, Zhang Fuming , Linhardt Robert J, Dudeja Pradeep K, Tobacman Joanne K. Toll-like Receptor 4 Mediates Induction of the Bcl10-NFB-Interleukin-8 Inflammatory Pathway by Carrageenan in Human Intestinal Epithelial Cells. *J Biol Chem* Apr 2008;283(16)10550–10558

WHO Food Additives Series: 59. "Safety evaluation of certain food additives and contaminants." June 2007. Print.

CHAPTER 21: FINE-TUNING FOR SPECIAL POPULATIONS

Diabetes: Lindeberg S, Jönsson T, Granfeldt Y, Borgstrand E, Soffman J, Sjöström K, Ahrén B. A Palaeolithic diet improves glucose tolerance more than a Mediterranean-like diet in individuals with ischaemic heart disease. *Diabetologia* 2007;50(9):1795-1807

Eggs: Cordain Loren. Lysozyme From Egg Whites. *The Paleo Diet Update*, Mar 2010;6(4):3-6

Nightshades: Akbar A, Yiangou Y, Facer P, Walters J R F, Anand P, Ghosh S. Increased capsaicin receptor TRPV1-expressing sensory fibres in irritable bowel syndrome and their correlation with abdominal pain. *Gut* 2008;57:923-929

Childers N.F. A relationship of arthritis to the Solanaceae (nightshades). *J Intern Acad Prev Med* 1979;7:31-37

Smith Garrett. "Nightshades." *westonaprice.org*, The Weston A. Price Foundation. March 29 2010. Web.

Dairy: Dip J B. The distribution of multiple sclerosis in relation to the dairy industry and milk consumption. *New Zealand Med J* 1976;83:427–430

Monetini L, Cavallo M G, Stefanini L, et al. Bovine beta-casein antibodies in breast- and bottle-fed infants: their relevance in Type 1 diabetes. *Diabetes Metab Res Rev* 2001;17:51–54

Agranoff B W, Goldberg D. Diet and the geographical distribution of multiple sclerosis. *Lancet* 2 Nov 1974;2(7888):1061–1066

Malosse D, Perron H, Sasco A et al. Correlation between milk and dairy product consumption and multiple sclerosis prevalence: a worldwide study. *Neuroepidemiology* 192;11:304–312

NSAID: Bjarnason I, Williams P, Smethurst P, Peters T J, Levi J. Effect of non-steroidal anti-inflammatory drugs and prostaglandins on the permeability of the human small intestine. *Gut* 1986;27:1292-1297

IBS/IBD: Interview with Chad Potteiger, D.O., Smoky Mountain Gastroenterology, Maryville, TN. November 2011.

Abraham Clara, Cho Judy H. IL-23 and Autoimmunity: New Insights into the Pathogenesis of Inflammatory Bowel Disease. *Ann Rev Med* Feb 2009;60:97-110

Fruit and IBS/IBD: Gibson P R, Newnham E, Barrett J S, Shepherd S J, Muir J G. Fructose malabsorption and the bigger picture. *Aliment Pharma Ther* Feb 2007;25(4):349–363

Coffee and IBS/IBD: Alun Jones V, Mclaughlin P, Shorthouse M et al. Food intolerance: a major factor in the pathogenesis of irritable bowel syndrome. *Lancet* 1982;2(8308):1115-1117

Parker T J, Naylor S J, Riordan A M et al. Management of patients with food intolerance in irritable bowel syndrome: the development and use of an exclusion diet. *J Hum Nutr Diet* 1995;8:159-66

Fish oil and IBD: Stenson W F, Cort D, Rodgers J, Burakoff R, DeSchryver-Kecskemeti K, Gramlich T L, Beeken W. Dietary supplementation with fish oil in ulcerative colitis. *Ann Intern Med* Apr 1992;116(8):609-14

Allergies: Campbell-McBride Natasha. Food Allergy. *J Orthomol Med* 2009;24(1):31-41

High intensity: Dunbar C C, Kalinski M I. Using RPE to regulate exercise intensity during a 20-week training program for postmenopausal women: a pilot study. *Percept Mot Skills* Oct 2004;99(2):688-90

Duncan G E, Sydeman S J, Perri M G, Limacher M C, Martin A D. Can sedentary adults accurately recall the intensity of their physical activity? *Prev Med* Jul 2001;33(1):18-26

Pregnancy and protein: Goldman HI et al. Clinical effects of two different levels of protein intake on low-birth-weight infants. *J Pediatr* Jun 1969;74(6):881-9

Goldman H I et al. Effects of early dietary protein intake on low-birth-weight infants: evaluation at 3 years of age. *J Pediatr* Jan 1971;78(1):126-9

Goldman H I et al. Late effects of early dietary protein intake on low-birth-weight infants. *J Pediatr* Dec 1974;85(6):764-9

Koletzko B et al. Lower protein in infant formula is associated with lower weight up to age 2 y: a randomized clinical trial. *Am J Clin Nutr* Jun 2009;89(6):1836-45

Speth J D. Protein selection and avoidance strategies of contemporary and ancestral foragers: unresolved issues. *Philos Trans R Soc Lond B Biol Sci* 29 Nov 1991;334(1270):265-270

Omega-3 and pregnancy: Coletta J M, Bell S J, Roman A S. Omega-3 fatty acids and pregnancy. *Rev Obstet Gynecol* 2010;3(4):163-171

Simopoulos Artemis P, Leaf Alexander, Salem Jr. Norman. Essentiality of and Recommended Dietary Intakes for Omega-6 and Omega-3 Fatty Acids. *Ann Nutr Metab* 1999;43:127-130

Prenatal vitamins: Kresser Chris. Episode 7 - Nutrition for Fertility, Pregnancy & Breastfeeding. *chriskresser.com*, Chris Kresser L.Ac. April 12, 2011. Web.

Interview with Chris Kresser, L.Ac. via email. February 16, 2012.

Breast milk beenfits: Jackson Kelly M, Nazar Andrea M. Breastfeeding, the Immune Response, and Long-term Health. *J Am Osteopath Assoc* 1 Apr 2006;106(4);203-207

Cordain Loren. Cereal grains: humanity's double-edged sword. *World Rev Nutr Diet* 1999;84:19-73

Virtanen S M, Räsänen L, Ylönen K, Aro A, Clayton D, Langholz B, Pitkäniemi J, Savilahti E, Lounamaa R, Toumilehto J. Early introduction of dairy products associated with increased risk of IDDM in Finnish children. The Childhood in Diabetes in Finland Study Group. *Diabetes* Dec 1993;42(12):1786-1790

CHAPTER 22: SUPPLEMENT YOUR HEALTHY DIET

Nutrients delivered by food: Jacobs Jr David R, Gross Myron D, Tapsell Linda C. Food synergy: an operational concept for understanding nutrition. *Am J Clin Nutr* May 2009;(89)5:1543S-1548S

Studies show: Martin Suzy. "Some vitamin supplements don't protect against lung cancer." *eurekaalert.org*, Eureka Alert. 2007. Web.

Anthes, Emily. "The Vita Myth: Do supplements really do any good?" *slate.com*, Slate. January 6 2010. Web.

El-Kadiki Alia, Sutton Alexander J. Role of multivitamins and mineral supplements in preventing infections in elderly people: systematic review and meta-analysis of randomised controlled trials. *BMJ* 16 Apr 2005;330(7496):871

Neuhouser M L, Wassertheil-Smoller S, Thomson C, Aragaki A, Anderson GL, Manson J E, Patterson R E, Rohan T E, van Horn L, Shikany J M, Thomas A, LaCroix A, Prentice R L. Multivitamin use and risk of cancer and cardiovascular disease in the Women's Health Initiative cohorts. *Arch Intern Med* 9 Feb 2009;169(3):294-304

Lonn E, Bosch J, Yusuf S, Sheridan P, Pogue J, Arnold JM, Ross C, Arnold A, Sleight P, Probstfield J, Dagenais GR.Effects of long-term vitamin E supplementation on cardiovascular events and cancer: a randomized controlled trial. *JAMA* 16 Mar 2005;293(11):1338-47

Cook NR, Albert CM, Gaziano JM, et al. A randomized factorial trial of vitamins C and E and beta carotene in the secondary prevention of cardiovascular events in women: results from the Women's Antioxidant Cardiovascular Study. Archives of Internal Medicine. 2007;167(15):1610–1618.

Vitamin C: "Dietary Supplement Fact Sheet: Vitamin C." *ods.od.nih.gov*, National Institutes of Health. n.d. Web.

Antioxidant supplements: "Antioxidant Supplements For Health: An Introduction." *nccam.nih.gov*, The National Center for Complimentary and Alternative Medicine. October 2011. Web.

Hodis Howard N., Mack Wendy J, Sevanian Alex. Antioxidant Vitamin Supplementation and Cardiovascular Disease. *Nutrition and Health* 2005;(III):245-277

Jacobs Jr. David R, Gross Myron D, Tapsell Linda C. Food synergy: an operational concept for understanding nutrition. *Am J Clin Nutr* May 2009;89:(5)1543S-1548S

Bjelakovic Goran, Nikolova Dimitrinka, Gluud Lise Lotte, Simonetti Rosa G, Gluud Christian. Mortality in Randomized Trials of Antioxidant Supplements for Primary and Secondary Prevention Systematic Review and Meta-analysis. *JAMA* 2007;297(8):842-857

Bjelakovic Goran, Nikolova Dimitrinka, Simonetti Rosa G, Gluud Christian. Antioxidant supplements for prevention of gastrointestinal cancers: a systematic review and meta-analysis. *The Lancet* Oct 2004;364(9441)1219-1228

Kritharides Leonard, Stocker Roland.The use of antioxidant supplements in coronary heart disease. *Atherosclerosis* Oct 2002;164(2)211-219

Bjelakovic G, Nikolova D, Gluud L L, Simonetti R G, Gluud C. Antioxidant supplements for prevention of mortality in healthy participants and patients with various diseases. *Cochrane Database of Systematic Reviews* 2008;2:CD007176

Fish oil: Kris-Etherton Penny M, Harris William S, Appel Lawrence J. Fish Consumption, Fish Oil, Omega-3 Fatty Acids, and Cardiovascular Disease. *Circulation* 2002;106:2747-2757

Herold PM, Kinsella JE. Fish oil consumption and decreased risk of cardiovascular disease: a comparison of findings from animal and human feeding trials. *Am J Clin Nutr* Apr 1986;43(4)566-598

Wang Chenchen, Harris William S, Chung Mei, Lichtenstein Alice H, Balk Ethan M, Kupelnick Bruce, Jordan Harmon S, Lau Joseph. n–3 Fatty acids from fish or fish-oil supplements, but not α-linolenic acid, benefit cardiovascular disease outcomes in primary- and secondary-prevention studies: a systematic review. *Am J Clin Nutr* Jul 2006;84(1):5-17

Rissanen Tina, Voutilainen Sari, Nyyssönen Kristina, Lakka Timo A, Salonen Jukka T. Fish Oil–Derived Fatty Acids, Docosahexaenoic Acid and Docosapentaenoic Acid, and the Risk of Acute Coronary Events. *Circulation* 2000;102:2677-2679

Nestel Paul J. Fish oil attenuates the cholesterol induced rise in lipoprotein cholesterol. *Am J Clin Nutr* May 1986;43(5):52-757

Nestel Paul J. Fish oil and cardiovascular disease: lipids and arterial function. *Am J Clin Nutr* Jan 2000;71(1):228S-231S

Connor William E, Connor Sonja L. The importance of fish and docosahexaenoic acid in Alzheimer disease. *Am J Clin Nutr* Apr 2007;85(4):929-930

"Fish Oil." *nlm.nih.gov,* National Library of Medicine, National Institutes for Health. December 2011. Web.

Vitamin D$_3$: Holick MF. Vitamin D: importance in the prevention of cancers, type 1 diabetes, heart disease, and osteoporosis. *Am J Clin Nutr* 2004;79(3):362-371

Giovannucci Edward, Liu Yan, Hollis Bruce W, Rimm Eric B. 25-Hydroxyvitamin D and Risk of Myocardial Infarction in Men. *Arch Intern Med* 2008;168(11):1174-1180

Guyton K Z, Kensler T W, Posner G H. Vitamin D and vitamin D analogs as cancer chemopreventive agents. *Nutr Rev* 2003;61(7):227-238

Vieth R, Chan P C, MacFarlane G D. Efficacy and safety of vitamin D3 intake exceeding the lowest observed adverse effect level. *Am J Clin Nutr* 2001;73(2):288-294

Heaney R P, Davies K M, Chen T C, Holick M F, Barger-Lux M J. Human serum 25-hydroxycholecalciferol response to extended oral dosing with cholecalciferol. *Am J Clin Nutr* 2003;77(1):204-210

Magnesium: King Dana E, Mainous III Arch G, Geesey Mark E, Woolson Robert F. Dietary Magnesium and C-reactive Protein Levels. *J Am Coll Nutr* Jun 2005;24(3):166-171

Ford E S, Mokdad A H. Dietary magnesium intake in a national sample of US adults. *J Nutr* Sep 2003;133(9):2879-82

Cotruvo J, Bartram J, eds. "Calcium and Magnesium in Drinking-water : Public health significance." Geneva, World Health Organization, 2009.

Digestive enzymes: Balch Phyllis, Balch James. *Prescription for Natural Healing.* New York: Avery Trade, 2010. Print.

Gut dysbiosis: Lipski Elizabeth. *Digestive Wellness.* New York: Mc-Graw Hill. 2005. Print.

Steinhoff U. Who controls the crowd? New findings and old questions about the intestinal microflora. *Immunol Lett* Jun 2005;99(1):12–6

Probiotics: Interview with Dr. Timothy Gerstmar, N.D. Aspire Natural Health, Redmond WA. February 16, 2012.

INDEX